Ear, Nose, and Throat Disorders

SOURCEBOOK

THIRD EDITION

Ear, Nose, and Throat Disorders
SOURCEBOOK

THIRD EDITION

Basic Consumer Health Information about the Causes, Symptoms, Diagnosis, and Treatment of Diseases and Disorders That Affect the Ears, Nose, Sinuses, Throat, and Voice, Including Ear Infections, Otosclerosis, Cholesteatoma, Hearing Loss, Ototoxicity, Tinnitus, Vertigo, Ménière Disease, Perilymph Fistula, Sinusitis, Deviated Septum, Sleep Apnea, Sore Throat, Laryngitis, Tonsillitis, Swallowing Disorders, Otolaryngologic Cancers, Laryngeal Cancer, and More

Along with Reports on Current Research Initiatives, a Glossary of Related Medical Terms, and a Directory of Sources for Further Help and Information

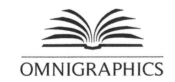

OMNIGRAPHICS

615 Griswold, Ste. 520, Detroit, MI 48226

Library of Congress Cataloging-in-Publication Data

Title: Ear, nose, and throat disorders sourcebook : basic consumer health information about disorders of the ears, hearing loss, vestibular disorders, nasal and sinus problems, throat and vocal cord disorders, and otolaryngologic cancers, including facts about ear infections and injuries, genetic and congenital deafness, sensorineural hearing disorders, tinnitus, vertigo, Ménière disease, rhinitis, sinusitis, snoring, sore throats, hoarseness, and more, along with reports on current research initiatives, a glossary of related medical terms, and a dictionary of sources for further help and information / Lauren Parrott, managing editor.

Description: 3rd edition. I Detroit, MI : Omnigraphics, Inc., [2019] I Includes index.

Identifiers: LCCN 2019013652 (print) I LCCN 2019014578 (ebook) I ISBN 9780780817029 (ebook) I ISBN 9780780817012 (hard cover : alk. paper)

Subjects: LCSH: Otolaryngology--Popular works.

Classification: LCC RF59 (ebook) I LCC RF59 .E18 2019 (print) I DDC 617.5/1--dc23

LC record available at https://lccn.loc.gov/2019013652

Table of Contents

Part III: Hearing Disorders

Part IV: Vestibular Disorders

Part V: Disorders of the Nose and Sinuses

Part VI: Disorders of the Throat and Vocal Cords

Part VII: Cancers of the Ears, Nose, and Throat

Part VIII: Additional Help and Information

Preface

About This Book

The ear, nose, and throat are important organs of the human body as they perform several vital functions on a daily basis. Anatomically, they are located close to each other, and their functions are also closely related. Ailments of these vital organs are some of the most common illnesses troubling Americans today.

- 2 to 3 children out of every 1000 in the United States are born with a detectable level of hearing loss.

- About 30.8 million adults in the United States are suffering from sinusitis.

- About 7.5 million people in the United States have voice disorders.

Ear, Nose, and Throat Disorders Sourcebook, Third Edition provides readers with updated health information about the causes, symptoms, diagnosis, and treatment of diseases and disorders that affect the ears, nose, sinuses, throat, and voice, including ear infections, otosclerosis, cholesteatoma, hearing loss, ototoxicity, tinnitus, vertigo, Ménière disease, perilymph fistula, sinusitis, deviated septum, sleep apnea, sore throat, laryngitis, tonsillitis, swallowing disorders, otolaryngologic cancers, laryngeal cancer, and so on. Current research initiatives are also described, along with a glossary of related terms and directory of resources for further help and information.

How to Use This Book

This book is divided into parts and chapters. Parts focus on broad areas of interest. Chapters are devoted to single topics within a part.

Part I: Structure and Functions of Ear, Nose, and Throat begins with an introduction to the anatomy of the ear, nose, and throat. It also explains how the functionalities of these vital organs are closely related.

Part II: Disorders of the Ears describes in detail the disorders that commonly affect the ear, including ear infections and injuries. It also discusses the most frequently used diagnostic tests.

Part III: Hearing Disorders provides a detailed look at the most common types of hearing loss. It explains how hearing loss is diagnosed and looks at ways to protect hearing. The part concludes with facts about electronic hearing devices, including hearing aids and cochlear implants, and methods of communicating with people who are deaf or hard of hearing.

Part IV: Vestibular Disorders looks at disorders affecting the sense of balance and the diagnostic tests commonly used to detect them. The ways in which aging, allergies, and other environmental factors impact the vestibular system are explained. The impact of vestibular disorders and the methods of vestibular rehabilitation are also discussed.

Part V: Disorders of the Nose and Sinuses describes nasal and sinus anatomy, and it details the disorders that most commonly affect the nose and sinuses. Frequently used diagnostic tests and surgical procedures are also explained.

Part VI: Disorders of the Throat and Vocal Cords offers information about sore throats, disorders of the tonsils and adenoids, laryngitis and other laryngeal problems, swallowing disorders, and disorders of the voice and vocal cords.

Part VII: Cancers of the Ears, Nose, and Throat provides a detailed look at nasopharyngeal, esophageal, laryngeal, and other cancers that affect the ears, nose, and throat. Each cancer-related chapter includes a discussion of risk factors, symptoms, diagnosis, staging, and treatment. This part concludes with a summary of recent research findings regarding cancers of the ear, nose, and throat.

Part VIII: Additional Help and Information provides a glossary of terms related to the ears, nose, and throat and a directory of organizations that can provide further information.

Bibliographic Note

This volume contains documents and excerpts from publications issued by the following U.S. government agencies: Centers for Disease Control and Prevention (CDC); Effective Health Care Program; Federal Aviation Administration (FAA); Genetic and Rare Diseases Information Center (GARD); Genetics Home Reference (GHR); National Cancer Institute (NCI); National Center for Complementary and Integrative Health (NCCIH); National Council on Disability (NCD); National Eye Institute (NEI); National Heart, Lung, and Blood Institute (NHLBI); National Institute on Aging (NIA); National Institute on Deafness and Other Communication Disorders (NIDCD); National Institutes of Health (NIH); *NIH News in Health*; Rehabilitation Research & Development Service (RR&D); U.S. Consumer Product Safety Commission (CPSC); U.S. Department of Veterans Affairs (VA); and U.S. Food and Drug Administration (FDA).

It may also contain original material produced by Omnigraphics and reviewed by medical consultants.

About the Health Reference Series

The *Health Reference Series* is designed to provide basic medical information for patients, families, caregivers, and the general public. Each volume takes a particular topic and provides comprehensive coverage. This is especially important for people who may be dealing with a newly diagnosed disease or a chronic disorder in themselves or in a family member. People looking for preventive guidance, information about disease warning signs, medical statistics, and risk factors for health problems will also find answers to their questions in the *Health Reference Series*. The *Series*, however, is not intended to serve as a tool for diagnosing illness, in prescribing treatments, or as a substitute for the physician/patient relationship. All people concerned about medical symptoms or the possibility of disease are encouraged to seek professional care from an appropriate healthcare provider.

A Note about Spelling and Style

Health Reference Series editors use *Stedman's Medical Dictionary* as an authority for questions related to the spelling of medical terms and the *Chicago Manual of Style* for questions related to grammatical structures, punctuation, and other editorial concerns. Consistent adherence is not always possible, however, because the individual volumes within the *Series* include many documents from a wide variety of different producers, and the editor's primary goal is to present material from each source as accurately as is possible. This sometimes means that information in different chapters or sections may follow other guidelines and alternate spelling authorities. For example, occasionally a copyright holder may require that eponymous terms be shown in possessive forms (Crohn's disease vs. Crohn disease) or that British spelling norms be retained (leukaemia vs. leukemia).

Medical Review

Omnigraphics contracts with a team of qualified, senior medical professionals who serve as medical consultants for the *Health Reference Series*. As necessary, medical consultants review reprinted and originally written material for currency and accuracy. Citations including the phrase "Reviewed (month, year)" indicate material reviewed by this team. Medical consultation services are provided to the *Health Reference Series* editors by:

Dr. Vijayalakshmi, MBBS, DGO, MD
Dr. Senthil Selvan, MBBS, DCH, MD
Dr. K. Sivanandham, MBBS, DCH, MS (Research), PhD

Our Advisory Board

We would like to thank the following board members for providing initial guidance on the development of this series:

- Dr. Lynda Baker, Associate Professor of Library and Information Science, Wayne State University, Detroit, MI

- Nancy Bulgarelli, William Beaumont Hospital Library, Royal Oak, MI

- Karen Imarisio, Bloomfield Township Public Library, Bloomfield Township, MI

- Karen Morgan, Mardigian Library, University of Michigan-Dearborn, Dearborn, MI

- Rosemary Orlando, St. Clair Shores Public Library, St. Clair Shores, MI

Health Reference Series *Update Policy*

The inaugural book in the *Health Reference Series* was the first edition of *Cancer Sourcebook* published in 1989. Since then, the *Series* has been enthusiastically received by librarians and in the medical community. In order to maintain the standard of providing high-quality health information for the layperson the editorial staff at Omnigraphics felt it was necessary to implement a policy of updating volumes when warranted.

Medical researchers have been making tremendous strides, and it is the purpose of the *Health Reference Series* to stay current with the most recent advances. Each decision to update a volume is made on an individual basis. Some of the considerations include how much new information is available and the feedback we receive from people who use the books. If there is a topic you would like to see added to the update list, or an area of medical concern you feel has not been adequately addressed, please write to:

Managing Editor
Health Reference Series
Omnigraphics
615 Griswold, Ste. 520
Detroit, MI 48226

Part One

Structure and Functions of Ear, Nose, and Throat

Chapter 1

Anatomy and Functions of the Ear

Structure and Parts of the Ear

The ear has three major parts: the outer ear, the middle ear, and the inner ear. The outer ear, also called the "pinna," includes everything we see on the outside—the curved flap of the ear leading down to the earlobe—but it also includes the ear canal, which begins at the opening to the ear and extends to the eardrum. The eardrum is a membrane that separates the outer ear from the middle ear.

The middle ear—which is where ear infections occur—is located between the eardrum and the inner ear. Within the middle ear are three tiny bones called the "malleus," "incus," and "stapes" that transmit sound vibrations from the eardrum to the inner ear. The bones of the middle ear are surrounded by air.

The inner ear contains the labyrinth, which help us keep our balance. The cochlea, a part of the labyrinth, is a snail-shaped organ that converts sound vibrations from the middle ear into electrical signals. The auditory nerve carries these signals from the cochlea to the brain.

This chapter contains text excerpted from the following sources: Text under the heading "Structure and Parts of the Ear" is excerpted from "Ear Infections in Children," National Institute on Deafness and Other Communication Disorders (NIDCD), May 12, 2017; Text under the heading "How Do We Hear?" is excerpted from "How Do We Hear?" National Institute on Deafness and Other Communication Disorders (NIDCD), January 3, 2018.

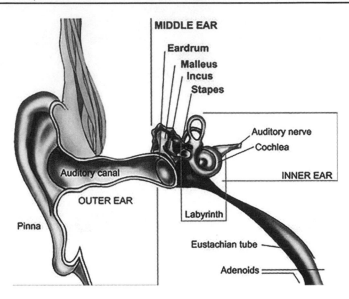

Figure 1.1. *Parts of the Ear*

Other nearby parts of the ear also can be involved in ear infections. The eustachian tube is a small passageway that connects the upper part of the throat to the middle ear. Its job is to supply fresh air to the middle ear, drain fluid, and keep air pressure at a steady level between the nose and the ear.

Adenoids are small pads of tissue located behind the back of the nose, above the throat, and near the eustachian tubes. Adenoids are mostly made up of immune system cells. They fight off infection by trapping bacteria that enter through the mouth.

How Do We Hear?

Hearing depends on a series of complex steps that change sound waves in the air into electrical signals. Our auditory nerve then carries these signals to the brain.

1. Sound waves enter the outer ear and travel through a narrow passageway called the "ear canal," which leads to the eardrum.

2. The eardrum vibrates from the incoming sound waves and sends these vibrations to the malleus, incus, and stapes.

3. The bones in the middle ear amplify, or increase, the sound vibrations and send them to the cochlea in the inner ear.

An elastic partition runs from the beginning to the end of the cochlea, splitting it into an upper and lower part. This partition is called the "basilar membrane" because it serves as the base, or ground floor, on which key hearing structures sit.

4. Once the vibrations cause the fluid inside the cochlea to ripple, a traveling wave forms along the basilar membrane. Hair cells—sensory cells sitting on top of the basilar membrane—ride the wave. Hair cells near the wide end of the snail-shaped cochlea detect higher-pitched sounds, such as an infant crying. Those closer to the center detect lower-pitched sounds, such as a large dog barking.

5. As the hair cells move up and down, microscopic hair-like projections (known as "stereocilia") that perch on top of the hair cells bump against an overlying structure and bend. Bending causes pore-like channels, which are at the tips of the stereocilia, to open up. When that happens, chemicals rush into the cells, creating an electrical signal.

6. The auditory nerve carries this electrical signal to the brain, which turns it into a sound that we recognize and understand.

Chapter 2

Anatomy and Functions of the Nose

Structure and Parts of the Nose

The normal anatomy of the nose is shown in Figure 2.1 to Figure 2.3. The various terms used for nasal structures and dimensions are shown in Figure. 2.1. The cartilaginous components of the nose and terms for regions is shown in Figure 2.2, and, in Figure 2.3, the cross section is shown.

Some anatomical landmarks deserve specific mention, as these are not always used with standard meaning.

Nasal root: The most depressed, superior part of the nose along the nasal ridge.

Nasion: The midline point, just superior to the nasal root, overlying the nasofrontal suture.

Nasal bridge: A saddle-shaped area that includes the nasal root and the lateral aspects of the nose. It lies between the glabella and the inferior boundary of the nasal bone and extends laterally to the inner canthi.

This chapter contains text excerpted from the following sources: Text beginning with the heading "Structure and Parts of the Nose" is excerpted from "Anatomy of the Nose," National Institutes of Health (NIH), January 23, 2009. Reviewed April 2019; Text under the heading "How Does Your Sense of Smell Work?" is excerpted from "Smell Disorders," National Institute on Deafness and Other Communication Disorders (NIDCD), May 12, 2017.

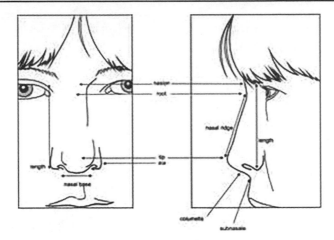

Figure 2.1. *Nasal Structures and Dimensions*

Nasal ridge: The midline prominence of the nose, extending from the nasal root to the tip (also called the "dorsum of the nose").

Nasal base: An imaginary line between the most lateral points of the external inferior attachments of the alae nasi to the face.

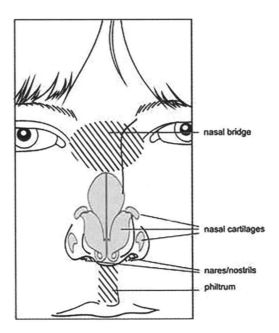

Figure 2.2. *Cartilaginous Components of the Nose*

Nasal tip: The junction of the inferior margin of the nasal ridge and the columella. Commonly, it is the part of the nose furthest from the plane of the face. In rare circumstances, such as markedly prominent and convex nasal profiles, other parts of the ridge may be further removed from the facial plane.

Ala: The tissue comprising the lateral boundary of the nose, inferiorly, surrounding the nostril.

Columella: The tissue that links the nasal tip to the nasal base, and separates the nares. It is the inferior margin of the nasal septum.

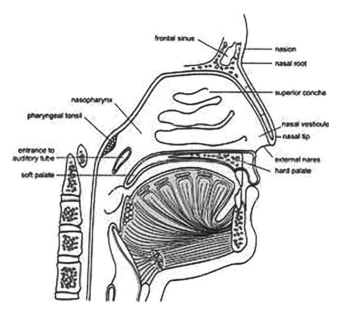

Figure 2.3. *Cross Section of the Nose*

Measurements of the Nose

Measurements of the nose are possible by using sliding calipers. The reliability of measurements taken with a tape measure is poor. Furthermore, the actual position of several of the landmarks may preclude accurate measurement. For example, if the nasal tip overhangs the upper lip, the position of subnasale is difficult to define. Nasal length and width are the most common measurements taken in practice. A short description of how to measure each dimension is provided as the various terms are defined.

Growth of the nose does not end at puberty; the nose continues to increase in size with age. There are no normal standards for nasal size in adulthood.

Anatomical Variation

Anomalies of the nose may be classified into quantitative traits and qualitative features:

1. **Variations in length:** long; short

2. **Variations in width:** wide nose, narrow nose, broad nasal base, narrow nasal base, broad nasal tip, narrow nasal tip, wide nasal ridge, narrow nasal ridge, wide nasal bridge, narrow nasal bridge, broad columella.

3. **Variations in length and width:** prominent nose, absent nasal cartilage, absent nose.

4. **Variations in shape or position:** depressed nasal bridge, depressed nasal ridge, depressed nasal tip, bulbous nose, bifid nasal tip, bifid nose, overhanging nasal tip, deviated nasal tip, fullness of paranasal tissue, prominent nasal bridge, convex nasal ridge, concave nasal ridge, low insertion of the columella, low hanging columella, short columella, high insertion of the columella, thick ala nasi, underdeveloped ala nasi, cleft ala nasi, enlarged naris, narrow naris, single naris, proboscis, supernumerary naris, anteverted nares.

How Does Your Sense of Smell Work?

Your sense of smell—similar to your sense of taste—is part of your chemosensory system, or the chemical senses.

Your ability to smell comes from specialized sensory cells, called "olfactory sensory neurons," which are found in a small patch of tissue high inside the nose. These cells connect directly to the brain. Each olfactory neuron has one odor receptor. Microscopic molecules released by substances around us—whether it is coffee brewing or pine trees in a forest—stimulate these receptors. Once the neurons detect the molecules, they send messages to your brain, which identifies the smell. There are more smells in the environment than there are receptors, and any given molecule may stimulate a combination of receptors, creating a unique representation in the brain. These representations are registered by the brain as a particular smell.

Smells reach the olfactory sensory neurons through two pathways. The first pathway is through your nostrils. The second pathway is through a channel that connects the roof of the throat to the nose. Chewing food releases aromas that access the olfactory sensory neurons through the second channel. If the channel is blocked, such as when your nose is stuffed up by a cold or flu, odors cannot reach the sensory cells that are stimulated by smells. As a result, you lose much of your ability to enjoy a food's flavor. In this way, your senses of smell and taste work closely together.

Without the olfactory sensory neurons, familiar flavors, such as chocolate or oranges, would be hard to distinguish. Without smell, foods tend to taste bland and have little or no flavor. Some people who go to the doctor because they think they have lost their sense of taste are surprised to learn that they have lost their sense of smell instead.

Your sense of smell is also influenced by something called the "common chemical sense." This sense involves thousands of nerve endings, especially on the moist surfaces of the eyes, nose, mouth, and throat. These nerve endings help you sense irritating substances, such as the tear-inducing power of an onion or the refreshing coolness of menthol.

Chapter 3

Anatomy and Functions of the Throat

Structure and Parts of the Throat
Pharynx

The pharynx, commonly called the "throat," is a passageway that extends from the base of the skull to the level of the sixth cervical vertebra. It serves both the respiratory and digestive systems by receiving air from the nasal cavity and air, food, and water from the oral cavity. Inferiorly, it opens into the larynx and esophagus. The pharynx is divided into three regions according to location: the nasopharynx, the oropharynx, and the laryngopharynx (hypopharynx).

The nasopharynx is the portion of the pharynx that is posterior to the nasal cavity and extends inferiorly to the uvula. The oropharynx is the portion of the pharynx that is posterior to the oral cavity. The most inferior portion of the pharynx is the laryngopharynx that extends from the hyoid bone down to the lower margin of the larynx.

The upper part of the pharynx (throat) lets only air pass through. Lower parts permit air, foods, and fluids to pass.

This chapter contains text excerpted from the following sources: Text under the heading "Structure and Parts of the Throat" is excerpted from "Pharynx," Surveillance, Epidemiology, and End Results Program (SEER), National Cancer Institute (NCI), July 1, 2002. Reviewed April 2019; Text under the heading "How Do We Swallow?" is excerpted from "Dysphagia," National Institute on Deafness and Other Communication Disorders (NIDCD), March 6, 2017.

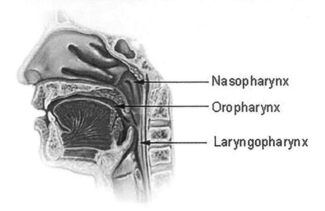

Figure 3.1. *Illustration of the Pharynx*

The pharyngeal, palatine, and lingual tonsils are located in the pharynx. They are also called "Waldereyer's ring." The retromolar trigone is the small area behind the wisdom teeth.

Larynx

The larynx, commonly called the "voice box" or "glottis," is the passageway for air between the pharynx above and the trachea below. It extends from the fourth to the sixth vertebral levels. The larynx is often divided into three sections: sub larynx, larynx, and supralarynx. It is formed by nine cartilages that are connected to each other by muscles and ligaments.

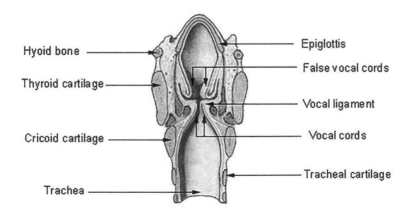

Figure 3.2. *Larynx*

The larynx plays an essential role in human speech. During sound production, the vocal cords close together and vibrate as air expelled from the lungs passes between them. The false vocal cords have no role in sound production, but help close off the larynx when food is swallowed.

The thyroid cartilage is the Adam's apple. The epiglottis acts as a trap door to keep food and other particles from entering the larynx.

Trachea

The trachea, commonly called the "windpipe," is the main airway to the lungs. It divides into the right and left bronchi at the level of the fifth thoracic vertebra, channeling air to the right or left lung.

The hyaline cartilage in the tracheal wall provides support and keeps the trachea from collapsing. The posterior soft tissue allows for expansion of the esophagus, which is immediately posterior to the trachea.

The mucous membrane that lines the trachea is ciliated pseudostratified columnar epithelium similar to that in the nasal cavity and nasopharynx. Goblet cells produce mucus that traps airborne particles and microorganisms, and the cilia propel the mucus upward, where it is either swallowed or expelled.

How Do We Swallow?

Swallowing is a complex process. Some 50 pairs of muscles and many nerves work to receive food into the mouth, prepare it, and move it from the mouth to the stomach. This happens in three stages. During the first stage, called the "oral phase," the tongue collects the food or liquid, making it ready for swallowing. The tongue and jaw move solid food around in the mouth so it can be chewed. Chewing makes solid food the right size and texture to swallow by mixing the food with saliva. Saliva softens and moistens the food to make swallowing easier. Normally, the only solid we swallow without chewing is in the form of a pill or caplet. Everything else that we swallow is in the form of a liquid, a puree, or a chewed solid.

The second stage begins when the tongue pushes the food or liquid to the back of the mouth. This triggers a swallowing response that passes the food through the pharynx, or throat (see figure 3.3). During this phase, called the "pharyngeal phase," the larynx closes tightly and breathing stops to prevent food or liquid from entering the airway and lungs.

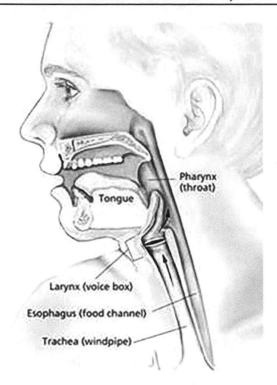

Figure 3.3. *Parts of Mouth and Neck Involved in Swallowing*

The third stage begins when food or liquid enters the esophagus, the tube that carries food and liquid to the stomach. The passage through the esophagus, called the "esophageal phase," usually occurs in about three seconds, depending on the texture or consistency of the food, but can take slightly longer in some cases, such as when swallowing a pill.

Chapter 4

Ear, Nose, and Throat Examination

Ear, nose, and throat (ENT) specialty centers provide a wide range of services. Evaluation and management of ear problems, including chronic otitis, hearing loss, and dizziness, are offered. Nasal and endoscopic sinus surgery with computerized image guidance are available. Video stroboscopy and transnasal esophagoscopy are available for the complete evaluation of disorders of voice and swallowing. The diagnosis, treatment, and surveillance of malignancies of the skin (including melanoma), the throat, airways, lymph nodes, thyroid, and parathyroids are a large part of the services offered. Sentinel node mapping and biopsy, as well as extensive neck dissections, are offered. Reconstruction of traumatic and postsurgical defects of the face and neck and surgery for obstructive sleep apnea are available. Evaluation and care from an ENT specialist requires a consultation request.

During the course of the physical examination of each child, a comprehensive examination of the ear, nose, and oral pharynx was performed. Prior to examining a child, the physician would have reviewed each examinee's medical history and would have become familiar with

This chapter contains text excerpted from the following sources: Text in this chapter begins with excerpts from "Otolaryngology (Ear, Nose and Throat or ENT)," U.S. Department of Veterans Affairs (VA), July 20, 2017; Text under the heading "Ear, Nose, and Throat Tests" is excerpted from "Hearing Sensitivity and Related Medical Findings among Children," Centers for Disease Control and Prevention (CDC), n.d.

the child's history in regard to speech; ear pathology, including otitis media; or problems related to hearing, as indicated by his or her parents. Thus the physician, at the time of the examination, was aware if the child was known to have a specific disturbance of the ear, nose, or throat.

Ear, Nose, and Throat Tests

The ENT examination itself consisted of an inspection of the external ears, auditory canals, tympanic membranes, anterior nasal cavity, and oral pharynx.

Inspection of the external ears focused on congenital or acquired defects and the presence of scars, adenopathy, or fistulae of the pinna.

The otoscopic examination involved an evaluation of the auditory canals for polyps, exostoses, foreign bodies, and inflammation, and of the tympanic membranes for mobility, dullness, abnormal transparency, opacity, scars, perforations, and exudates. When the canals were either partially or completely blocked by cerumen or cellular debris, no attempt was made to remove the obstruction, and the physician indicated that the particular canal was "occluded" and noted the appropriate reason or material causing the occlusion.

At the time of this otoscopic examination, tympanic drum mobility was tested by means of pneumatic otoscopy.

The nose was examined by speculum, with notation made of the presence of turbinate hypertrophy, polyps, septal deviation, foreign body, or obstruction by swollen tissue or exudate. No attempt was made in this or other parts of the ENT examination to delineate whether tissue swelling or exudates were related to an allergic reaction as opposed to another cause.

The subtle clinical judgment necessary for the recognition of the former was not possible in the survey with the time limitations and the brief specialized training that could be provided the medical examiners.

The oral pharynx was evaluated by inspection for the presence of cleft palate (repaired or unrepaired), hypertrophic lymphoid tissue on the posterior pharyngeal wall, and postnasal mucopurulent discharge. An evaluation of the adenoid tissue in the nasopharynx and the eustachian tubes were not included because of the time and additional expertise required to perform these more difficult evaluations.

Tonsils were evaluated as to presence or absence, and, if present, were further graded according to size, employing the following system: Grade I–tonsils present, within the tonsillar pillars; Grade II–present, with tissue extending beyond the boundaries of the tonsillar pillars but not meeting in the midline; Grade III–tonsils greatly enlarged and meeting in the midline.

To ensure skillful examinations by the staff physician and standardization of observations among the many different physicians employed during the course of the survey, two specific training methods were employed. Prior to reporting to the field from the medical center at which he or she was in training, each field examining physician received four half-days of special training, under the supervision of an otolaryngologist, in the specific examination of the ear, nose, and throat to be used in the survey. These sessions included a review of the regional anatomy, refinement of the individual physician's examining skills, and training in the technique of pneumatic otoscopy. In addition, during the first several days of examinations at a location where a new staff physician was in attendance, senior medical advisers of the Health Examination Survey were present to review examination procedures, to perform replicate examinations, and to ensure the minimization of interobserver variation in grading and reporting.

Part Two

Disorders of the Ears

Chapter 5

Disorders of Pinna (The External Ear)

Chapter Contents

Section 5.1

Anotia (Born without Ears) and Microtia (Small Ear)

This section includes text excerpted from "Facts about Anotia/Microtia," Centers for Disease Control and Prevention (CDC), April 10, 2018.

What Are Anotia and Microtia?

Anotia and microtia are birth defects of a baby's ear. Anotia happens when the external ear (the part of the ear that can be seen) is missing completely. Microtia happens when the external ear is small and not formed properly.

Anotia/microtia usually happens during the first few weeks of pregnancy. These defects can vary from being barely noticeable to being a major problem with how the ear formed. Most of the time, anotia/microtia affects how the baby's ear looks, but usually the parts of the ear inside the head (the inner ear) are not affected. However, some babies with this defect also will have a narrow or missing ear canal.

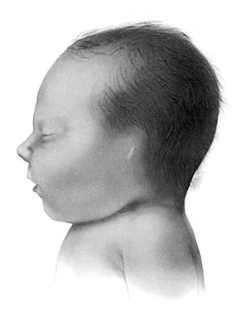

Figure 5.1. *Baby with Anotia*

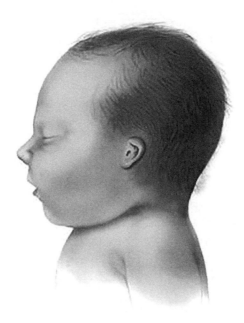

Figure 5.2. *Baby with Microtia*

Types of Microtia

There are four types of microtia, ranging from Type 1 to Type 4. Type 1 is the mildest form, where the ear retains its normal shape, but is smaller than usual. Type 4 is the most severe type, where all external ear structures are missing—anotia. This condition can affect one or both ears. However, it is more common for babies to have only one affected ear.

Occurrence

Because the severity of microtia ranges from mild to severe, researchers have a hard time estimating how many babies in the United States are affected. State birth-defects tracking systems have estimated that anotia/microtia range from less than 1 in 10,000 live births to about 5 in 10,000 live births.

Causes and Risk Factors

The causes of anotia/microtia among most infants are unknown. Some babies have anotia/microtia because of a change in their genes.

In some cases, anotia/microtia occurs because of an abnormality in a single gene, which can cause a genetic syndrome. Another known cause for anotia/microtia is the mother taking a medicine called "isotretinoin" (Accutane®) during pregnancy. This medicine can lead to a pattern of birth defects, which often includes anotia/microtia. These defects also are thought to be caused by a combination of genes and other factors, such as the things the mother comes in contact with in the environment or what the mother eats or drinks or certain medicines she uses during pregnancy.

Like many families of children with a birth defect, the Centers for Disease Control and Prevention (CDC) wants to find out what causes them. Understanding the factors that are more common among babies with a birth defect will help us learn more about the causes. The CDC funds the Centers for Birth Defects Research and Prevention (CBDRP), which collaborate on large studies, such as the National Birth Defects Prevention Study (NBDPS; births 1997-2011) and the Birth Defects Study To Evaluate Pregnancy exposureS (BD-STEPS; began with births in 2014), to understand the causes of and risks for birth defects, including anotia/microtia.

The CDC reported on important findings about some factors that increase the risk of having a baby with anotia or microtia:

- Diabetes? Women who have diabetes before they get pregnant have been shown to be more at risk for having a baby with anotia/microtia, compared to women who did not have diabetes.

- Maternal diet—Pregnant women who eat a diet lower in carbohydrates and folic acid might have an increased risk for having a baby with microtia, compared to all other pregnant women.

The CDC continues to study birth defects, such as anotia/microtia, and how to prevent them. If you are pregnant or thinking about becoming pregnant, talk with your doctor about ways to increase your chances of having a healthy baby.

Diagnosis

Anotia/microtia are visible at birth. A doctor will notice the problem by just examining the baby. A computed tomography (CT or CAT) scan (special X-ray test) of the baby's ear can provide a detailed picture of the ear. This will help the doctor see if the bones or other structures in the ear are affected. A doctor will also perform a thorough physical exam to look for any other birth defects that may be present.

Treatment

Treatment for babies with anotia/microtia depends on the type or severity of the condition. A healthcare provider or hearing specialist called an "audiologist" will test the baby's hearing to determine any hearing loss in the ear(s) with the defect. Even a hearing loss in one ear can hurt school performance. All treatment options should be discussed, and early action may provide better results. Hearing aids may be used to improve a child's hearing ability and to help with speech development.

Surgery is used to reconstruct the external ear. The timing of surgery depends on the severity of the defect and the child's age. Surgery is usually performed between 4 and 10 years of age. Further treatment may be necessary if the child has other birth defects present.

In the absence of other conditions, children with anotia/microtia can develop normally and lead healthy lives. Some children with anotia/microtia may have issues with self-esteem if they are concerned with visible differences between themselves and other children. Parent-to-parent support groups can prove to be useful for new families of babies with birth defects of the head and face, including anotia/microtia.

Section 5.2

Cauliflower Ear

"Cauliflower Ear," © 2019 Omnigraphics. Reviewed April 2019.

Know about Cauliflower Ear

Blunt trauma causing permanent disfigurement of the outer ear, such as a wrinkled, bulged, curled up, and pale appearance with loss of stiffness, is collectively called "cauliflower ear."

Other names of this condition include:

- Boxer's ear

- Wrestler's ear

- Athletes' ears

- Perichondrial hematoma

The external ear—the outer ear (i.e., what we see)—is not made of bones. It is made of cartilage, which gives shape and support to the ear. It has no nerve cells or blood vessels on its own, but is surrounded by a flexible connective tissue called "perichondrium." The perichondrium serves as a passage through which the blood reaches the cartilage from the skin. The blood, in turn, provides essential oxygen and nutrients for its endurance; in other words, without blood flow, the cartilage will die. In any manner, the cartilage depends entirely on the attached skin for its survival.

The blood flow can be blocked due to any one of the following reasons:

- Direct trauma, leading to a skin tear (disconnection of skin and the cartilage) caused by:

  - Accidental ear injury, such as hitting the ear or hitting the side of the head

  - Getting repeated hits to the ear as a part of boxing, wrestling, mixed martial arts (MMA), water polo, or other sports activities

- Inflammation (reddening and swelling) of the cartilage due to infection. On occasion, cosmetic conch piercing can lead to a cartilage infection called "auricular perichondritis."

- Severe bruising, if not treated immediately, results in the collection of fluid called "seroma" and the formation of a blood clot (solidification of blood). This buildup of clots is called "hematomas." Both the seromas and hematomas can block the blood flow.

Ultimately, if the cartilage dies due to no blood supply, the risk of infection increases, and a new fibrous tissue forms, surrounding the dead cartilage, giving the ear a cauliflower-like texture; hence the name "cauliflower ear," a condition that causes the ears to lose its stiffness and firm shape. Once this happens, it is not reversible However, cauliflower ear can be prevented if symptoms are observed and treated immediately after injury.

Symptoms

Common symptoms of cauliflower ear include:

- Redness and swelling

- Pain

- Bruising

- Seroma

- Hematoma

- Visible changes in size and shape (curvature) of the ear

If the symptoms mentioned above are left untreated, it can lead to severe symptoms, such as:

- Excessive bleeding

- Facial swelling

- Headaches

- Blurred vision

- Tinnitus (ringing in the ear)

- Loss of hearing (mild to moderate)

- Increased risk of infections

Treatment

Prompt treatment after an injury can prevent the formation of cauliflower ear.

- **Cold compression**—application of ice at the site of injury in 15-minute intervals can reduce swelling.

- **Drainage**—a surgical procedure done by doctors to drain seroma/hematoma by making an incision at the site of injury. If drained rapidly after an injury, scarring can be prevented.

- **Dressing**—the application of a compression dressing postdrainage to ensure that the injury heals in a normal shape.

- **Antibiotics**—healthcare professionals prescribe antibiotics either to prevent infection after injury or to avoid further infection.

Without immediate medical attention, or if all the above measures fail, the appearance of a cauliflower-like texture emerges. The cartilage becomes thick and is followed by scar formation, which is irreversible.

To correct this cauliflower-like texture, a surgery called "otoplasty" can be done. This surgical procedure is done under general or local anesthesia, in which the doctor makes a cut (incision) behind the ear to expose the cartilage, shaves some of the cartilage to reshape the ear, and closes the incision using stitches. The doctor applies compression dressings to ensure that the area heals in a normal shape and prescribes antibiotics to prevent infection. In some cases, otoplasty can reverse the cauliflower-like appearance. One should be able to resume their normal activities in six weeks or within a timeframe otherwise suggested by their healthcare provider, with regards to their degree of response and improvement to the treatment.

Prevention

- The best preventative measure is to prevent trauma.

- During participation or the learning of high-risk or contact sports—such as wrestling, martial arts, MMA, water polo, etc.—wear a helmet or protective headgear with ear guards to avoid injury.

- Avoid blood thinners before participating in any contact sports.

- On occasion, any delay in diagnosis after an injury can also lead to the development of cauliflower ear, which causes difficulty for the healthcare provider in managing the condition while attempting to normalize ear structure. Therefore, prompt diagnosis should also be considered as a preventative measure.

References

1. Gardner, Stephanie S. MD. "Cauliflower Ear," WebMD, January 22, 2018.

2. Gupta, Rupal Christine. MD. "What's Cauliflower Ear?" The Nemours Foundation/KidsHealth®, April 15, 2005.

3. Biggers, Alana. MD; Madormo, Carrie RN, MPH. "Everything You Should Know about Cauliflower Ear," Healthline.com, June 1, 2017.

Section 5.3

Otoplasty (Ear Plastic Surgery)

"Otoplasty (Ear Plastic Surgery)," © 2019
Omnigraphics. Reviewed April 2019.

Otoplasty is a cosmetic ear surgery performed to alter the shape, size, position, and proportion of the pinna or outer ear. It is a reconstructive surgery that involves correcting a deformity and improving the appearance of the ear, thereby enhancing one's self-image. The surgery can be done at any age after the ears have grown to their full size. However, it is considered to work best on children between 4 and 14 years of age.

Why Otoplasty Is Done

Otoplasty can optimize the symmetry of ears and bring more natural shape to the face. The surgery typically treats conditions such as:

- Protruding ears
- Macrotia—a condition where the ear lobes are abnormally large
- Lop ear—a condition in which the ear tips are folded
- Shell ear—a condition with missing ear features, such as natural curves and folds
- Ears that stick out far from the head
- Ear defects resulting from injuries

How Otoplasty Is Done
Before the Surgery

Medical advancements have greatly simplified otoplasty procedure. Before the surgery, a plastic surgeon will review your medical history and do a physical examination of your ears. You may explain what you are expecting in terms of ear appearance after the surgery with your surgeon. Some precautions to be taken before the surgery are listed below.

- Avoid smoking, as it can slow down the healing process.
- Avoid taking aspirin and nonsteroidal anti-inflammatory drugs (NSAIDs) a few days before the date of your surgery.

- Do not eat or drink anything six hours prior to the surgery. Filling up your stomach before the surgery may increase the chances of anesthetic complications.

During the Surgery

In general, otoplasty is performed in the surgeon's office or any outpatient facility. Adults can undergo the surgery with local anesthesia. Whereas general anesthesia is used for children in order to make sure that they do not move around during the surgery. Following the anesthesia, the surgeon makes incisions to remove the excess skin and cartilage from the ears. The incisions are made either on the back of the ears or within the inner creases, depending on the type of correction required. Once the correction is made, the cartilage is folded to its proper position, stitched, and covered with bandages for protection. The procedure usually lasts about two to three hours. But, based on the complexity of the situation, it may take even longer.

After the Surgery

Here are a few steps you need to take after the otoplasty to attain a speedy recovery.

- Take medications regularly and as prescribed by your doctor.
- Keep your head elevated while you sleep. This may reduce swelling.
- Avoid rubbing or scratching your ears, either consciously or unconsciously.
- Eat lighter foods in the first few days after the surgery since it may be difficult to chew harder foods. Also, make sure to follow a healthy diet because the body needs enough vitamins and minerals to heal properly.
- Avoid smoking for a couple of weeks after the surgery.
- Avoid prolonged exposure to sun or extreme temperatures for at least a couple of months after the surgery. Also, avoid using hair dryers.
- Stay away from pools for at least six weeks after the surgery.
- Once the bandages are removed, wear a headband that covers the ears completely. The headband can remove the tension from the ears and keep them in place in case of accidental bumps.

- Notify your doctor immediately if you develop fever or experience excessive bleeding during the period of recovery.

Risks and Complications of Otoplasty

As with any surgery, there are risks involved in otoplasty too. The following are some of the commonly reported risks and complications of otoplasty.

- Ear infection

- Permanent scars or a keloid formation at the back of the ear or within the creases

- Numbness of the ear and facial skin

- Prolonged or extreme pain

- Excessive bleeding or a blood clot

- Narrowing of the external ear canal

- Overcorrection, leading to unnatural contours

- Asymmetrical ear placement, due to the changes occurring during the healing process

References

1. "Otoplasty," Mayo Clinic, August 14, 2018.

2. Walsh, Margaret. "Cosmetic/Reconstructive Surgery of the Ears (Otoplasty Surgical Instructions)," MedicineNet, July 27, 2016.

3. Grayson, Charlotte E. "Ear Reshaping (Otoplasty)," MedicineNet, September 2003.

4. Kasrai, Leila. "Top 8 Things You Have to Do after Otoplasty," My Plastic Surgeon, April 4, 2016.

Chapter 6

Ear Infections

Chapter Contents

Section 6.1

Ear Infection: An Overview

This section includes text excerpted from "Ear Infection," Centers for
Disease Control and Prevention (CDC), January 27, 2017.

What Is an Ear Infection?

Ear infections can affect the ear canal or the middle ear.

Acute otitis externa (AOE) is the scientific name for an infection of
the ear canal, which is also called "swimmer's ear."

Middle ear infections are called "otitis media," and there are two
types of middle ear infections:

- Otitis media with effusion (OME) occurs when fluid builds up
  in the middle ear without pain, pus, fever, or other signs and
  symptoms of infection.

- Acute otitis media (AOM) occurs when fluid builds up in the
  middle ear and is often caused by bacteria, but can also be
  caused by viruses.

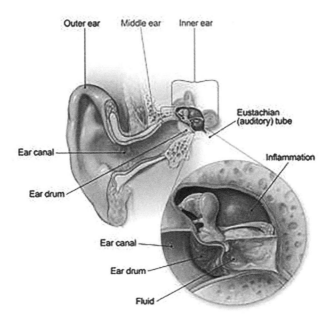

Figure 6.1. *Ear Infection*

How Are Ear Infections Caused and How Can They Be Prevented?

Bacteria

AOM is often caused by bacteria, and Streptococcus pneumoniae is a common bacterial cause of AOM.

Ensure your child is up-to-date on vaccinations, including the pneumococcal vaccination which protects against Streptococcus pneumoniae. Breastfeeding exclusively until your baby is 6 months old and continuing to breastfeed for at least 12 months can protect your baby from infections, including AOM.

Cold and Flu Season

AOM often occurs after a cold. Viruses cause OME, and then bacteria can grow in the fluid, leading to AOM.

- Ensure your child is up-to-date on vaccinations and gets a flu vaccine every year.

Injury to the Ear

Foreign objects, such as cotton swabs and bobby pins, can cause cuts and bruises in the ear canal that can get infected, causing AOE.

- Avoid putting foreign objects in the ear.

Cigarette Smoke

Exposure to cigarette smoke can lead to more colds and more AOM.

- Avoid smoking and exposure to secondhand smoke.

Family History

The tendency to develop AOM can run in families.

- Family history is not preventable. Instead, focus on other prevention methods, such as staying up-to-date on vaccinations, breastfeeding, and avoiding smoke.

Normal Tympanic Membrane

- Pneumococcal polysaccharide-protein conjugate vaccine (PCV7) should be administered in children between 2 and 23 months of age. This vaccine has been a key player in the reduction of bacterial ear infections. Since the emergence of the PCV7 vaccine, the virus H. Influenzae has become a more widespread cause of AOM.

- In the United States, viral and bacterial ear infections are the most common childhood illnesses treated with antibiotics. Early detection and treatment of ear infections is vital because it can significantly reduce the negative effects on public and personal wellbeing.

Normal Eardrum

- Early childhood vaccinations can help to prevent bacterial ear infections.

- Most ear infections are viral and can get better on their own without antibiotic treatment.

Section 6.2

Otitis Externa (Swimmer's Ear)

This section includes text excerpted from "Ear Infections," Centers for Disease Control and Prevention (CDC), May 4, 2016.

Ear infections can be caused by leaving contaminated water in the ear after swimming. This infection, known as "swimmer's ear" or "otitis externa," is not the same as the common childhood middle ear infection. The infection occurs in the outer ear canal and can cause pain and discomfort for swimmers of all ages. In the United States, swimmer's ear results in an estimated 2.4 million healthcare visits every year and nearly half a billion dollars in healthcare costs.

Below are answers to the most common questions regarding ear infections, swimmer's ear, and healthy swimming.

What Are the Symptoms of Swimmer's Ear?

Symptoms of swimmer's ear usually appear within a few days of swimming and include:

- Itchiness inside the ear

- Redness and swelling of the ear

- Pain when the infected ear is tugged or when pressure is placed on the ear

- Pus draining from the infected ear

Although all age groups are affected by swimmer's ear, it is more common in children and can be extremely painful.

How Is Swimmer's Ear Spread at Recreational Water Venues?

Swimmer's ear can occur when water stays in the ear canal for long periods of time, providing the perfect environment for germs to grow and infect the skin. Germs found in pools and at other recreational water venues are one of the most common causes of swimmer's ear.

Swimmer's ear cannot be spread from one person to another.

If you think you have swimmer's ear, consult your healthcare provider. Swimmer's ear can be treated with antibiotic ear drops.

Is There a Difference between a Childhood Middle Ear Infection and Swimmer's Ear?

Yes. Swimmer's ear is not the same as the common childhood middle ear infection. If you can wiggle the outer ear without pain or discomfort, then your ear condition is probably not swimmer's ear.

How Do I Protect Myself and Family?

To reduce the risk of swimmer's ear:
Do keep your ears as dry as possible.

- Use a bathing cap, earplugs, or custom-fitted swim molds when swimming.

Do dry your ears thoroughly after swimming or showering.

- Use a towel to dry your ears well.

- Tilt your head to hold each ear facing down to allow water to escape the ear canal.

- Pull your earlobe in different directions while your ear is faced down to help water drain out.

- If you still have water left in your ears, consider using a hair dryer to move air within the ear canal.

  - Put the dryer on the lowest heat and speed/fan setting.

  - Hold the dryer several inches from your ear.

Do not put objects in your ear canal (including cotton-tip swabs, pencils, paperclips, or fingers).

Do not try to remove ear wax. Ear wax helps protect your ear canal from infection.

- If you think that your ear canal is blocked by earwax, consult your healthcare provider.

Consult your healthcare provider about using ear drops after swimming.

- Drops should not be used by people with ear tubes, damaged eardrums, outer ear infections, or ear drainage (pus or liquid coming from the ear).

Consult your healthcare provider if you have ear pain, discomfort, or drainage from your ears.

Ask your pool/hot tub operator if disinfectant and pH levels are checked at least twice per day—hot tubs and pools with proper disinfectant and pH levels are less likely to spread germs.

Use pool test strips to check the pool or hot tub yourself for adequate disinfectant (chlorine or bromine) levels.

Section 6.3

Otitis Media

This section includes text excerpted from "Otitis Media," National
Institute on Deafness and Other Communication Disorders (NIDCD),
October 2000. Reviewed April 2019.

What Is Otitis Media?

Otitis media is an infection or inflammation of the middle ear. This
inflammation often begins when infections that cause sore throats,
colds, or other respiratory or breathing problems spread to the middle
ear. These can be viral or bacterial infections. 75 percent of children
experience at least 1 episode of otitis media by their third birthday.
Almost half of these children will have 3 or more ear infections during
their first 3 years. It is estimated that medical costs and lost wages
because of otitis media amount to $5 billion* a year in the United
States. Although otitis media is primarily a disease of infants and
young children, it can also affect adults.

** Gates GA, Cost-effectiveness considerations in otitis media treatment, Otolaryngol
Head Neck Surg, 114 (4), April 1996, 525–530.*

Why Are More Children Affected by Otitis Media than Adults?

There are many reasons why children are more likely to suffer from
otitis media than adults. First, children have more trouble fighting
infections. This is because their immune systems are still developing.
Another reason has to do with the child's eustachian tube. The eustachian tube is a small passageway that connects the upper part of the
throat to the middle ear. It is shorter and straighter in the child than
in the adult. It can contribute to otitis media in several ways. The
eustachian tube is usually closed but opens regularly to ventilate or
replenish the air in the middle ear. This tube also equalizes middle ear
air pressure in response to air pressure changes in the environment.

However, a eustachian tube that is blocked by swelling of its lining
or plugged with mucus from a cold or for some other reason cannot
open to ventilate the middle ear. The lack of ventilation may allow
fluid from the tissue that lines the middle ear to accumulate. If the
eustachian tube remains plugged, the fluid cannot drain and begins
to collect in the normally air-filled middle ear.

One more factor that makes children more susceptible to otitis media is that adenoids in children are larger than they are in adults. Adenoids are composed largely of cells (lymphocytes) that help fight infections. They are positioned in the back of the upper part of the throat near the eustachian tubes. Enlarged adenoids can, because of their size, interfere with the eustachian tube opening. In addition, adenoids themselves may become infected, and the infection may spread into the eustachian tubes.

Bacteria reach the middle ear through the lining or the passageway of the eustachian tube and can then produce infection, which causes swelling of the lining of the middle ear, blocking of the eustachian tube, and migration of white cells from the bloodstream to help fight the infection. In this process, the white cells accumulate, often killing bacteria and dying themselves, leading to the formation of pus, a thick yellowish-white fluid in the middle ear. As the fluid increases, the child may have trouble hearing because the eardrum and middle ear bones are unable to move as freely as they should. As the infection worsens, many children also experience severe ear pain. Too much fluid in the ear can put pressure on the eardrum and eventually tear it.

How Can Someone Tell If a Child Has Otitis Media?

Otitis media is often difficult to detect because most children affected by this disorder do not yet have sufficient speech and language skills to tell someone what is bothering them. Common signs to look for are:

- Unusual irritability
- Difficulty sleeping
- Tugging or pulling at one or both ears
- Fever
- Fluid draining from the ear
- Loss of balance
- Unresponsiveness to quiet sounds or other signs of hearing difficulty, such as sitting too close to the television or being inattentive

What Are the Effects of Otitis Media?

Otitis media not only causes severe pain but may result in serious complications if it is not treated. An untreated infection can travel from the middle ear to the nearby parts of the head, including the brain. Although the hearing loss caused by otitis media is usually temporary, untreated otitis media may lead to permanent hearing impairment. Persistent fluid in the middle ear and chronic otitis media can reduce a child's hearing at a time that is critical for speech and language development. Children who have early hearing impairment from frequent ear infections are likely to have speech and language disabilities.

Can Anything Be Done to Prevent Otitis Media?

Specific prevention strategies applicable to all infants and children, such as immunization against viral respiratory infections or specifically against the bacteria that cause otitis media, are not currently available. Nevertheless, it is known that children who are cared for in group settings, as well as children who live with adults who smoke cigarettes, have more ear infections.

Therefore, a child who is prone to otitis media should avoid contact with sick playmates and environmental tobacco smoke. Infants who nurse from a bottle while lying down also appear to develop otitis media more frequently. Children who have been breastfed often have fewer episodes of otitis media. Research has shown that cold and allergy medications, such as antihistamines and decongestants, are not helpful in preventing ear infections.

The best hope for avoiding ear infections is the development of vaccines against the bacteria that most often cause otitis media. Scientists are currently developing vaccines that show promise in preventing otitis media. Additional clinical research must be completed to ensure their effectiveness and safety.

How Does a Child's Physician Diagnose Otitis Media?

The simplest way to detect an active infection in the middle ear is to look in the child's ear with an otoscope, a light instrument that allows the physician to examine the outer ear and the eardrum. Inflammation of the eardrum indicates an infection. There are several ways that a physician checks for middle ear fluid. The use of a special type of otoscope called a "pneumatic otoscopy," allows the physician to blow a puff of air onto the eardrum to test eardrum movement. An eardrum with fluid behind it does not move as well as an eardrum with air behind it.

A useful test of middle ear function is called "tympanometry." This test requires insertion of a small soft plug into the opening of the child's ear canal. The plug contains a speaker, a microphone, and a device that is able to change the air pressure in the ear canal, allowing for several measures of the middle ear. The child feels air pressure changes in the ear or hears a few brief tones. While this test provides information on the condition of the middle ear, it does not determine how well the child hears. A physician may suggest a hearing test for a child who has frequent ear infections to determine the extent of hearing loss. The hearing test is usually performed by an audiologist, a person who is specially trained to measure hearing.

How Is Otitis Media Treated?

Many physicians recommend the use of an antibiotic (a drug that kills bacteria) when there is an active middle ear infection. If a child is experiencing pain, the physician may also recommend a pain reliever. Following the physician's instructions is very important. Once started, the antibiotic should be taken until it is finished. Most physicians will have the child return for a follow-up examination to see if the infection has cleared. Unfortunately, there are many bacteria that can cause otitis media, and some have become resistant to some antibiotics. This happens when antibiotics are given for coughs, colds, flu, or viral infections where antibiotic treatment is not useful. When bacteria become resistant to antibiotics, those treatments are then less effective against infections. This means that several different antibiotics may have to be tried before an ear infection clears. Antibiotics may also produce unwanted side effects, such as nausea, diarrhea, and rashes.**

*** There is ongoing scientific discussion about the use and potential overuse of antibiotic therapy for otitis media.*

Once the infection clears, fluid may remain in the middle ear for several months. Middle ear fluid that is not infected often disappears after 3 to 6 weeks. Neither antihistamines nor decongestants are recommended as helpful in the treatment of otitis media at any stage in the disease process. Sometimes physicians will treat the child with an antibiotic to hasten the elimination of the fluid. If the fluid persists for more than 3 months and is associated with a loss of hearing, many physicians suggest the insertion of "tubes" in the affected ears. This operation, called a "myringotomy," can usually be done on an outpatient basis by a surgeon, who is usually an otolaryngologist (a physician who specializes in the ears, nose, and throat). While the child is asleep under general anesthesia, the surgeon makes a small opening in the child's eardrum. A small metal or plastic tube is placed into the opening in the eardrum. The tube ventilates the middle ear and helps keep the air pressure in the middle ear equal to the air pressure in the environment. The tube normally stays in the eardrum for 6 to 12 months, after which it usually comes out spontaneously. If a child has enlarged or infected adenoids, the surgeon may recommend removal of the adenoids at the same time the ear tubes are inserted. Removal of the adenoids has been shown to reduce episodes of otitis media in some children, but not those who are under 4 years of age. Research, however, has shown that removal of a child's tonsils does not reduce occurrences of otitis media. Tonsillotomy and adenoidectomy may be appropriate for reasons other than middle ear fluid.

Hearing should be fully restored once the fluid is removed. Some children may need to have the operation again if the otitis media returns after the tubes come out. While the tubes are in place, water should be kept out of the ears. Many physicians recommend that a child with tubes wear special earplugs while swimming or bathing so that water does not enter the middle ear.

Section 6.4

Ear Infections in Children

This section includes text excerpted from "Ear Infections in Children," National Institute on Deafness and Other Communication Disorders (NIDCD), May 12, 2017.

What Is an Ear Infection?

An ear infection is an inflammation of the middle ear, usually caused by bacteria, that occurs when fluid builds up behind the eardrum. Anyone can get an ear infection, but children get them more often than adults. Five out of six children will have at least one ear infection by their third birthday. In fact, ear infections are the most common reason parents bring their child to a doctor. The scientific name for an ear infection is otitis media (OM).

What Are the Symptoms of an Ear Infection?

There are three main types of ear infections. Each has a different combination of symptoms.

- **Acute otitis media (AOM)** is the most common ear infection. Parts of the middle ear are infected and swollen and fluid is trapped behind the eardrum. This causes pain in the ear—commonly called an "earache." Your child might also have a fever.

- **Otitis media with effusion (OME)** sometimes happens after an ear infection has run its course and fluid stays trapped behind the eardrum. A child with OME may have no symptoms, but a doctor will be able to see the fluid behind the eardrum with a special instrument.

- **Chronic otitis media with effusion (COME)** happens when fluid remains in the middle ear for a long time or returns over and over again, even though there is no infection. COME makes it harder for children to fight new infections and also can affect their hearing.

How Can I Tell If My Child Has an Ear Infection?

Most ear infections happen to children before they have learned how to talk. If your child is not old enough to say, "my ear hurts," here are a few things to look for:

- Tugging or pulling at the ear(s)

- Fussiness and crying

- Trouble sleeping

- Fever (especially in infants and younger children)

- Fluid draining from the ear

- Clumsiness or problems with balance

- Trouble hearing or responding to quiet sounds

What Causes an Ear Infection

An ear infection usually is caused by bacteria and often begins after a child has a sore throat, cold, or other upper respiratory infection. If the upper respiratory infection is bacterial, these same bacteria may spread to the middle ear; if the upper respiratory infection is caused by a virus, such as a cold, bacteria may be drawn to the microbe-friendly environment and move into the middle ear as a secondary infection. Because of the infection, fluid builds up behind the eardrum.

Why Are Children More Likely than Adults to Get Ear Infections?

There are several reasons why children are more likely than adults to get ear infections.

Eustachian tubes are smaller and more level in children than they are in adults. This makes it difficult for fluid to drain out of the ear, even under normal conditions. If the eustachian tubes are swollen or blocked with mucus, due to a cold or other respiratory illness, fluid may not be able to drain.

A child's immune system is not as effective as an adult's because it is still developing. This makes it harder for children to fight infections.

As part of the immune system, the adenoids respond to bacteria passing through the nose and mouth. Sometimes, bacteria get trapped in the adenoids, causing a chronic infection that can then pass on to the eustachian tubes and the middle ear.

How Does a Doctor Diagnose a Middle Ear Infection?

The first thing a doctor will do is ask you about your child's health. Has your child had a head cold or sore throat recently? Is she or he having trouble sleeping? Is she or he pulling at her ears? If an ear infection seems likely, the simplest way for a doctor to tell is to use a lighted instrument, called an "otoscope," to look at the eardrum. A red, bulging eardrum indicates an infection.

A doctor also may use a pneumatic otoscope, which blows a puff of air into the ear canal, to check for fluid behind the eardrum. A normal eardrum will move back and forth more easily than an eardrum with fluid behind it.

Tympanometry, which uses sound tones and air pressure, is a diagnostic test a doctor might use if the diagnosis still is not clear. A tympanometer is a small, soft plug that contains a tiny microphone and speaker as well as a device that varies air pressure in the ear. It measures how flexible the eardrum is at different pressures.

How Is an Acute Middle Ear Infection Treated?

Many doctors will prescribe an antibiotic, such as amoxicillin, to be taken over 7 to 10 days. Your doctor also may recommend over-the-counter pain relievers, such as acetaminophen or ibuprofen, or eardrops, to help with fever and pain. (Because aspirin is considered a major preventable risk factor for Reye syndrome, a child who has a fever or other flu-like symptoms should not be given aspirin unless instructed to by your doctor.)

If your doctor is not able to make a definite diagnosis of OM and your child does not have severe ear pain or a fever, your doctor might ask you to wait a day or two to see if the earache goes away. The American Academy of Pediatrics (AAP) issued guidelines in 2013 that encourage doctors to observe and closely follow these children with ear infections that cannot be definitively diagnosed, especially those between the ages of 6 months to 2 years. If there is no improvement within 48 to 72 hours from when symptoms began, the guidelines recommend doctors start antibiotic therapy. Sometimes ear pain is not caused by infection, and some ear infections may get better without antibiotics. Using antibiotics cautiously and with good reason helps prevent the development of bacteria that become resistant to antibiotics.

If your doctor prescribes an antibiotic, it is important to make sure your child takes it exactly as prescribed and for the full amount of time. Even though your child may seem better in a few days, the infection still has not completely cleared from the ear. Stopping the medicine too soon could allow the infection to come back. It is also important to return for your child's follow-up visit, so that the doctor can check if the infection is gone.

How Long Will It Take My Child to Get Better?

Your child should start feeling better within a few days after visiting the doctor. If it has been several days and your child still seems sick, call your doctor. Your child might need a different antibiotic. Once the infection clears, fluid may still remain in the middle ear but usually disappears within three to six weeks.

What Happens If My Child Keeps Getting Ear Infections?

To keep a middle ear infection from coming back, it helps to limit some of the factors that might put your child at risk, such as not being around people who smoke and not going to bed with a bottle. In spite of these precautions, some children may continue to have middle ear infections, sometimes as many as five or six a year. Your doctor may want to wait for several months to see if things get better on their own, but, if the infections keep coming back and antibiotics are not helping, many doctors will recommend a surgical procedure that places a small ventilation tube in the eardrum to improve air flow and prevent fluid backup in the middle ear. The most commonly used tubes stay in place for six to nine months and require follow-up visits until they fall out.

If placement of the tubes still does not prevent infections, a doctor may consider removing the adenoids to prevent infection from spreading to the eustachian tubes.

Can Ear Infections Be Prevented?

Currently, the best way to prevent ear infections is to reduce the risk factors associated with them. Here are some things you might want to do to lower your child's risk for ear infections.

- Vaccinate your child against the flu. Make sure your child gets the influenza, or flu, vaccine every year.

- It is recommended that you vaccinate your child with the 13-valent pneumococcal conjugate vaccine (PCV13). The PCV13 protects against more types of infection-causing bacteria than the previous vaccine, the PCV7. If your child already has begun PCV7 vaccination, consult your physician about how to transition to PCV13. The Centers for Disease Control and Prevention (CDC) recommends that children under the age of two be vaccinated, starting at two months of age. Studies have shown that vaccinated children get far fewer ear infections than children who are not vaccinated. The vaccine is strongly recommended for children in day care.

- Wash hands frequently. Washing hands prevents the spread of germs and can help keep your child from catching a cold or the flu.

- Avoid exposing your baby to cigarette smoke. Studies have shown that babies who are around smokers have more ear infections.

- Never put your baby down for a nap, or for the night, with a bottle.

- Do not allow sick children to spend time together. As much as possible, limit your child's exposure to other children when your child or your child's playmates are sick.

What Research Is Being Done on Middle Ear Infections?

Researchers sponsored by the National Institute on Deafness and Other Communication Disorders (NIDCD) are exploring many areas to improve the prevention, diagnosis, and treatment of middle ear infections. For example, finding better ways to predict which children are at higher risk of developing an ear infection could lead to successful prevention tactics.

Another area that needs exploration is why some children have more ear infections than others. For example, Native American and Hispanic children have more infections than do children in other ethnic groups. What kinds of preventive measures could be taken to lower the risks?

Doctors also are beginning to learn more about what happens in the ears of children who have recurring ear infections. They have identified colonies of antibiotic-resistant bacteria, called "biofilms," that are present in the middle ears of most children with chronic ear infections. Understanding how to attack and kill these biofilms would be one way to successfully treat chronic ear infections and avoid surgery.

Understanding the impact that ear infections have on a child's speech and language development is another important area of study. Creating more accurate methods to diagnose middle ear infections would help doctors prescribe more targeted treatments. Researchers also are evaluating drugs currently being used to treat ear infections and developing new, more effective and easier ways to administer medicines.

The NIDCD-supported investigators continue to explore vaccines against some of the most common bacteria and viruses that cause middle ear infections, such as nontypeable Haemophilus influenzae (NTHi) and Moraxella catarrhalis. One team is conducting studies on a method for delivering a possible vaccine without a needle.

Section 6.5

Ear Tubes

"Ear Tubes," © 2019 Omnigraphics. Reviewed April 2019.

Natural Ear Tubes (Eustachian Tubes)

The middle ear normally ventilates using the tubes that run from the middle ear to the back of the throat called "eustachian tubes," which opens and closes at the end of the throat. The functions include:

- Regulating/equalizing the pressure inside the ear with regards to the outside environment

- Refreshing the air inside the ear

- Removing secretions or draining the fluid that gets collected in the middle ear

Inflammation, swelling, or mucus in the eustachian tubes as a result of upper respiratory infection or allergy can block the tubes, causing fluid accumulation in the middle ear. This occurs mostly in children, partly due to their eustachian tubes being narrow and small, and partly due to other factors that cause clogging. When this happens, the need for artificial/synthetic ear tubes arises.

Synthetic Ear Tubes

Tiny cylindrical tube-like structures made of plastic or metal that are inserted into the ears for treatment purposes are called "ear tubes." The other names of ear tubes are:

- Tympanostomy tubes

- Myringotomy tubes

- Ventilation tubes

- Pressure equalization (PE) tubes
The benefits of the ear tubes include:

- Restoring ventilation

- Reducing risk of infection

- Preventing collection of fluid into the eardrum

- Restoring hearing loss caused by infection

- Decreasing sleep disruption caused by an ear infection

Ear tubes act as an alternative for eustachian tubes. The tubes are often recommended for children who have trapped fluid due to fluid buildup (effusion) in the middle ear, which is caused by any of the following:

- Eustachian tube blockage or dysfunction

- Perforation or tearing of eardrum

- Viral or bacterial infection of the middle ear (otitis media)

- Long-term middle ear infections that do not respond or improve with antibiotic treatments. This condition leads to hearing loss, which delays speech development in children.

Ear Tube Insertion

This procedure of insertion of ear tubes is termed as "tympanostomy" or "myringotomy," which is done under surgical setting for individuals who develop fluid buildup behind the eardrum--which occurs predominantly in children than adults. Ear tube insertion is one of the treatment options for persistent or recurrent ear infections.

Before the Procedure—Instructions and Inquires

The healthcare professional may ask you the following details:

- List of medications that you take (regular, as well as as-needed)

- Personal and family history of allergies or adverse reactions if any (especially to anesthesia)

- Known allergies to medications/drugs (especially antibiotics), food, or agents, if any

Points to note include:

- The stomach should be empty during the procedure, and, for that purpose, one should follow the instructions of the doctor on what to eat or drink.

- Follow the doctor's advice if any medication changes are suggested, such as temporary stoppage of certain medications.

- Clarify with the professional regarding the check-in time, type of anesthesia they are planning to administer (face mask, intravenous (IV) line, or injection), duration of surgery, recovery time, do's and don'ts, etc., if any.

For children, the setup may be scary even though it is a minor procedure; therefore, preparing children is important to avoid or reduce fear tantrums. Here are some tips:

- Start speaking about the hospital environment and what they can expect some days before the procedure.
- Ensure them that you will be with them before, during, and after the procedure.
- Explain to them that the procedure is done to make their ear feel better.
- Inform that they will be given a sleep medicine during the procedure.
- Allow them to take their toys and favorite pillow to keep near to them during the pre-surgery period.

What Happens during the Procedure

- Before entering into the operative room, a premedication will be given to help relax the individual.
- In the operative room, the anesthesiologist will first put the patient under a sleep-like state. Once the individual is safely and comfortably asleep, the ear, nose, and throat (ENT) surgeon will start the procedure:
- A small cut (incision) is made in the eardrum through the outer ear canal (myringotomy).
- The removal of fluid from the middle ear (in the eardrum) will be done using suction.
- A small plastic/metal tube is inserted through the incision (tympanotomy).
- Ear drops, along with a cotton plug, will be placed in the ear.
- The individual will be sent to the recovery room.
- This procedure takes around 15 minutes, and an overnight stay is not required.
- There will be no visible cuts or stitches.

What Happens Immediately after Surgery

- Once the patient fully recovers from anesthesia (usually less than one hour), they will be sent home.

- To prevent post-operative nausea and vomiting, it is best to resume a normal diet after an hour or two.

- Ear drops are normally administered three times a day, with three to four drops in each ear.

- Drainage of a clear yellow or mucousy fluid can occur immediately after the procedure or anytime as the tubes are in—which is normal.

Follow-Up Care

- If there are no complications, then the follow-up checkup is done usually in the first two to four weeks after the procedure. The ENT specialist (otolaryngologist) will inspect the placement and function of the tubes. If drainage persists, then the continuation of using ear drops until the next follow-up visit will be recommended. An audiogram will be obtained to check if the ear has healed completely.

- Do not resume swimming until the healthcare provider advises you to. If a patient dives into more than 6 feet of water in a chlorinated pool, lake, or pond, they are at increased risk of infection. Follow the doctor's advice for water precautions.

- Most of the ear tubes fall out over a period of six to nine months, and the holes heal and shut on their own. However, some tubes get stuck. In that case, removal of tubes and closing the hole with stitches will be done surgically.

- It is important to have checkup about every six months if tubes stay in place for a long time.

Risks and Complications of Ear Tubes

- Failure to resolve infections

- Thickening of eardrum over time, which affects hearing at a minor degree

- Perforation becomes permanent after the tube falls out of the eardrum

- Drainage that occurs for a longer period of time
- Scarring of eardrum
- The need for keeping the ear dry and using earplugs for a longer period of time
- Allergic reaction to the material of tubes (plastic or metal). This is rare, but if it occurs, removal of tubes is needed.
- Skin tissues in the ear canal or material getting trapped inside the eardrum

When to Contact the Doctor

- If any allergic reaction occurs, such as a skin rash or intolerable pain after using ear drops, discontinue the drops and contact the doctor immediately.
- If the drainage is foul-smelling or if bloody, yellow, or brown discharge (otorrhea) occurs even after using ear drops, then it is a sign of infection. Contact your doctor.
- If there is persistent pain, hearing problems, or balance issues after surgery, contact your doctor.

References

1. Cunha, John P. DO, FACOEP; Stöppler, Melissa Conrad MD. "Ear Tubes (Myringotomy and Tympanostomy Tubes)," MedicineNet, July 9, 2018.

2. Brennan, Dan MD. "Why Does My Child Need Tubes for Ear Infections?" WebMD, August 1, 2018.

3. Ben-Joseph, Elana Pearl MD. "Ear Tube Surgery," The Nemours Foundation/KidsHealth®, January 2019.

Section 6.6

Treating Ear Infections

This section contains text excerpted from the following sources: Text in this section begins with excerpts from "Ear Infection Treatment Shouldn't Be Shortened," *NIH News in Health*, National Institutes of Health (NIH), February 2017; Text beginning with the heading "Normal Tympanic Membrane" is excerpted from "Middle Ear Infections: What to Expect and Treatment Options," Effective Health Care Program, Agency for Healthcare Research and Quality (AHRQ), November 15, 2010. Reviewed April 2019.

Middle ear infections are common in kids. The illness is often caused by bacteria, and can be treated with antibiotics. But bacteria can become resistant to antibiotics. That is why it is important to take these medications as directed. Scientists have wondered if shorter treatments might reduce the risk of bacteria becoming resistant to antibiotics. Shorter treatments might also reduce other side effects. A National Institutes of Health (NIH)-funded study provides some answers—at least for children under the age of two.

The study enrolled 520 children, between the ages of 6 and 23 months, who had middle ear infections diagnosed using stringent criteria. Kids were randomly assigned to receive either a standard 10-day course of antibiotics or a shorter (5-day) treatment.

The scientists found that 77 of the 229 children (34%) in the 5-day treatment group did not improve or had worsening symptoms and signs of infection, compared to 39 of 238 (16%) who received the 10-day treatment.

After treatment, the researchers examined bacteria from the kids noses and throats. They expected the shorter treatment to reduce the development of drug-resistant bacteria. However, they found no significant differences between the two groups. Both treatment groups also had similar levels of side effects.

"The results of this study clearly show that for treating ear infections in children between 6 and 23 months of age, a 5-day course of antibiotic offers no benefit in terms of adverse events or antibiotic resistance," says study lead Dr. Alejandro Hoberman of the University of Pittsburgh School of Medicine. The findings confirm that standard antibiotics prescribed for an ear infection should be taken the full 10 days in young children.

Normal Tympanic Membrane

- Pneumococcal polysaccharide-protein conjugate vaccine (PCV7) should be administered in children between the ages of 2 and 23 months. This vaccine has been a key player in the reduction of bacterial ear infections. Since the emergence of the PCV7 vaccine, the virus H. Influenzae has become a more widespread cause of acute otitis media (AOM).

- In the United States, viral and bacterial ear infections are the most common childhood illnesses treated with antibiotics. Early detection and treatment of ear infections is vital because it can significantly reduce the negative effects on public and personal well-being.

Normal Eardrum

- Early childhood vaccinations can help to prevent bacterial ear infections.
- Most ear infections are viral and can get better on their own without antibiotic treatment.

Acute Otitis Media
Diagnostic Criteria

1. Rapid onset of signs and symptoms
2. Middle ear effusion
3. Middle-ear inflammation

Signs and Symptoms

1. Bulging tympanic membrane (TM)
2. Decreased mobility of TM
3. Fluid behind TM
4. Otorrhea
5. Erythematous TM
6. Otalgia

Risk Factors

1. Bottle-fed versus breast-fed

2. Passive cigarette smoking exposure

3. Day care attendance

Treatment

Antimicrobial agents have typically been used to manage AOM, but a "wait and see" approach is increasingly used, given concerns about medication resistance.

Amoxicillin is frequently suggested as the first-line medication treatment in children.

1. Amoxicillin

2. Amoxicillin-Clavulanate

3. Cephalosporins (e.g., ceftriaxone, cefdinir, cefixime)

Potential negative outcomes of antibiotic use:

1. Antibiotic resistance

2. Allergic reactions

3. Diarrhea/vomiting

Ear Infection
Signs of an Ear Infection

1. Fever

2. Earache (child tugging or pulling on ear is a sign)

3. Irritability

4. Liquid draining from the ear

5. Hearing difficulty

Treatment

1. "Wait and see" approach

    i. Does ear pain decrease?

    ii. Is the fever gone?

2. Prescription medications may be needed to:

   i. Decrease ear pain

   ii. Reduce fever

   iii. Treat ear infection

Parent / Guardian Follow Up

- Follow up as directed by your healthcare provider

- Use and complete all of the medications as prescribed

- Keep ears clean and dry

Otitis Media with Effusion

- Treatment can vary based on child's age and severity of symptoms. For uncomplicated AOM, the existing research suggests the "wait and see" approach.

Parent / Guardian Instructions

- Keep ears clean and dry

- Follow up with provider for symptoms of fever, ear pain, drainage from the ear

- Follow up with provider as directed

Fluid in the Eardrum

- With this type of an ear infection, clear fluid builds up or collects behind the eardrum. Often, the fluid will go away on its own without medication.

- "Wait and see" approach

Parent / Guardian Instructions

1. Keep ears clean and dry.

2. Follow up with provider for symptoms of fever, ear pain, drainage from the ear.

3. Follow up with provider as directed.

Otitis Media with Perforation

- Topical antibiotic drops are the first-line treatment for AOM with perforation.

- Fluoroquinolone antibiotics are preferred due to their lack of ototoxicity. If the infection appears to be more than just localized, then oral and sometimes even parenteral antibiotics may be needed.

- Surgery may be needed to repair a perforation if it persists for more than six weeks.

Ear Infection with Ruptured Eardrum

- Sometimes severe ear infections can cause the eardrum to burst. This opening in the eardrum can:

  1. Make it difficult to hear

  2. Cause ear infections

  3. Cause other serious problems

- If you have a ruptured eardrum, you may notice:

  1. Decrease or loss of ear pain

  2. Drainage from your ear

  3. Loss of hearing

  4. Ringing sound in your ears

  5. Dizziness

  6. Nausea and/or vomiting

- It is important that you seek medical attention right away if you have any of these signs or symptoms.

- Follow-up visits may also be needed in order to ensure that the ruptured eardrum has healed after being treated.

Tympanostomy Tubes

Recurrent otitis media (ROM) is defined as 3 or more diagnosed occurrences of AOM within 6 months or 4 episodes within 12 months.

Tympanostomy tube insertion can substantially reduce the rate of ear infections after the first six months of tube insertion in children with ROM.

Outcomes with Tympanostomy Tubes

1. Improved fluid drainage

2. Reduced pressure in tympanic membrane (TM)

3. Improved equilibrium maintenance

Treatment for Infection with Tympanostomy Tube

1. Ciprofloxacin 0.3 percent-dexamethasone 0.1 percent otic drops

2. Amoxicillin-Clavulanate

3. Cephalosporins (e.g., ceftriaxone, cefuroxime)

4. Quinolones

5. Antibiotic prophylaxis

Ear Tubes
Are Ear Tubes an Option for My Child?

Ear tubes may be an option for children who suffer from recurrent ear infections. (More than 3 in 6 months, or 4 in 12 months).

Ear Tubes Help To

1. Reduce pressure in the eardrum (that may cause ear pain)

2. Drain fluid from the eardrum

3. Decrease the number of ear infections

Parent/Guardian Care

1. Keep ears clean and dry

2. Wear earplugs when swimming

3. Do not put anything into the ear (e.g., Q-tips)

4. Call your provider if there is discolored drainage, fever, red ears, irritability/ear tugging occurs

5. Follow up with provider as directed

Chapter 7

Ear Injuries

Chapter Contents

Section 7.1

Perforated Eardrum

A perforated eardrum—also called a "ruptured eardrum" or "perforated tympanic membrane"—is a tear in the thin membrane that separates the outer ear from the middle ear. The function of this cone-shaped membrane is to transmit sound waves gathered by the outer ear to the ossicles (three small bones) in the middle ear and then to the oval window, the port to the fluid-filled inner ear. Structures in the inner ear stimulate auditory nerves, which then transmit impulses that the brain interprets as sound.

Perforated eardrums generally result in some degree of hearing loss, and in rare cases, this could be permanent. Most of the time, the tear will heal on its own in a few weeks, but in more serious instances, surgery or another type of medical intervention may be necessary. And until the perforation heals or is repaired, the normally sterile middle ear is subject to infection.

Causes

There are numerous potential causes for a perforated eardrum, some pathological (caused by disease) and some traumatic (caused by injury). These can include:

- Middle ear infections

- Damage from foreign objects, such as cotton swabs, inserted into the ear

- Injury to the ear from a powerful slap or other impact

- Barotrauma, damage caused by a change in pressure, as with air travel or scuba diving

- Very loud noise, such as a gunshot or explosion, close to the ear

- Severe head trauma, such as a skull fracture

Symptoms

The primary symptom of a perforated eardrum is pain, which might initially seem like a common earache but then increases in severity. It can be extremely sharp and sudden, dull and steady, or intermittent. Other symptoms may include:

- Partial or complete hearing loss in the affected ear
- Ringing or buzzing in the ear
- Drainage from the ear, which may be pus, blood, or clear liquid
- Facial weakness
- Dizziness
- Repeated ear infections

Diagnosis

A physician—either a family doctor or an ear, nose, and throat (ENT) specialist—will generally begin by taking a medical history of the patient and his or her family. This will likely be followed by a series of questions about symptoms of the ailment and any medications taken by the patient. The physical examination is done with an otoscope, a specialized instrument with a light that will allow the doctor to see into the ear and determine whether or not the eardrum has been ruptured.

Other tests that may be performed include:

- Audiology test, which uses generated sound to assess the extent of hearing loss
- Tuning-fork test, a less technical but still effective method of assessing hearing loss
- Tympanometry, an examination that tests the eardrum's response to pressure changes.
- Laboratory tests of fluid draining from the ear, if any

Treatment

Many ear infections heal on their own over the course of a few weeks or, at most, a few months. In such cases, the doctor may prescribe antibiotics, either pills or ear drops, to help prevent infection, as well as pain medicine, usually over-the-counter (OTC) medications, such as acetaminophen or ibuprofen. Warm compresses might also be recommended to relieve discomfort.

If the perforation does not begin to heal on its own, and if the hole is not too large, the ENT specialist may apply a special patch to the eardrum. This is done with a very thin, medicated material that both protects the wound and encourages healing of the membrane. The procedure takes only 15 to 30 minutes and can usually be done in the doctor's office using a local anesthetic.

If the eardrum does not heal on its own, and the rupture is too large for a patch, a surgical repair called a "tympanoplasty" might be required. In this procedure, the surgeon makes the repair through the ear canal itself or through an incision behind the ear. After cleaning and preparing the damaged area, the surgeon will take a small piece of tissue from elsewhere on the body and graft it onto the eardrum to seal the perforation.

Tympanoplasty is generally performed in a hospital with the patient under general anesthetic. It usually lasts up to one hour if the procedure is done through the ear canal, or up to three hours if an incision behind the ear is required.

In cases in which the ossicles—the tiny bones in the middle ear—have been damaged by injury or infection, an ossiculoplasty might need to be performed. This procedure, which is also done in a hospital under general anesthetic, involves the replacement of the damaged bones with bones from a donor or with an artificial substitute.

Complications

Most perforated eardrums heal well with simple treatment, and even patients with more extensive ruptures can achieve a good result with proper medical attention. However, left untreated, a punctured eardrum can lead to potentially serious complications, including:

- Fever

- Severe pain

- Dizziness

- Hearing loss, usually temporary but possibly permanent

- Middle ear infections, caused by bacteria entering through the opening

- Damage to the bones of the middle ear

- Middle ear cholesteatoma, a cyst composed of skin cells and other debris

- In rare cases, infection may spread to the brain

Prevention

One of the most effective ways to prevent a perforated eardrum is to keep foreign objects out of the ear. And if an object does become lodged in the ear canal, it is best to have it removed by a medical professional. Another important prevention method is to get treatment for ear infections before they become serious enough to damage the eardrum.

A few other ways to prevent ruptured eardrums include:

- Keep ears dry to help avoid infection.
- If susceptible to ear infections, wear earplugs when swimming or bathing.
- Protect ears while flying (yawn or chew gum to equalize pressure).
- Avoid flying with a cold or sinus infection.
- Wear earplugs or earmuffs to protect against loud noises.

References

1. Derrer, David T., MD. "Ruptured Eardrum: Symptoms and Treatments," WebMD, August 17, 2014.

2. "Eardrum Rupture," Healthline.com, August 25, 2016.

3. Kacker, Ashutosh, MD, BS. "Ruptured Eardrum," MedLincPlus. gov, May 18, 2014.

4. "Ruptured Eardrum," Mount Sinai Hospital, August 10, 2015.

5. "Ruptured Eardrum (Perforated Eardrum)," Mayo Clinic, January 4, 2014

Section 7.2

Tympanoplasty and Mastoidectomy

This section includes text excerpted from "Ear Surgery:
Tympanoplasty, Mastoidectomy," U.S. Department of Veterans
Affairs (VA), July 2013. Reviewed April 2019.

Reasons for Surgery

Your eardrum is called the "tympanic membrane." If there is a hole in your eardrum, you may get an infection. This can affect your hearing. You may also get a cholesteatoma. This is a cyst made up of trapped skin cells. The cyst can invade the inner ear, brain, or facial nerve. For this reason, a cholesteatoma must be completely removed.

Ossicles

These are bones in the middle ear. They send sound from the eardrum to the inner ear. These may be eroded from repeated infections or from cholesteatoma. They may need to be replaced with a human-made part (called a "prosthesis") when you have surgery. This may help you hear better.

Tympanoplasty and Mastoidectomy

Your doctor will make a cut (an incision) behind your ear or inside the ear canal. A small amount of tissue will be taken from the muscle above your ear. This is done through the same incision. You may also have a small skin graft removed from the back of your ear. The doctor may use cartilage from your ear canal to rebuild your eardrum. Then, your ear will be sewn back in place. The doctor will pack your ear canal with a spongy material.

You will go home the same day of surgery. You will need someone to drive you home. It is normal to feel a little dizzy for a few days after surgery. If the dizziness is very bad, call your doctor. It is normal to hear funny noises inside your ear for weeks to months after surgery.

Postoperative Instructions
Ear Surgery

1. If you have a plastic cup ear dressing, remove it after 24 hours. You do not have to wear it any longer. You may replace the

gauze in the cup with clean gauze and use it at night to sleep if your ear is more comfortable that way. Or you can throw it away.

2. When you remove the plastic cup dressing, take off the nonstick gauze that is over the incision behind your ear. Begin applying an antibiotic ointment, such as Polysporin or Bacitracin, to the incision two times a day. Do this for four days. Gently clean the incision with a mixture of half hydrogen peroxide and half water on a Q-tip to remove dried blood. The stitches will go away on their own.

3. After three days, you can wash your hair and pat dry your incision. Keep water out of your ear canal until your postoperative appointment. You can do this by placing a cotton ball in your ear canal, covering it with Vaseline, and removing it after bathing.

4. If you have a gauze ear dressing, cut it off when told to by your doctor.

5. After 24 hours, take out the cotton ball from your ear canal. Use the antibiotic drops the way your doctor told you to. Most often, you will place 4 to 5 drops in your ear canal two times a day until you return for your postoperative visit. This will lessen your risk of infection. It will also keep the sponge packing in your ear canal wet. This will make it much easier to clean out at your next visit.

6. After 24 hours, you can put in another cotton ball if your ear is draining. If you do not have drainage, you do not need to do this.

7. You may have some drainage and mild bleeding from your ear canal for the first few days after surgery. If you need to change more than 12 cotton balls in a 24 hour period because they are bloody, this is too much. You will need to be seen by your doctor.

8. Some of the packing that is placed in your ear canal may fall out after surgery. Sometimes, it looks like a tiny wet sponge. Other times, it looks like a tiny piece of meat. Do not worry about this. Do not try to put the packing back in.

9. Do not place anything in your ear canal. Do not insert a Q-tip into your ear canal.

10. Do not blow your nose for at least two weeks after surgery. You may gently wipe the front of your nose. Blowing the nose could dislodge your new eardrum.

11. Sneeze with your mouth open for two weeks. Pressure from a sneeze could dislodge your new eardrum.

12. If you wear eyeglasses, you can use them once the dressing is removed, but place a gauze pad or a Band-aid to keep the rims from irritating the incision.

Activity

Do not do any heavy lifting, straining, or vigorous activity for three weeks after surgery. Such activities could dislodge your new eardrum. Do not swim until your doctor tells you that you can. You can often return to work one to two weeks after surgery, but ask your doctor first.

Diet

You may eat your regular diet after surgery, as long as your stomach is not upset from the anesthesia. If it is, wait until you feel better before you start eating solid foods.

Pain

Pain is usually mild to moderate for the first 24 to 48 hours. Then it will decrease. You may not need strong narcotic medicine. The sooner you reduce your narcotic pain medication use, the faster you will recover. As your pain lessens, try using extra-strength acetaminophen (Tylenol) instead of your narcotic medication. It is best to reduce your pain to a level that you can manage, rather than to get rid of the pain completely. Start at a lower of narcotic pain medicine dosage, and increase the dose only if the pain remains uncontrolled. Decrease the dose if the side effects are too severe.

Do not drive, operate dangerous machinery, or do anything dangerous if you are taking narcotic pain medication (examples are oxycodone, hydrocodone, and morphine,) These drugs affect your reflexes and responses, just like alcohol.

When to Call Your Doctor, If You Have

1. Any concerns.

2. A fever over 101.5°F that does not go away

3. A large amount of bleeding from your ear or from your incision

4. Headaches

5. Leakage of a lot of clear fluid from your nose or ear canal

6. Severe dizziness

7. Weakness of your facial muscles

8. Excessive swelling of the incision behind your ear

9. Redness or warmth around your incision

10. Foul-smelling discharge from the ear or from the incision

11. Pain that continues to increase instead of decrease

12. Problems urinating

13. Chest pain or problems breathing. Do not call ahead—go to the emergency room right away.

Call Your Doctor

If it is urgent, call 911 or go directly to the closest emergency room without calling ahead.

Postoperative Appointment

You will need to have your ear canal cleaned out at your postoperative visit.

Section 7.3

Barotrauma/Barotitis Media

This section contains text excerpted from the following sources:
Text in this section begins with excerpts from "Barotrauma,"
MedlinePlus, National Institutes of Health (NIH), February 7, 2019;
Text under the heading "Management" is excerpted from "Airman
Education Programs," Federal Aviation Administration (FAA),
November 18, 2010. Reviewed April 2019.

Barotrauma means injury to your body because of changes in barometric (air) or water pressure. One common type happens to your ear. A change in altitude may cause your ears to hurt. This can happen if you are flying in an airplane, driving in the mountains, or scuba diving. Divers can also get decompression sickness, which affects the whole body.

Common symptoms of ear barotrauma include:

- Pain

- A feeling that your ears are stuffed

- Hearing loss

- Dizziness

Treatments for ear barotrauma include chewing gum and yawning to relieve the pressure. Medications, such as decongestants, may also help.

Management

An ear block is usually preceded by a fullness in the ear, gradual loss of hearing, and, eventually, pain. Most ear blocks are a result of not knowing how to properly equalize the pressure in the middle ear or trying to fly with a cold.

Normally, there is little difficulty equalizing pressure during descent; by occasionally swallowing, yawning, or tensing the muscles of the throat, the pressure will equalize. Infants should be given a bottle or pacifier to aid in equalization. Small children can avoid difficulty by chewing gum.

If these actions fail to equalize the pressure, a Valsalva maneuver should be performed. The Valsalva maneuver is performed by closing the mouth, pinching the nostrils closed and blowing air through the nose. This will force air up the eustachian tube and into the middle ear. This is not a dangerous procedure and should not be delayed until the pressure in the ears becomes painful, otherwise it may be extremely difficult to open the eustachian tube. Painful ear blocks generally occur when the descent rate is too rapid. This should be followed by a slower descent, if possible.

Along with the lack of improper equalization maneuvers, flying with a cold can be just as much a problem, if not more so. Equalization of the middle ear can be impaired when the eustachian tube, or its opening, becomes restricted as the result of inflammation, upper respiratory infection, sore throat, infection of the middle ear, or sinusitis. It may be possible to equalize the middle ear by a forceful Valsalva, but this may result in the infected material being carried into the eustachian tube along with the air, causing infection of the middle ear. Since the resulting infection may result in a longer grounding than the cold, it may be advisable not to fly if you suspect you have a cold.

The sinuses most often affected by pressure change are the frontal and the maxillary sinuses. These air-filled, rigid, bony cavities lined with mucous membrane are connected with the nasal cavity by means of one or more small openings. When these openings into the sinuses are normal, air passes through these cavities without difficulty and can accommodate any moderate rate of ascent or descent. If the openings of the sinuses are obstructed by the swelling of the mucous membrane lining, ready equalization of pressure becomes difficult, and the possibility of a sinus block will increase. This is another example of what could happen as a result of flying, or diving with a cold. Keep in mind that most sinus blocks occur on descent and will give little or no warning.

When the maxillary sinuses are affected, the pain will probably be felt on either side of the nose, under the cheekbones. Maxillary sinusitis may produce pain referred to the teeth of the upper jaw, and may be mistaken for a toothache.

When the frontal sinuses are affected, the pain will be located above the eyes and usually is quite severe. This type of sinus problem is the most common.

Equalization of pressure to relieve pain in the sinuses is best accomplished by use of the Valsalva procedure, and/or inhalants, previously mentioned in conjunction with ear blocks. Again, you should be very cautious in your use of any over-the-counter medication. Reversing the direction of pressure change as rapidly as possible may be necessary to clear severe sinus blocks.

Section 7.4

Foreign Object in the Ear

"Foreign Object in the Ear," © 2019 Omnigraphics.
Reviewed April 2019.

Getting a foreign object stuck in the ear canal is a relatively common ear problem. Since the ear canal is very sensitive, one can easily know if an object is stuck. However, young children may find it difficult to feel or express the presence of foreign objects within their ears. Even though having a foreign object in the ear canal is rarely an emergency, it can sometimes cause serious threats, such as pain, infection, and bleeding, and it may even lead to hearing loss.

What Objects Can Get into the Ears

A vast majority of foreign objects that are put into the ears are voluntarily placed into the ears by the person themselves. Toddlers and young children get into this sort of trouble very often as they place various items in their ears out of curiosity. The most common things that get stuck in the ear canal are:

- Food particles
- Beads
- Marbles
- Shells
- Small toys
- Cotton swabs
- Batteries
- Insects

At times, a buildup of earwax (cerumen) can also be considered problematic. Although it is technically not a foreign object, excess accumulation of earwax can cause discomfort and decrease hearing ability.

Symptoms of Having Foreign Object in the Ear

The symptoms of having a foreign object in the ear may vary, depending on the shape, size, and type of the object involved. The most common symptoms are:

- Sense of heaviness inside the ear

- Redness, inflammation, and pain in the area surrounding the ear

- Discharge of pus

- Bleeding, if the object inside the ear is sharp or pointed

- Irritation in the ear canal, leading to nausea or vomiting

- Reduced hearing on the side of the blockage

- A buzzing sound, if there is a live insect inside the ear canal

Small children will not be able to verbalize when something is stuck in their ears. In such cases, parents or guardians can look for visible symptoms, such as redness, swelling, bleeding, or pus formation. When children rub or scratch their ears continuously, it can also act as a sign of the presence of foreign objects.

How to Remove a Foreign Object from the Ear

Whenever a foreign object is put in the ear, people tend to probe the area with tools, such as cotton swabs, pins, matchsticks, etc. But, these tools may push the object even farther into the ear canal and cause more damage.

The following are some home remedies to dislodge foreign objects from the ear.

- Tilt your head towards the affected side, and try to get the foreign object out. If the object does not come out, gently pull the pinna (external ear), so that the ear canal will straighten out and make more room for the object to roll out.

- If the eardrum is intact, irrigate the ear with warm water. This can wash the object out of the ear.

- If the foreign object is a live insect, pour a few drops of warm oil into the ear and tilt your head, so that the insect will float out.

If the above methods fail, visit an ear, nose, and throat (ENT) doctor immediately. The doctor can remove the object successfully by using the appropriate tools and equipment, such as forceps and suction tubes. If you are experiencing pain after the removal of the object, consult your doctor and take proper medications.

References

1. "Foreign Object in the Ear: First Aid," Mayoclinic, September 12, 2017.

2. Buccino, Kenneth. "Foreign Body in Ear," eMedicineHealth, February 1, 2002.

3. Cunha, John P. "Foreign Body in the Ear: Symptoms and Causes," MedicineNet, April 7, 2017.

Section 7.5

Stay Away from Ear Candles

This section includes text excerpted from "Don't Get Burned: Stay Away From Ear Candles," U.S. Food and Drug Administration (FDA), December 15, 2017.

A lit candle that can drip hot wax into your ear, usually as you lie on your side.

Sound dangerous? The U.S. Food and Drug Administration (FDA) thinks so, and is warning consumers to steer clear of products being sold as ear candles.

These candles—hollow cones that are about 10 inches long and made from a fabric tube soaked in beeswax, paraffin, or a mixture of the two—are being marketed as treatments for a variety of conditions. These conditions include ear wax buildup, sinus infections, hearing loss, headaches, colds, flu, and sore throats.

Marketers of ear candles claim that warmth created by the lit device produces suction that draws wax and other impurities out of the ear canal.

"Some ear candles are offered as products that purify the blood, strengthen the brain, or even 'cure' cancer," says Eric Mann, M.D., Ph.D., clinical deputy director of the FDA's Division of Ophthalmic, Neurological, and Ear, Nose, and Throat Devices.

He adds that some firms claim the candles are appropriate for use on children.

But the FDA warns that ear candles can cause serious injuries, even when used in accordance to manufacturers' directions. "Also," says Mann, "the FDA believes that there is no valid scientific evidence for any medical benefit from their use."

Burns and Other Risks

Mann says that ear candling—the procedure is also called "ear coning" and "thermal auricular therapy"—exposes the recipient to risks such as:

- Starting a fire

- Burns to the face, ear canal, eardrum, and middle ear

- Injury to the ear from dripping wax

- Ears plugged by candle wax

- Bleeding

- Puncture of the eardrum

- Delay in seeking needed medical care for underlying conditions, such as sinus and ear infections, hearing loss, cancer, and temporomandibular joint (TMJ) disorders. TMJ disorders often cause headache and painful sensations in the area of the ear, jaw, and face.

Even many promoters of ear candles warn potential users to have the procedure done by an experienced "candler," and to not use the candles on themselves.

Ear candling involves placing the candle in the outer ear, usually while the recipient lies on his or her side. It is also done with the recipient sitting upright.

Often, before being lit, the candle is placed through a hole located in the center of a plate. The plate is supposed to protect against hot wax or ash coming down the side of the device and onto the recipient.

Enforcement

The FDA and Health Canada, the Canadian health regulatory agency, have acted against manufacturers of ear candles. These actions have included import alerts, seizures, injunctions, and warning letters. The FDA import alerts identify products that are suspected of violating the law so that agency field personnel and U.S. Customs and Border

Protection (CBP) staff can stop these entries at the border prior to distribution in the United States.

In February 2010, the FDA issued warning letters to three large manufacturers of ear candles. These firms were informed that the FDA had determined that there was no agency approval or clearance, no manufacturing facility registration or device listing, and no adverse-event reporting systems in place in regard to their ear candles.

The FDA will continue to take enforcement action when appropriate.

Concern for Children

Claims that ear candling is appropriate for kids have caused great concern at the FDA. "Children of any age, including babies, are at increased risk for injuries and complications if they are exposed to ear candles," says Mann.

He adds that small children and infants may move while the device is being used, increasing the likelihood of wax burns and ear candle wax plugging the ear canal. "Also, their smaller ear canal size may make children more susceptible than adults to injuries from ear candles," he says.

Since the FDA views ear candles as medical devices, manufacturers seeking approval to sell them must submit evidence to the FDA that the products are safe and effective.

Reports of Injuries

The FDA believes that injuries associated with ear candles are likely underreported, and encourages consumers and healthcare professionals to report such injuries to MedWatch: The FDA Safety Information and Adverse Event Reporting Program.

Over the past decade, the FDA has received reports of burns, punctured eardrums, and blockage of the ear canal that required outpatient surgery from the use of ear candles.

In its testing, Health Canada found that ear candles produce no measurable effect in the ear and have no therapeutic value.

And in a survey published in 1996, the medical journal Laryngoscope reported 13 cases of burns of the ear, 7 cases of ear canal blockage due to wax, and 1 case of a punctured eardrum.

That study also reported that ear candles produced no measurable vacuum pressure or suction on a model of the ear, and that burning ear candles dripped candle wax onto the eardrum of test subjects.

Chapter 8

Ear Secretions and Growths

Chapter Contents

Section 8.1

Earwax (Cerumen)

This section contains text excerpted from the following sources: Text
in this section begins with excerpts from "Why You Shouldn't Use
Cotton Swabs to Clean Your Ears," National Institute on Deafness
and Other Communication Disorders (NIDCD), July 27, 2017; Text
beginning with the heading "Risk Factors" is excerpted from "Earwax
Blockage," U.S. Department of Veterans Affairs (VA), March 2017.

Have you ever been tempted to clean out your ears (or your children's ears) with cotton swabs? Experts have one word of advice: do not.

Earwax (cerumen) is supposed to be in your ears. It has a mission: to keep your ears healthy by trapping dust and dirt so that they do not travel deeper into your ear. Having a waxy coating on your delicate ear canal skin also helps to protect it. The inside of your ear does not need to be cleaned because earwax is the cleaner.

Your body already has a way to deal with earwax it no longer needs. Chewing, other jaw movements, and skin growing inside your ear will push old earwax out naturally. Using cotton swabs, however, can push the wax deeper into your ear canal. You might also seriously damage sensitive ear-canal skin or your eardrum.

Earwax buildup is not very common. According to the American Academy of Otolaryngology—Head and Neck Surgery (AAO—HNS), only 1 in 10 children and 1 in 20 adults have this problem. Some people may be more susceptible to earwax buildup. About 3 in 10 elderly adults and developmentally disabled adults might have more of a problem with earwax.

Signs of too much earwax or earwax that is stuck and blocking the ear canal include:

- Pain or itching

- A feeling that your ear is full

- Ringing in the ear (tinnitus)

- Hearing loss (or a change in how well hearing aids work, for those who use them)

- Odor or discharge

If you have any of these symptoms, see a doctor or other healthcare provider.

Risk Factors

- Using cotton swabs to clean the ear can compress wax and block the ear canal.

General Measures

- Do not use Q-tips or other objects to remove wax. You may cause damage to the eardrum or infection in the ear canal.

Medication

- Using nonprescription wax-softening ear drops, such as Debrox, can help remove the wax from your ear with less pain.

- If you are scheduled for the ear wash clinic, begin using the drops three days before your appointment. Follow the directions on the box.

- Take acetaminophen (unless advised against use) for minor pain.

If symptoms still persist, then the patient may need removal by a healthcare provider.

Section 8.2

Otosclerosis

This section includes text excerpted from "Otosclerosis,"
National Institute on Deafness and Other Communication
Disorders (NIDCD), July 17, 2018.

What Is Otosclerosis?

Otosclerosis is a term that comes from two ancient words: "oto," which means "from the ear" and "sclerosis," which means "the abnormal hardening of body tissue." Otosclerosis is the result of abnormal remodeling of the bones in the middle ear. The remodeling of the bones is a permanent process in which the bone tissue is renewed by replacing old tissue with a new one. In otosclerosis, abnormal remodeling disrupts the ability of sound to travel from the middle ear to the inner ear. Otosclerosis affects more than three million people in the United States. It is believed that many of the cases of otosclerosis are hereditary. White women of middle age are at the greatest risk.

What Causes Otosclerosis

Otosclerosis usually occurs when one of the bones of the middle ear, the stapes, gets stuck in place. When this bone cannot vibrate, sound cannot travel through the ear, and hearing deteriorates.

It is still unclear why this happens, but scientists believe it could be related to previous measles infection, stress fractures in the bone tissue that surrounds the inner ear, or immune system disorders. Otosclerosis also tends to be hereditary.

It could also be caused by the interaction of three different cells of the immune system known as "cytokines." Researchers believe that the proper balance of these three substances is necessary for the remodeling of healthy bone. Also, researchers believe that an imbalance in their levels could cause the type of abnormal remodeling that occurs in otosclerosis.

What Are the Symptoms of Otosclerosis?

Hearing loss is the symptom of otosclerosis that is reported the most. It usually begins in one ear and then passes to the other. This loss can appear very gradually. Many people with otosclerosis first realize that they can not hear low tones or hear a whisper. Some people may also have dizziness, balance problems, or tinnitus. Tinnitus is a roaring, clicking, whistling, or buzzing in the ears or in the head that sometimes occurs with hearing loss.

How Is Otosclerosis Diagnosed?

Health professionals who specialize in hearing are those who diagnose otosclerosis. These professionals include an otolaryngologist, who is a doctor who specializes in disorders of the ear, nose, throat, and neck (ENT); an otologist, a doctor who specializes in diseases of the ears; or an audiologist, a trained healthcare professional that identifies, measures, and treats hearing disorders. The first step in the diagnosis is to rule out other diseases or health problems that can cause the same symptoms as otosclerosis. The following steps include hearing tests that measure hearing sensitivity (audiogram) and sound conduction in the middle ear (tympanogram). Sometimes, diagnostic images are also used.

What Is the Treatment for Otosclerosis?

Currently, there is no effective pharmacological treatment for otosclerosis. There is hope that the research being done on the remodeling of the bones could identify new potential therapies. Mild otosclerosis can be treated with a hearing aid that amplifies sound, but often requires surgery. In a procedure known as a "stapedectomy," the surgeon inserts a prosthesis into the middle ear that passes around the abnormal bone and allows the sound waves to travel to the inner ear, thus restoring hearing.

It is important to discuss any surgical procedure with an ear specialist to clarify the potential risks and limitations of the operation. For example, some hearing loss may remain after stapedectomy, and in rare cases, surgery may even worsen hearing loss.

What Research Is Being Done on Otosclerosis?

The complicated architecture of the inner ear makes it difficult for scientists to study this part of the body. Because researchers cannot remove and analyze a sample from the inner ear of someone with otosclerosis (or with other hearing disorders), they must study ear bone samples from cadavers donated for research. These samples, which are called "temporary bone," are scarce. To encourage further research on otosclerosis, the National Institute on Deafness and Other

Communication Disorders (NIDCD) supports national collections of temporary bones, such as the Otopathology Research Collaboration Network at Massachusetts Eye and Ear Infirmary. This effort coordinates the collection and exchange of temporary bone tissue between laboratories. It also encourages scientists to incorporate modern technologies in the fields of biology, computer science, and imaging with information from the patient's medical history and pathology reports. In this way, we hope to find new clues and solutions for ear disorders caused by bone abnormalities.

The NIDCD also funds genetic studies and research on bone remodeling to better understand the causes of otosclerosis and investigate possible new treatments. Currently, researchers funded by the NIDCD are testing the effectiveness of an implantable device on animals. This device could directly administer a medication in the inner ear that inhibits the growth of bones to correct the abnormalities of the bones that cause otosclerosis. If the results are promising, studies will be conducted on people in the future.

Section 8.3

Cholesteatoma

This section includes text excerpted from "Cholesteatoma," Genetic and Rare Diseases Information Center (GARD), National Center for Advancing Translational Sciences (NCATS), April 28, 2017.

Cholesteatoma is an abnormal growth of skin in the middle ear behind the eardrum. It can be congenital (present from birth), but it more commonly occurs as a complication of chronic ear infections. Individuals with this condition usually experience a painless discharge from the ear. Hearing loss, dizziness, and facial muscle paralysis are rare but can result from continued cholesteatoma growth. Treatment usually involves surgery to remove the growth.

Symptoms

Early symptoms may include fluid drainage from the ear, sometimes with a foul odor. As the cholesteatoma enlarges, it can lead to:

- A full feeling, or pressure in the ear

- Hearing loss

- Dizziness

- Pain

- Numbness or muscle weakness on one side of the face

Occasionally, individuals may experience complications of the central nervous system, including:

- A blood clot in certain veins within the skull, including the sigmoid sinus

- A collection of infected material between the outer covering of brain and skull (epidural abscess)

- Inflammation of the tissue that surrounds the brain and spinal cord (meningitis)

Cause

A cholesteatoma usually occurs because of poor eustachian tube function in combination with infection in the middle ear. When the eustachian tube is not working correctly, the pressure within the middle ear can pull part of the eardrum the wrong way, creating a sac or cyst that fills with old skin cells. If the cyst gets bigger, some of the middle ear bones may break down, affecting hearing. Rarely, a congenital form of cholesteatoma can occur in the middle ear and elsewhere, such as in the nearby skull bones.

Treatment

Initial treatment may involve careful cleaning of the ear, antibiotics, and eardrops. Therapy aims to stop drainage in the ear by controlling the infection. Large or more complicated cholesteatomas may require surgery. Cholesteatomas very often continue to grow if they are not removed. Surgery is usually successful.

Prognosis

Cholesteatomas usually continue to grow if not removed. Surgery is typically successful, but occasional ear cleaning by a healthcare provider may be necessary. Additional surgery may be needed if the cholesteatoma comes back.

In rare cases, complications may arise. These include:

- A collection of pus and other material in the brain (brain abscess)
- Hearing loss in one ear
- Dizziness (vertigo)
- A breakdown of the facial nerves, leading to facial paralysis
- Meningitis
- Persistent ear drainage
- Spread of the cyst into the brain

Part Three

Hearing Disorders

Chapter 9

Hearing Loss: The Basics

Chapter Contents

Section 9.1

Hearing and Hearing Loss: Explained

This section contains text excerpted from the following sources: Text in this section begins with excerpts from "Understanding Hearing Loss," Centers for Disease Control and Prevention (CDC), April 11, 2018; Text beginning with the heading "How Do We Hear?" is excerpted from "How Does Loud Noise Cause Hearing Loss?" Centers for Disease Control and Prevention (CDC), December 11, 2018; Text under the heading "Understanding Hearing Loss: About Sound" is excerpted from "Understanding Hearing Loss: About Sound," Centers for Disease Control and Prevention (CDC), April 11, 2018.

Many different things can happen in the ear to cause hearing loss. Our ear and hearing are made up of many parts:

- The outer ear
- The middle ear
- The inner ear
- The ear (auditory) nerve—the hearing (auditory) system pathway in the brain

These terms describe hearing loss where the part of the ear that is not working in a usual way:

- **Conductive loss**—hearing loss caused by something that stops sounds from getting through the outer or middle ear.
- **Sensorineural loss**—hearing loss that occurs when there is a problem in the way the inner ear or hearing nerve works.
- **Mixed hearing loss**—hearing loss that includes a conductive and a sensorineural hearing loss.
- **Auditory neuropathy spectrum disorder (ANSD)**—hearing loss that occurs when sound enters the ear normally, but because of damage to the inner ear or the hearing nerve, sound is not organized in a way that the brain can understand.

These terms describe the degree or the amount of hearing loss a child has:

- **Mild hearing loss**—a person with mild hearing loss may hear some speech sounds, but soft sounds are hard to hear.

- **Moderate hearing loss**—a person with moderate hearing loss may hear almost no speech when another person is talking at a normal level.
- **Severe hearing loss**—a person with severe hearing loss will hear no speech of a person talking at a normal level and only some loud sounds.
- **Profound hearing loss**—a person with profound hearing loss will not hear any speech and only very loud sounds.

These terms describe when the hearing loss happened:

- **Prelingual**—the hearing loss occurred before the child learned to talk.
- **Postlingual**—the hearing loss occurred after the child learned to talk.

These terms describe the side or sides on which the hearing loss occurs:

- **Unilateral**—there is a hearing loss in one ear.
- **Bilateral**—there is a hearing loss in both ears.

Parents and professionals will use these terms to describe a child's unique type of hearing loss when talking to others.

If professionals and other parents use terms that you do not understand, please ask questions.

How Do We Hear?

We hear sound because of vibrations (sound waves) that reach our ears. We recognize those vibrations as speech, music, or other sounds.

Outer Ear

The outer ear—the part of the ear you see—funnels sound waves into the ear canal. The sound waves travel through the ear canal to reach the eardrum.

Middle Ear

The eardrum vibrates from the incoming sound waves and sends these vibrations to three tiny bones in the middle ear. These bones amplify, or increase, the sound vibrations and send them to the inner ear.

Inner Ear

The inner ear contains a snail-shaped structure filled with fluid called the "cochlea." Sound vibrations create waves in the cochlear fluids. As the waves peak, they cause tiny hair cells (types of receptors that can detect sound) to bend, which converts the vibrations into electrical signals.

Auditory Nerve

The auditory nerve carries the electrical signals from the inner ear to the brain, which interprets the signals as sound that you recognize and understand.

Damaged Hair Cells in Your Ears Can Lead to Hearing Loss

The average person is born with about 16,000 hair cells within their cochlea. These cells allow your brain to detect sounds. Up to 30 to 50 percent of hair cells can be damaged or destroyed before changes in your hearing can be measured by a hearing test. By the time you notice hearing loss, many hair cells have been destroyed and cannot be repaired.

After leaving a very loud event, such as a concert or football game, you may notice that you don't hear as well as before. You might not hear whispers, sound might seem muffled, or you may hear ringing in your ears. Normal hearing usually returns within a few hours to a few days. This is because the hair cells, similar to blades of grass, will bend more if the sound is louder. But they will become straight again after a recovery period.

However, if loud noise damaged too many of the hair cells, some of them will die. Repeated exposures to loud noises will eventually destroy many hair cells. This can gradually reduce your ability to understand speech in noisy environments. Eventually, if hearing loss continues, it can become hard to understand speech, even in quieter places.

Noise Can Also Damage Nerves in Your Ears

In addition to damaging hair cells, noise can also damage the auditory nerve that carries information about sounds to your brain. Early damage may not show up on your hearing test, but can create a "hidden hearing loss" that may make it difficult for you to understand speech in noisy environments. The cumulative effect of noise affects how well you might hear later in life and how quickly you might develop hearing problems, even after exposure has stopped.

Understanding Hearing Loss: About Sound

In order to understand hearing loss, it helps to understand how we hear. Sounds are described in terms of their frequency, known as "pitch," and intensity, known as "loudness."

Sound Frequency (Pitch)

Frequency is measured in hertz (Hz). A person who has the ability to hear within the normal range can hear sounds that have frequencies between 20 and 20,000 Hz. The most important sounds we hear every day are in the 250 to 6,000 Hz range.

Speech includes a mix of low and high-frequency sounds:

- Vowel sounds—such as a short "o," as in the word "hot"—have low frequencies (250 to 1,000 Hz) and are usually easier to hear.

- Consonants, such as "s," "h," and "f," have higher frequencies (1,500 to 6,000 Hz) and are harder to hear. Consonants convey most of the meaning of what we say. Someone who cannot hear high-frequency sounds will have a hard time understanding speech and language.

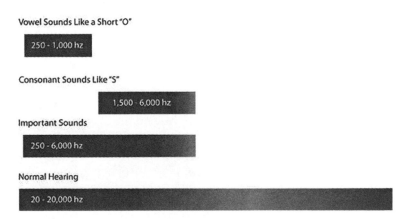

Figure 9.1. *Frequency Chart for Hearing Loss*

Frequency of sounds (measured in hertz (Hz))

Sound Intensity (Loudness)

Sound intensity, or loudness, is measured in decibels (dB).

- A person with hearing within the normal range can hear sounds ranging from 0 to 140 dB.

- A whisper is around 25 to 30 dB.

- Conversations are usually 45 to 60 dB.

- Sounds that are louder than 90 dB can be uncomfortable to hear.

- A loud rock concert might be as loud as 110 dB.

- Sounds that are 120 dB or louder can be painful and can result in temporary or permanent hearing loss.

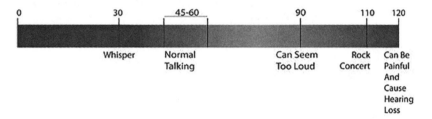

Figure 9.2. *Hearing Loss Chart in Decibels*

Intensity of sounds (measured in decibels (dB))

Different groups and organizations use decibels to define the degree of hearing loss differently.

Section 9.2

Mechanism Underlying Stereocilia

This section contains text excerpted from the following sources:
Text in this section begins with excerpts from "Researchers Discover
Mechanism Underlying Stereocilia Self-Renewal," National Institute
on Deafness and Other Communication Disorders (NIDCD), June 7,
2010. Reviewed April 2019; Text under the heading "Proteins Linked
to Congenital Deafness Help Build, Maintain Stereocilia in the Inner
Ear" is excerpted from "Proteins Linked to Congenital Deafness Help
Build, Maintain Stereocilia in the Inner Ear," National Institute on
Deafness and Other Communication Disorders (NIDCD),
March 16, 2009. Reviewed April 2019.

Size is important. This is according to the National Institute
on Deafness and Other Communication Disorders (NIDCD) scientists investigating the internal mechanisms that underlie the hearing process and how the structures responsible for hearing rebuild
themselves.

Hearing happens at the level of the hair cells of the ear—the basic
sensory elements of hearing—where sound energy is transformed
into electrical energy by tiny hairlike projections jutting from the
top of cells in bundles called "stereocilia." The cells are called "hair
cells" because of their appearance, and these structures can only be
seen with powerful microscopes. Stereocilia are arranged in varying
lengths, similar to a stack of soda straws graded in height forming a
staircase-like bundle, to accommodate the different energies found in
different frequencies of sound waves. When stimulated, the stereocilia bundle moves and the individual hair cells splay apart, which
creates an electrical signal that travels to the brain by way of the
auditory nerve, allowing hearing to take place. The bending action
can cause damage to the stereocilia, but a delicate mechanism of turnover replaces the components of stereocilia in an orderly manner to
minimize injury.

Researchers have looked at various factors that control and regulate the rate of repair or turnover that takes place in stereocilia. In
this study, they found that the turnover rate is determined by size—
longer stereocilia are replaced at a faster rate than shorter ones. The
stereocilia, which are largely made up of the building block protein,
actin, rebuilds itself continuously, maintaining the overall structure.
The scientists theorize that this activity may help maintain function
over the course of a lifetime.

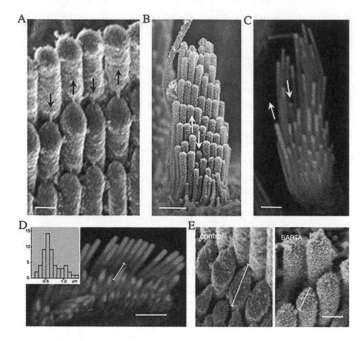

Figure 9.3. *Stereocilia*

Dynamic regulation of stereocilia structure. (A-C) Scanning electron microscope (SEM) images of the organ of Corti (A) and vestibular (B) hair bundles demonstrate slight irregularities in stereocilia lengths within the characteristically packed rows of the hair bundle. Arrows pointing down show slightly shorter stereocilia, whereas arrows pointing up to show longer stereocilia in the same row. In the actin-green fluorescent protein (GFP)-transfected vestibular hair cell, the incorporation and treadmill rates (C) reflect the slight length variations within stereocilia of the same row in the bundle. The actin treadmill rates are faster in stereocilia that are taller than their neighbors in the same row (upward arrow) and slower in stereocilia that are shorter than their peers of the same row (downward arrow). Bars: (A) 250 micrometre (μm); (B) 1 μm; (C) 2 μm. (D) Natural variability in stereocilia tip shape and rate of actin-GFP incorpo-ration. The stereocilia of the tallest row in a bundle have uniform oblate tips, whereas the stereocilia from the second and lower rows exhibit prolate tips that can be slightly pointed to very elongated. The rate of actin-GFP incorporation is increased in the more elongated tips. Bar, 2 μm. Inset shows the frequency distribution of tip length measured as indicated by the measuring bar in the figure. (E) Remodeling of ste-reocilia tips exposed to 1,2-bis (o-aminophenoxy) ethane-N,N,N',N'-tetraacetic acid (BAPTA). SEM images of the stereocilia after 5-min incubation with 5 mM BAPTA in calcium-free L-15 media and 30-min recovery (right) reveal that tip links are disrupted and stereocilia tips become rounded when compared with control (left). The length of the tip defined as shown on the figure was 0.51 ± 0.05 μm for control and 0.34 ± 0.02 μm for BAPTA-treated stereocilia (n = 50). Bar, 250 nm.

How this turnover mechanism is regulated remains unknown, but the researchers noted that the levels and activity of another protein, myosin, are correlated with stereocilia length in genetically-altered mice. Mutations in the gene for myosin are known to prevent stereocilia elongation. The investigators say they will continue to look for other proteins in order to identify key players in the self-renewal mechanism and interactions between them. They believe that understanding how malfunctions occur regarding the ability of the hair cell bundle to make fine changes in their lengths may account for subtle changes in hearing. Moreover, long-term applications of this research may prove important in the development of treatments for temporary and permanent hearing loss due to stereocilia injury.

Proteins Linked to Congenital Deafness Help Build and Maintain Stereocilia in the Inner Ear

If the inner ear were a city, then stereocilia could be considered the flashy, high-rise buildings making up the skyline. Protruding from the tops of hair inside the inner ear, stercocilia are composed of long filaments of actin, a robust protein that also assists in muscle contraction, cell division, and other cellular activities. They are also the site at which sound vibrations entering the ear are converted into electrical signals that travel to the brain, so scientists want to know more about how stercocilia are constructed.

Researchers from the NIDCD, one of the National Institutes of Health (NIH), and others have now learned that two proteins that have been implicated in some forms of inherited deafness are responsible for building and maintaining these exquisitely formed structures.

Stereocilia are arranged in tiered bundles, with one bundle topping each hair cell. Tiny filaments connect the shorter stereocilia to their taller neighbors so that, when stimulated by sound, the entire hair bundle moves as a unit. Moreover, each hair bundle is fine-tuned to respond to a specific sound frequency, with the length of its projections correlated to its preferred pitch. The lower the pitch, the longer the stereocilia need to be; the higher the pitch, the shorter the stereocilia.

In earlier studies, NIDCD scientist Bechara Kachar, M.D. and others found that, throughout our lives, our stereocilia operate as constantly moving treadmills in which new actin is added to the tip of the filament and older actin is pushed downward until it reaches the bottom, at which point it can be recycled and added to the tip again. Exactly how the stereocilia are assembled remained unclear, however.

Using immunofluorescence (IF) techniques, Dr. Kachar and others in NIDCD's Laboratory of Cell Structure and Dynamics (LCSD), along with researchers at the University of Maryland, University of North Carolina, and University of California, Berkeley, found myosin IIIa and espin 1 colocalize at the tips of the stereocilia. However, they noted that the two proteins were present in a more graded fashion along the length of the stereocilium, with the highest concentration at the tip. This indicated that the two proteins are continuously climbing from the bottom to the tip as opposed to being stationed there permanently.

When the researchers coaxed hair cells, as well as other nonsensory cells, to express more of the two proteins through the insertion of DNA, the filaments grew longer than they did when only one of the two proteins was added.

Based on these and other confirming biochemical and molecular biology techniques, the scientists concluded that myosin IIIa transports espin 1 from the base of the stereocilium to the tip, where espin 1 begins its task of adding more actin to the filament. Myosin IIIa is a motor protein, a protein that burns energy to move materials within cells. Although individual actin monomers—the bricks, so to speak—are smaller and can diffuse up the stereocilia on their own, espin 1—the machinery required to lay the bricks—is much larger and requires a lift to the top. Once the stereocilia reach their required height, the length is dynamically maintained.

Dr. Kachar likens the scenario to a home builder who suddenly decides to build a skyscraper instead. The builder would need a whole new set of tools and equipment to do that. So these two molecules, which are the products of genes whose mutations result in deafness, seem to be involved in the mechanism to build and maintain high-rises.

Dr. Kachar points out that, although a mutation in the gene that produces espin 1 results in hearing loss in newborns, mutations in the gene that produces myosin IIIa cause late-onset deafness, which can begin when a person reaches her or his twenties. This raises a new question: if myosin IIIa is so important to building and maintaining stereocilia, why isn't the hearing loss immediate? His team is currently studying whether a similar myosin present in stereocilia—myosin IIIb—compensates for the lack of myosin IIIa before a person reaches early adulthood. These and other findings could enable researchers to consider new tools for replacing or compensating for defective proteins, thus opening up additional opportunities for the development of therapeutic strategies for hearing loss.

Section 9.3

Types of Hearing Loss

This section includes text excerpted from "Types of Hearing Loss," Centers for Disease Control and Prevention (CDC), April 11, 2018.

Parts of the Ear

A hearing loss can happen when any part of the ear or auditory (hearing) system is not working in the usual way.

Outer Ear

The outer ear is made up of:

- The part we see on the sides of our heads, known as "pinna"
- The ear canal
- The eardrum, sometimes called the "tympanic membrane," which separates the outer and middle ear

Middle Ear

The middle ear is made up of:

- The eardrum
- Three small bones, called "ossicles," that send the movement of the eardrum to the inner ear

Inner Ear

The inner ear is made up of:

- The snail-shaped organ for hearing known as the "cochlea"
- The semicircular canals that help with balance
- The nerves that go to the brain

Auditory (Ear) Nerve

This nerve sends sound information from the ear to the brain.

Auditory (Hearing) System

The auditory pathway processes sound information as it travels from the ear to the brain so that our brain pathways are part of our hearing.

Types of Hearing Loss
Conductive Hearing Loss

Hearing loss caused by something that stops sounds from getting through the outer or middle ear. This type of hearing loss can often be treated with medicine or surgery.

Sensorineural Hearing Loss

Hearing loss that occurs when there is a problem in the way the inner ear or hearing nerve works.

Mixed Hearing Loss

Hearing loss that includes both a conductive and a sensorineural hearing loss.

Auditory Neuropathy Spectrum Disorder

Hearing loss that occurs when sound enters the ear normally, but because of damage to the inner ear or the hearing nerve, the sound is not organized in a way that the brain can understand.

The Degree of Hearing Loss Can Range from Mild to Profound
Mild Hearing Loss

A person with a mild hearing loss may hear some speech sounds, but soft sounds are hard to hear.

Moderate Hearing Loss

A person with a moderate hearing loss may hear almost no speech when another person is talking at a normal level.

Severe Hearing Loss

A person with severe hearing loss will hear no speech when a person is talking at a normal level and only some loud sounds.

Profound Hearing Loss

A person with a profound hearing loss will not hear any speech and only very loud sounds.

Hearing Loss Can Also Be Described As
Unilateral or Bilateral

Hearing loss is in one ear (unilateral) or both ears (bilateral).

Prelingual or Postlingual

Hearing loss happened before a person learned to talk (prelingual) or after a person learned to talk (postlingual)

Symmetrical or Asymmetrical

Hearing loss is the same in both ears (symmetrical) or is different in each ear (asymmetrical).

Progressive or Sudden

Hearing loss worsens over time (progressive) or happens quickly (sudden).

Fluctuating or Stable

Hearing loss gets either better or worse over time (fluctuating) or stays the same over time (stable).

Congenital or Acquired / Delayed Onset

Hearing loss is present at birth (congenital) or appears sometime later in life (acquired or delayed onset).

Section 9.4

Statistics about Hearing Disorders, Ear Infections, and Deafness

This section includes text excerpted from "Quick Statistics about Hearing," National Institute on Deafness and Other Communication Disorders (NIDCD), December 15, 2016.

The following are statistics for hearing disorders, ear infections, and deafness in United States.

- About 2 to 3 out of every 1,000 children in the United States are born with a detectable level of hearing loss in one or both ears.

- More than 90 percent of deaf children are born to hearing parents.

- Approximately 15 percent of American adults (37.5 million) 18 years of age and over reported some trouble hearing.

- Among adults between the ages of 20 and 69, the overall annual prevalence of hearing loss dropped slightly from 16 percent (28.0 million) in the 1999–2004 period to 14 percent (27.7 million) in the 2011–2012 period.

- Age is the strongest predictor of hearing loss among adults between the ages of 20 and 69, with the greatest amount of hearing loss in the 60 to 69 age group.

- Men are almost twice as likely as women to have hearing loss among adults between the ages of 20 and 69.

- Non-Hispanic White adults are more likely than adults in other racial/ethnic groups to have hearing loss; non-Hispanic Black adults have the lowest prevalence of hearing loss among adults between the ages of 20 and 69.

- About 18 percent of adults between the ages of 20 and 69 have speech-frequency hearing loss in both ears from among those who report 5 or more years of exposure to very loud noise at work, as compared to 5.5 percent of adults with speech-frequency hearing loss in both ears who report no occupational noise exposure.

- 1 in 8 people in the United States (13%, or 30 million) 12 years of age or older has hearing loss in both ears, based on standard hearing examinations.

- About 2 percent of adults between the ages of 45 and 54 have disabling hearing loss. The rate increases to 8.5 percent for adults between the ages of 55 and 64. Nearly 25 percent of those between the ages of 65 and 74 and 50 percent of those who are 75 years of age and older have disabling hearing loss.

- Roughly 10 percent of the U.S. adult population, or about 25 million Americans, has experienced tinnitus lasting at least 5 minutes in the past year.

- About 28.8 million U.S. adults could benefit from using hearing aids.

- Among adults 70 years of age and older with hearing loss who could benefit from hearing aids, fewer than 1 in 3 (30%) has ever used them. Even fewer adults between the ages of 20 and 69 (approximately 16%) who could benefit from wearing hearing aids have ever used them.

- As of December 2012, approximately 324,200 cochlear implants have been implanted worldwide. In the United States, roughly 58,000 devices have been implanted in adults and 38,000 in children.

- Five out of six children experience ear infection (otitis media) by the time they are three years old.

Chapter 10

Hearing Loss in Varying Ages

Chapter Contents

Section 10.1

Hearing Loss in Children

This section includes text excerpted from "What Is
Hearing Loss in Children?" Centers for Disease
Control and Prevention (CDC), April 11, 2018.

Hearing loss can affect a child's ability to develop speech, language, and social skills. The earlier children with hearing loss start getting services, the more likely they are to reach their full potential. If you think that a child might have hearing loss, ask the child's doctor for a hearing screening as soon as possible. Do not wait.

What Is Hearing Loss?

A hearing loss can happen when any part of the ear is not working in the usual way. This includes the outer ear, middle ear, inner ear, hearing (acoustic) nerve, and auditory system.

Signs and Symptoms

The signs and symptoms of hearing loss are different for each child. If you think that your child might have hearing loss, ask the child's doctor for a hearing screening as soon as possible.

Even if a child has passed a hearing screening before, it is important to look out for the following signs.

Signs in Babies

- Does not startle at loud noises

- Does not turn to the source of a sound after six months of age

- Does not say single words, such as "dada" or "mama" by one year of age

- Turns head when she or he sees you but not if you only call out her or his name. This sometimes is mistaken for not paying attention or just ignoring, but could be the result of a partial or complete hearing loss.

- Seems to hear some sounds but not others

Signs in Children

- Speech is delayed

- Speech is not clear

- Does not follow directions. This sometimes is mistaken for not paying attention or just ignoring, but could be the result of a partial or complete hearing loss.

- Often says, "Huh?"

- Turns the television volume up too high

Babies and children should reach milestones in how they play, learn, communicate, and act. A delay in any of these milestones could be a sign of hearing loss or other developmental problem.

Causes and Risk Factors

Hearing loss can happen any time during life—from before birth to adulthood.

Following are some of the things that can increase the chance that a child will have hearing loss:

- A genetic cause: About one out of two cases of hearing loss in babies is due to genetic causes. Some babies with a genetic cause for their hearing loss might have family members who also have a hearing loss. About one out of three babies with genetic hearing loss have a "syndrome." This means they have other conditions in addition to the hearing loss, such as Down syndrome or Usher syndrome.

- One out of four cases of hearing loss in babies is due to maternal infections during pregnancy, complications after birth, and head trauma. For example, the child:

  - Was exposed to infection before birth

  - Spent five days or more in a hospital neonatal intensive care unit (NICU) or had complications while in the NICU

  - Needed a special procedure, such as a blood transfusion to treat bad jaundice

  - Has head, face, or ears shaped or formed in a different way than usual

- Has a condition, such as a neurological disorder, that may be associated with hearing loss
- Had an infection around the brain and spinal cord; this is called "meningitis"
- Suffered a bad head injury that required a hospital stay
- For about one out of four babies born with hearing loss, the cause is unknown.

Screening and Diagnosis

A hearing screening can tell if a child might have hearing loss. Hearing screening is easy and is not painful. In fact, babies are often asleep while being screened. It takes a very short time—usually only a few minutes.

Babies

All babies should have a hearing screening no later than one month of age. Most babies have their hearing screened while still in the hospital. If a baby does not pass a hearing screening, it is very important to get a full hearing test as soon as possible, but no later than three months of age.

Children

Children should have their hearing tested before they enter school or any time there is a concern about the child's hearing. Children who do not pass the hearing screening need to get a full hearing test as soon as possible.

Treatments and Intervention Services

No single treatment or intervention is the answer for every person or family. Good treatment plans will include close monitoring, follow-ups, and any changes needed along the way. There are many different types of communication options for children with hearing loss and for their families. Some of these options include:

- Learning about other ways to communicate, such as sign language
- Technology to help with communication, such as hearing aids and cochlear implants

- Medicine and surgery to correct some types of hearing loss
- Family support services

Prevention

The following are tips for parents to help prevent hearing loss in their children:

- Have a healthy pregnancy
- Make sure your child gets all the regular childhood vaccines
- Keep your child away from high noise levels, such as from very loud toys

Get Help

- If your child does not pass a hearing screening, ask the child's doctor for a full hearing test as soon as possible.
- If your child has hearing loss, talk to the child's doctor about treatment and intervention services.

Hearing loss can affect a child's ability to develop speech, language, and social skills. The earlier children with hearing loss start getting services, the more likely they are to reach their full potential. If you are a parent and you suspect your child has hearing loss, trust your instincts and speak with your child's doctor.

Section 10.2

Hearing Loss and Older Adults

This section includes text excerpted from "Hearing Loss and Older Adults," National Institute on Deafness and Other Communication Disorders (NIDCD), July 17, 2018.

What Is Hearing Loss?

Hearing loss is a sudden or gradual decrease in how well you can hear. It is one of the most common conditions affecting older and elderly adults. Approximately 1 in 3 people between the ages of 65 and 74 have hearing loss, and nearly half of those older than 75 years of age have difficulty hearing. Having trouble hearing can make it hard to understand and follow doctor's advice, to respond to warnings, and to hear doorbells and alarms. It can also make it hard to enjoy talking with friends and family. All of this can be frustrating, embarrassing, and even dangerous.

What Should I Do If I Have Trouble Hearing?

Hearing problems can be serious. The most important thing you can do if you think you have a hearing problem is to seek professional advice. There are several ways to do this. You can start with your primary care physician, an otolaryngologist, an audiologist, or a hearing aid specialist. Each has a different type of training and expertise. Each can be an important part of your hearing healthcare.

An otolaryngologist is a doctor who specializes in diagnosing and treating diseases of the ear, nose, and throat. An otolaryngologist will try to find out why you are having trouble hearing and offer treatment options. She or he may also refer you to another hearing professional, an audiologist. An audiologist has specialized training in identifying and measuring the type and degree of hearing loss and recommending treatment options. Audiologists also may be licensed to fit hearing aids. Another source of hearing aids is a hearing aid specialist, who is licensed by a state to conduct and evaluate basic hearing tests, offer counseling, and fit and test hearing aids.

Why Am I Losing My Hearing?

Hearing loss happens for different reasons. Many people lose their hearing slowly as they age. This condition is known as "presbycusis."

Doctors do not know why presbycusis affects some people more than others, but it seems to run in families. Another reason for hearing loss with aging may be years of exposure to loud noise. This condition is known as "noise-induced hearing loss." Many construction workers, farmers, musicians, airport workers, yard and tree care workers, and people in the armed forces have hearing problems, even in their younger and middle years, because of too much exposure to loud noise.

Hearing loss can also be caused by viral or bacterial infections, heart conditions or stroke, head injuries, tumors, and certain medicines.

What Treatments and Devices Can Help?

Your treatment will depend on your hearing loss, so some treatments will work better for you than others. There are a number of devices and aids that can improve hearing loss. Here are the most common ones:

- **Hearing aids** are electronic instruments you wear in or behind your ear. They make sounds louder. Things sound different when you wear a hearing aid, but an audiologist or hearing aid specialist can help you get used to it. To find the hearing aid that works best for you, you may have to try more than one. Ask your audiologist or hearing specialist whether you can have a trial period with a few different hearing aids. Both of you can work together until you are comfortable.

- **Cochlear implants** are small electronic devices surgically implanted in the inner ear that help provide a sense of sound to people who are profoundly deaf or hard-of-hearing. If your hearing loss is severe, your doctor may recommend a cochlear implant in one ear or both.

- **Assistive listening devices** include telephone and cell phone amplifying devices, smartphone or tablet apps, and closed circuit systems (induction coil loops) in places of worship, theaters, and auditoriums.

- **Lip reading or speech reading** is another option that helps people with hearing problems follow the conversational speech. People who use this method pay close attention to others when they talk, by watching how the speaker's mouth and body move.

Are There Different Styles of Hearing Aids?

There are three basic styles of hearing aids. The styles differ by size, their placement on or inside the ear, and the degree to which they amplify sound.

Behind-the-ear (BTE) hearing aids consist of a hard plastic case worn behind the ear and connected to a plastic earmold that fits inside the outer ear. The electronic parts are held in the case behind the ear. Sound travels from the hearing aid through the earmold and into the ear. BTE aids are used by people of all ages for mild to profound hearing loss. A new kind of BTE aid is an open-fit hearing aid. Small, open-fit aids fit behind the ear completely, with only a narrow tube inserted into the ear canal, enabling the canal to remain open. For this reason, open-fit hearing aids may be a good choice for people who experience a buildup of earwax, since this type of aid is less likely to be damaged by such substances. In addition, some people may prefer the open-fit hearing aid because their perception of their voice does not sound "plugged up."

In-the-ear (ITE) hearing aids fit completely inside the outer ear and are used for mild to severe hearing loss. The case holding the electronic components is made of hard plastic. Some ITE aids may have certain added features installed, such as a telecoil. A telecoil is a small magnetic coil that allows users to receive sound through the circuitry of the hearing aid, rather than through its microphone. This makes it easier to hear conversations over the telephone. A telecoil also helps people hear in public facilities that have installed special sound systems, called "induction loop systems." Induction loop systems can be found in many churches, schools, airports, and auditoriums. ITE aids usually are not worn by young children because the casings need to be replaced often as the ear grows.

Canal aids fit into the ear canal and are available in two styles. The in-the-canal (ITC) hearing aid is made to fit the size and shape of a person's ear canal. A completely-in-canal (CIC) hearing aid is nearly hidden in the ear canal. Both types are used for mild to moderately severe hearing loss.

Because they are small, canal aids may be difficult for a person to adjust and remove. In addition, canal aids have less space available for batteries and additional devices, such as a telecoil. They usually are not recommended for young children or for people with severe to profound hearing loss because their reduced size limits their power and volume.

Are New Types of Aids Available?

Although they work differently than the hearing aids described above, implantable hearing aids are designed to help increase the transmission of sound vibrations entering the inner ear. A middle ear implant (MEI) is a small device attached to one of the bones of the middle ear. Rather than amplifying the sound traveling to the eardrum, an MEI moves these bones directly. Both techniques have the net result of strengthening sound vibrations entering the inner ear so that they can be detected by individuals with sensorineural hearing loss. A bone-anchored hearing aid (BAHA) is a small device that attaches to the bone behind the ear. The device transmits sound vibrations directly to the inner ear through the skull, bypassing the middle ear. BAHAs are generally used by individuals with middle ear problems or deafness in one ear. Because surgery is required to implant either of these devices, many hearing specialists feel that the benefits may not outweigh the risks.

Can My Friends and Family Help Me?

Yes. You and your family can work together to make hearing easier. Here are some things you can do:

- Tell your friends and family about your hearing loss. They need to know that hearing is hard for you. The more you tell the people you spend time with, the more they can help you.

- Ask your friends and family to face you when they talk so that you can see their faces. If you watch their faces move and see their expressions, it may help you to understand them better.

- Ask people to speak louder, but not shout. Tell them they do not have to talk slowly, just more clearly.

- Turn off the TV or the radio if you are not actively listening to it.

- Be aware of the noise around you that can make hearing more difficult. When you go to a restaurant, do not sit near the kitchen or near a band playing music. Background noise makes it hard to hear people talk.

Working together to hear better may be tough on everyone for a while. It will take time for you to get used to watching people as they talk and for people to get used to speaking louder and more clearly. Be patient and continue to work together. Hearing better is worth the effort.

113

Chapter 11

Recognizing and Diagnosing Hearing Loss

Chapter Contents

Section 11.1

Who Can I Turn To for Help with My Hearing Loss?

This section includes text excerpted from "Who Can I Turn To for Help with My Hearing Loss?" National Institute on Deafness and Other Communication Disorders (NIDCD), June 2, 2016.

Who Can I Turn To for Help?

If you or a family member might have hearing loss, consult a qualified health professional for early and appropriate care. Several types of professionals can help. Each has a different type of training and expertise, and each can be an important part of your hearing healthcare.

You may want to start by talking with your primary care provider. She or he will likely give you a medical exam to see if an infection, injury, or other condition (such as a buildup of earwax) might be causing your hearing loss. Your primary care provider might then refer you to an otolaryngologist or other hearing health provider for more specific tests and treatment.

Health Professionals to Help You with Hearing Loss

Listed below are the types of professionals who can help you with hearing loss.

A **primary care provider** is a physician, nurse practitioner, or physician assistant who provides general healthcare to patients by identifying and treating common medical conditions. Primary care providers often refer patients to medical specialists when necessary. Types of primary care providers include family practitioners or general practitioners, pediatricians, geriatricians, and internists.

An **otolaryngologist** is a physician who provides medical and surgical care, diagnosis, and treatment of the ear, nose, throat (ENT), and neck. Sometimes called an ENT, an otolaryngologist will work with you to find out why you are having trouble hearing and offer specific treatment options. She or he might also refer you to another hearing professional, such as an audiologist or hearing instrument specialist, to receive a hearing test and be fitted for a hearing aid.

An **audiologist** has specialized training to test your hearing and identify the type and degree of hearing loss. Audiologists are not physicians, but they have a doctor of audiology graduate degree (Au.D.), which typically requires four years to complete after earning a bachelor's degree. They must also pass an exam and complete a clinical fellowship. Audiologists are licensed to fit and dispense hearing aids; they can also work with you and your family to adapt to hearing loss and determine which devices, including hearing aids, would be most helpful.

A **hearing instrument** specialist, also known as a "hearing aid specialist," is a state-licensed professional who conducts basic hearing tests, fits and dispenses hearing aids, and educates individuals and their family members about their hearing loss. The licensure requirement varies among states; most states require completing a two-year apprenticeship.

Section 11.2

Diagnosing a Hearing Loss

This section includes text excerpted from "Screening and Diagnosis of Hearing Loss," Centers for Disease Control and Prevention (CDC), April 11, 2018.

Diagnosing hearing loss takes two steps:

- Hearing screening
- Full hearing test

Hearing Screening

Hearing screening is a test to tell if people might have hearing loss. Hearing screening is easy and not painful. In fact, babies are often asleep while being screened. It takes a very short time—usually only a few minutes.

Babies

- All babies should be screened for hearing loss no later than one month of age. It is best if they are screened before leaving the hospital after birth.

- If a baby does not pass a hearing screening, it is very important to get a full hearing test as soon as possible, but no later than three months of age.

Older Babies and Children

- If you think a child might have hearing loss, ask the doctor for a hearing screening as soon as possible.

- Children who are at risk for acquired, progressive, or delayed-onset hearing loss should have at least one hearing test by two to two and a half years of age. Hearing loss that gets worse over time is known as "acquired" or "progressive hearing loss." Hearing loss that develops after the baby is born is called "delayed-onset hearing loss."

- If a child does not pass a hearing screening, it is very important to get a full hearing test as soon as possible.

Full Hearing Test

All children who do not pass a hearing screening should have a full hearing test. This test is also called an "audiology evaluation." An audiologist, who is an expert trained to test hearing, will do the full hearing test. In addition, the audiologist will also ask questions about birth history, ear infection, and hearing loss in the family.

There are many kinds of tests an audiologist can do to find out if a person has hearing loss, how much of a hearing loss there is, and what type it is. The hearing tests are easy and not painful.

Some of the tests the audiologist might use include:

Auditory Brainstem Response Test or Brainstem Auditory Evoked Response Test

Auditory brainstem response (ABR) or brainstem auditory evoked response (BAER) is a test that checks the brain's response to sound. Because this test does not rely on a person's response behavior, the person being tested can be sound asleep during the test.

Otoacoustic Emissions

Otoacoustic emissions (OAEs) is a test that checks the inner ear response to sound. Because this test does not rely on a person's response behavior, the person being tested can be sound asleep during the test.

Behavioral Audiometry Evaluation

Behavioral audiometry evaluation will test how a person responds to sound overall. Behavioral audiometry evaluation tests the function of all parts of the ear. The person being tested must be awake and actively respond to sounds heard during the test.

With the parents' permission, the audiologist will share the results with the child's primary care doctor and other experts, such as:

- An ear, nose, and throat doctor, also called an "otolaryngologist"

- An eye doctor, also called an "ophthalmologist"

- A professional trained in genetics, also called a "clinical geneticist" or a "genetics counselor"

Get Help

- If a parent or anyone else who knows a child well thinks the child might have hearing loss, ask the doctor for a hearing screening as soon as possible. Do not wait.

- If the child does not pass a hearing screening, ask the doctor for a full hearing test.

- If the child is diagnosed with a hearing loss, talk to the doctor or audiologist about treatment and intervention services.

Hearing loss can affect a child's ability to develop communication, language, and social skills. The earlier children with hearing loss start getting services, the more likely they are to reach their full potential. If you are a parent and you suspect your child has hearing loss, trust your instincts and speak with your doctor.

Section 11.3

Newborn Hearing Screening

This section contains text excerpted from the following sources:
Text in this section begins with excerpts from "Your Baby's
Hearing Screening," National Institute on Deafness and Other
Communication Disorders (NIDCD), June 19, 2017; Text beginning
with the heading "Infants and Babies' Hearing Can Be Checked" is
excerpted from "Newborn Hearing Screening," Centers for Disease
Control and Prevention (CDC), April 11, 2018.

Most children hear and listen to sounds at birth. They learn to talk by imitating the sounds they hear around them and the voices of their parents and caregivers. But that is not true for all children. In fact, about 2 or 3 out of every 1,000 children in the United States are born with detectable hearing loss in one or both ears. More lose hearing later during childhood. Children who have hearing loss may not learn speech and language as well as children who can hear. For this reason, it is important to detect deafness or hearing loss as early as possible.

Because of the need for prompt identification of and intervention for childhood hearing loss, universal newborn hearing screening programs currently operate in all U.S. states and most U.S. territories. With help from the federal government, every state has established an early hearing detection and intervention program. As a result, more than 96 percent of babies have their hearing screened within 1 month of birth.

Why Is It Important to Have My Baby's Hearing Screened Early?

The most important time for a child to learn language is in the first three years of life, when the brain is developing and maturing. In fact, children begin learning speech and language in the first six months of life. Research suggests that children with hearing loss who get help early develop better language skills than those who do not.

When Will My Baby's Hearing Be Screened?

Your baby's hearing should be screened before she or he leaves the hospital or birthing center. If your baby's hearing was not tested within the first month of life, or if you have not been told the results of the hearing screening, ask your child's doctor today. Quick action will be important if the screening shows a possible problem.

How Will My Baby's Hearing Be Screened?

Two different tests are used to screen for hearing loss in babies. Your baby can rest or sleep during both tests.

- **Otoacoustic emissions (OAEs)** test whether some parts of the ear respond to sound. During this test, a soft earphone is inserted into your baby's ear canal. It plays sounds and measures an "echo" response that occurs in ears with normal hearing. If there is no echo, your baby might have hearing loss.

- **The auditory brainstem response (ABR)** tests how the auditory nerve and brainstem (which carry sound from the ear to the brain) respond to sound. During this test, your baby wears small earphones and has electrodes painlessly placed on her or his head. The electrodes adhere and come off like stickers, and should not cause discomfort.

What Should I Do If My Baby's Hearing Screening Reveals a Possible Problem?

If the results show that your baby may have hearing loss, make an appointment with a pediatric audiologist—a hearing expert who specializes in the assessment and management of children with hearing loss. This follow-up exam should be done by the time your baby is three months old. The audiologist will conduct tests to determine whether your baby has a hearing problem and, if so, the type and severity of that problem.

If you need help finding a pediatric audiologist, ask your pediatrician or the hospital staff who conducted your baby's screening. They may even be able to help you schedule an appointment. You can also try the directories provided by the American Academy of Audiology (AAA) or the American Speech-Language-Hearing Association (ASHA). If the follow-up examination confirms that your baby has hearing loss, he or she should begin receiving intervention services before the age of six months.

The pediatric audiologist may recommend that your baby visit a physician specializing in ear, nose, and throat disorders (an otolaryngologist), who can determine possible causes of hearing loss and recommend intervention options. If your child has siblings, the audiologist or otolaryngologist may also recommend that their hearing be tested.

The Follow-Up Exam Revealed That My Baby's Hearing Is Fine. Does That Mean We Do Not Need to Check Her or His Hearing Again?

Hearing loss can occur at any time of life. Some inherited forms of hearing loss do not appear until a child is older. In addition, illness, ear infection, head injury, certain medications, and loud noise are all potential causes of hearing loss in children. Use the baby's hearing and communicative development checklist, offered by the National Institute on Deafness and Other Communication Disorders (NIDCD), to monitor and track your child's communication milestones through five years of age. If you have concerns, talk to your pediatrician right away.

How Can I Help My Child Succeed If She or He Has Hearing Loss?

When interventions begin early, children with hearing loss can develop language skills that help them communicate freely and learn actively. The federal Individuals with Disabilities Education Act (IDEA) ensures that all children with disabilities have access to the services they need to get a good education. Your community may also offer additional services to help support your child.

Talk to and communicate with your child often. Other ways to support your child include:

- Keep all doctor's appointments
- Learn sign language or other strategies to support better communication
- Join a support group

Will My Child Be Successful in School?

Like all children, children who are deaf or hard-of-hearing can develop strong academic, social, and emotional skills and succeed in school. Find out how your school system helps children with hearing loss. With your input, your child's school will develop an Individualized Education Program (IEP) for your child, and you should ask if an educational audiologist is available to be part of the academic team. Explore programs outside of school that may help you and your child, and talk with other parents who have already dealt with these issues. The IDEA ensures that children with hearing loss receive free, appropriate, early-intervention services from birth through the school years.

Baby's Hearing Screening Timeline for Parents

Use this timeline to get started.

By One Month Old

Make sure that your baby's hearing is screened either before you leave the hospital or immediately afterward. After the screening, find out the results. If your newborn was not screened in the hospital, schedule a screening to occur by the time your baby is one month old.

By Three Months Old

If your baby does not pass the hearing screening, immediately schedule a follow-up appointment with a pediatric audiologist. Ask your doctor or hospital for a list of pediatric audiologists or use the directories provided by the American Academy of Audiology (AAA) and the American Speech-Language-Hearing Association (ASHA).

If you must cancel the follow-up appointment, reschedule it. Make sure you take your baby to a follow-up examination by age three months.

By Six Months Old

If the follow-up exam shows that your baby has hearing loss, start your baby in some form of intervention by the time she or he is six months old. Intervention can include hearing devices, such as hearing aids or cochlear implants; communication methods, including oral approaches (such as lipreading) or manual approaches (such as American Sign Language); or a combination of options, including assistive devices. Ask your healthcare team about the options.

Ongoing

- Remain active and involved in your child's progress.

- If you move, make sure that your child's doctors and specialists have your new address.

- Even if your child passed the follow-up exam, continue to monitor his or her communication development. If you have concerns, speak with your child's doctor. If your child has risk factors for childhood hearing loss, speak with an audiologist about how often her or his hearing should be monitored.

Infants and Babies' Hearing Can Be Checked

Do you know that your baby's hearing can be checked even before leaving the birth hospital? Many states, communities, and hospitals now offer hearing screening for babies. A baby's hearing can be screened using automated auditory brainstem response (AABR), otoacoustic emissions (OAEs), or both.

Babies usually have their hearing screened while still in the hospital, either in the nursery or in their mothers' room.

All Babies Should Have a Hearing Screening before They Are One Month Old

Hearing screening is easy and is not painful. In fact, babies are often asleep while being screened. It takes a very short time—usually only a few minutes. Sometimes the screening is repeated while the babies are still in the hospital or shortly after they leave the hospital.

Babies who do not pass hearing screening should be tested by an audiologist. An audiologist is a person trained to test hearing. This person will do additional testing to find out if there is a hearing loss. There are many kinds of tests an audiologist can do to find out if a baby has a hearing loss, how much of a hearing loss there is, and what type it is.

All Babies Who Do Not Pass the First Screening Should Have a Complete Hearing Test before Three Months of Age

Finding a hearing loss early and getting into a program that helps babies with hearing loss (beginning before a baby is six months old) helps a child to:

- Communicate better with others

- Do well in school

- Get along with other children

All Babies with Hearing Loss Should Begin Intervention Services before Six Months of Age

Intervention services are types of programs and resources available for children and their families. An intervention might be:

- Meeting with a professional (or team) who is trained to work with children who have a hearing loss, and their families

- Working with a professional (or team) who can help a family and child learn to communicate

- Fitting a baby with a hearing device, such as a hearing aid

- Joining family support groups

- Other resources available to children with a hearing loss and their families

Chapter 12

Genetic and Congenital Deafness

Chapter Contents

Section 12.1

The Genetics of Hearing Loss

This section contains text excerpted from the following
sources: Text in this section begins with excerpts from "Genetics of
Hearing Loss," Centers for Disease Control and Prevention (CDC),
April 11, 2018; Text beginning with the heading "What Causes
Hearing Loss" is excerpted from "A Parent's Guide to Genetics and
Hearing Loss," Centers for Disease Control and Prevention (CDC),
June 27, 2011. Reviewed April 2019.

Hearing loss has many causes. 50 to 60 percent of hearing loss in babies is due to genetic causes. There are also a number of things in the environment that can cause hearing loss. 25 percent or more of hearing loss in babies is due to environmental causes, such as maternal infections during pregnancy and complications after birth. Sometimes, both genes and environment work together to cause hearing loss. For example, there are some medicines that can cause hearing loss but only in people who have certain mutations in their genes.

Genes contain the instructions that tell the cells of people's bodies how to grow and work. For example, the instructions in genes control what color a person's eyes will be. There are many genes that are involved in hearing. Sometimes, a gene does not form in the expected manner. This is called a "mutation." Some mutations run in families and others do not. If more than one person in a family has hearing loss, it is said to be "familial." That is, it runs in the family. If only one person in the family has hearing loss, it is called "sporadic." That is, it does not run in the family.

About 70 percent of all mutations causing hearing loss are nonsyndromic. This means that the person does not have any other symptoms. About 30 percent of the mutations causing hearing loss are syndromic. This means that the person has other symptoms besides hearing loss. For example, some people with hearing loss are also blind.

The cochlea (the part of the ear that changes sounds in the air into nerve signals to the brain) is a very complex and specialized part of the body that needs many instructions to guide its development and function. These instructions come from genes. Changes in any one of these genes can result in hearing loss. The *GJB2* gene is one of the genes that contains the instructions for a protein called "connexin 26." This protein plays an important role in the functioning of the cochlea. In some populations, about 40 percent of newborns with a genetic hearing loss who do not have a syndrome have a mutation in the *GJB2* gene.

What Are the Types of Hearing Loss?

There are many different ways to talk about the different types of hearing loss.

- One way is based on whether or not a baby is born with hearing loss. If the baby is born with hearing loss, it is called "congenital." If the hearing loss occurs after the baby is born, it is called "acquired."

- Another way depends on whether or not the hearing loss gets worse over time. Hearing loss that gets worse over time is called "progressive." Hearing loss that does not change is called "nonprogressive."

- A third way depends on whether or not other symptoms are present; that is, is it syndromic or nonsyndromic?

- A fourth way depends on whether or not hearing loss runs in the family. If it does, it is called "familial," if it does not, it is sporadic.

- A fifth way is based on where in the ear the hearing loss occurs. If the loss occurs in the outer or middle ear, it is conductive. If it occurs in the inner ear, it is sensorineural. If the loss occurs in both areas, it is mixed.

What Causes Hearing Loss

Hearing loss can be caused by changes in genes, outside factors (such as injuries, illness or certain medications), or both. For many children with hearing loss, the cause is unknown.

Genes are passed from parents to children and cause certain traits to run in families. There are many genes that are involved in hearing. Sometimes, a gene does not form in the way it should and causes a mutation. Some mutations cause syndromic hearing loss and others cause nonsyndromic hearing loss. Even among some families with genetic hearing loss, a loss is not due to mutations in any of the known genes. Scientists are working to find all of the genes involved in hearing loss. Genes are described in more detail in the next section.

There are also a number of things that are not genetic that can cause hearing loss. For example, babies who are born too early and babies who need help breathing (for example, using a ventilator) are more likely to develop hearing loss than other babies. Some infections (such as cytomegalovirus) the mother has during her pregnancy can cause the baby to have hearing loss. Also, some infections (such as meningitis) that babies and children have can cause hearing loss.

Sometimes, both genes and the environment work together to cause hearing loss. For example, there are some medicines that can cause hearing loss but only among people who have certain mutations in their genes.

How Do Doctors Figure out What Caused a Person's Hearing Loss?

Doctors begin by looking at a person's physical features, medical history, and family history. Based on this, they classify the hearing loss in the ways described earlier (congenital or acquired, prelingual or postlingual, progressive or nonprogressive, conductive or sensorineural, syndromic or nonsyndromic, and familial or sporadic). The classifications often point to certain causes. The doctors might ask for more medical tests to look for signs of syndromic hearing loss, and they might ask for genetic tests.

About Genetic Testing
What Is Genetic Testing?

A genetic test involves looking at a person's DNA to see if certain mutations are present. A person's DNA sample usually is taken from one of two different sources: a small sample of a person's blood or cheek cells from a person's mouth. To get the cheek cells, a small, toothbrush-like swab is rubbed inside a person's mouth. The cheek swab is easy and painless, but the DNA obtained from this method is sometimes unstable and might not be usable.

Once a person's DNA sample is obtained, there are two different ways to look for mutations. The first way looks only for certain mutations. This mutation-specific testing will detect that one type of mutation if it is present, but it will not detect other mutations that also might be present. This type of testing is used when most of the people who have a genetic condition have the same mutation.

The other type of genetic testing is called "sequencing." In this method, the DNA sequence is determined for the entire gene or for a certain part of it. This method will detect any mutation that is present in the part of the gene looked at. This type of testing is harder and costs more. It usually is used when any one of several mutations in a gene could cause a condition.

What Are the Benefits of Genetic Testing?

If a mutation is found, it might explain why the person has a condition, such as hearing loss. In some cases, knowing what mutation a person has will allow doctors to predict how severe the condition might become and what other symptoms can be expected. Then, the person can get any other medical care that might be needed. Also, knowing the cause of a person's condition will let him or her know what the chances are of passing the condition on to his or her children. It also lets other family members know the chances that they might have a child with the same condition.

What Are the Limits of Genetic Testing?

- Not all of the genes that cause conditions are known. So, even if a condition runs in a family, it might not be possible to find the mutation that causes it.

- Some tests are hard to do. For example, the bigger a gene is, the harder it is to study the whole gene.

- Sometimes, it is not possible to tell if a mutation is the cause of a condition or just a coincidence.

Some mutations cause conditions among most people but not among all people who carry them. For each such mutation, a positive result (that is, a result showing that a person has one or more copies of a mutation) might not mean that the person will get the associated condition. Likewise, a negative result (that is, a result showing that a person does not carry a copy with that mutation) does not guarantee that the person will not get the associated condition. This is because the person might have a different mutation that was not detectable by the test used, or the person might have a mutation in a different gene that also causes the same condition.

What Are the Risks of Genetic Testing?

Some people have strong feelings when they get the results of a genetic test. Some people feel angry, sad, or guilty if they find out that they or their child has a mutation. It is important to remember that everyone carries mutations of some kind, and that a person's genes are no one's fault.

Genetic tests are different from other medical tests in that the results provide information about other members of the family and not just the person being tested. Some family members do not want to know that a mutation runs in their family. Also, because children get their genes from their parents, genetic tests that involve several family members can reveal personal information, such as a child having been adopted or having a different biological father.

Sometimes, people are concerned about keeping the results of their genetic tests private. For example, they do not want their friends, relatives, or coworkers to find out. Companies that offer genetic testing are very careful to make sure that test results are kept private. Test results cannot be seen by anyone who is not involved in the testing, unless the person tested or her or his parents or guardians give permission.

Section 12.2

Congenital Deafness with Vitiligo and Achalasia

This section includes text excerpted from "Congenital Deafness with Vitiligo and Achalasia," Genetic and Rare Diseases Information Center (GARD), National Center for Advancing Translational Sciences (NCATS), October 6, 2014. Reviewed April 2019.

Congenital deafness with vitiligo and achalasia is a syndrome characterized by deafness present from birth (congenital) and is associated with short stature, vitiligo, muscle wasting, and achalasia (swallowing difficulties). The condition was described in a brother and sister born to first cousin parents. It is believed to be inherited in an autosomal recessive manner.

Symptoms

Table 12.1 lists symptoms that people with this disease may have. For most diseases, symptoms will vary from person to person. People with the same disease may not have all the symptoms listed.

Table 12.1. Symptoms of Congenital Deafness with Vitiligo and Achalasia

Medical Terms	Other Names
80% to 99% of people have these symptoms	
Achalasia	
EEG abnormality	
Hypopigmented skin patches	Patchy loss of skin color
Sensorineural hearing impairment	
Severe short stature	Dwarfism Proportionate dwarfism Short stature, severe
Skeletal muscle atrophy	Muscle degeneration Muscle wasting
Percent of people who have these symptoms is not available through HPO	
Autosomal recessive inheritance	
Hearing impairment	Deafness Hearing defect
Short stature	Decreased body height Small stature
Vitiligo	Blotchy loss of skin color

Section 12.3

Usher Syndrome

This section includes text excerpted from "Facts about Usher Syndrome," National Eye Institute (NEI), April 2018.

What Is Usher Syndrome?

Usher syndrome is the most common condition that affects both hearing and vision; sometimes it also affects balance. The major symptoms of Usher syndrome are deafness or hearing loss and an eye disease called "retinitis pigmentosa" (RP).

Deafness or hearing loss in Usher syndrome is caused by abnormal development of hair cells (sound receptor cells) in the inner ear. Most children with Usher syndrome are born with moderate to profound hearing loss, depending on the type. Less commonly, hearing loss from Usher syndrome appears during adolescence or later. Usher syndrome can also cause severe balance problems due to abnormal development of the vestibular hair cells, sensory cells that detect gravity and head movement.

RP initially causes night blindness and a loss of peripheral (side) vision through the progressive degeneration of cells in the retina. The retina is the light-sensitive tissue at the back of the eye and is crucial for vision. As RP progresses, the field of vision narrows until only central vision remains, a condition called "tunnel vision." Macular holes (small breaks in the macula, the central part of the retina) and cataracts (clouding of the lens) can sometimes cause an early decline in central vision in people with Usher syndrome.

Who Is Affected by Usher Syndrome?

Usher syndrome affects approximately 4 to 17 per 100,000 people, and accounts for about 50 percent of all hereditary deaf-blindness cases. The condition is thought to account for 3 to 6 percent of all children who are deaf, and another 3 to 6 percent of children who are hard-of-hearing.

What Causes Usher Syndrome

Usher syndrome is inherited, which means that it is passed from parents to a child through genes. Each person inherits two copies of a gene, one from each parent. Sometimes genes are altered or mutated. Mutated genes may cause cells to develop or act abnormally.

Usher syndrome is inherited as an autosomal recessive disorder. "Autosomal" means that men and women are equally likely to have the disorder and equally likely to pass it on to a child of either sex. "Recessive" means that the condition occurs only when a child inherits two copies of the same faulty gene, one from each parent. A person with one abnormal Usher gene does not have the disorder but is a carrier who has a 50 percent chance of passing on the abnormal gene to each child. When two carriers with the same mutated Usher syndrome gene have a child together, each birth has a:

- One-in-four chance of having a child who neither has Usher syndrome nor is a carrier

- Two-in-four chance of having a child who is an unaffected carrier

- One-in-four chance of having Usher syndrome

The hearing, balance, and vision of carriers with one mutant Usher gene are typically normal. Carriers are often unaware of their carrier status.

What Are the Characteristics of the Three Types of Usher Syndrome?

There are three types of Usher syndrome. In the United States, types 1 and 2 are the most common. Together, they account for up to 95 percent of Usher syndrome cases.

Type 1: Children with type 1 Usher syndrome have profound hearing loss or deafness at birth and have severe balance problems. Many obtain little or no benefit from hearing aids but may be candidates for a cochlear implant—an electronic device that can provide a sense of sound to people with severe hearing loss or deafness. Parents should consult with their child's doctor and other hearing health professionals early to determine communication options for their child. Intervention should begin promptly, when the brain is most receptive to learning language, whether spoken or signed.

Balance problems associated with type 1 Usher syndrome delay sitting up without support. Walking rarely occurs prior to 18 months of age. Vision problems with type 1 Usher syndrome usually begin before the age of 10, starting with difficulty seeing at night and progressing to severe vision loss over several decades.

Type 2: Children with type 2 Usher syndrome are born with moderate to severe hearing loss but normal balance. Although the severity of hearing loss varies, most children with type 2 Usher syndrome can communicate orally and benefit from hearing aids. RP is usually diagnosed during late adolescence in people with type 2 Usher syndrome.

Type 3: Children with type 3 Usher syndrome have normal hearing at birth. Most have normal to near normal balance; however, some develop balance problems with age. The decline in hearing and vision varies. Children with type 3 Usher syndrome often develop hearing loss by adolescence, requiring hearing aids by mid-to-late adulthood. Night blindness also usually begins during adolescence. Blind spots appear by the late teens to early twenties. Legal blindness often occurs by midlife.

Table 12.2. Types of Usher Syndrome

	Type 1	Type 2	Type 3
Hearing	Profound hearing loss or deafness at birth.	Moderate to severe hearing loss at birth.	Progressive loss in childhood or early teens.
Vision	Decreased night vision by age 10, progressing to severe vision loss by midlife.	Decreased night vision by adolescence, progressing to severe vision loss by midlife.	Varies in severity and age of onset; night vision problems often begin in teens and progress to severe vision loss by midlife.
Balance (vestibular function)	Balance problems from birth.	Normal balance.	Normal to near-normal balance in childhood; chance of later problems.

How Is Usher Syndrome Diagnosed?

Diagnosis of Usher syndrome involves asking questions about the patient's medical history and testing of hearing, balance, and vision. Early diagnosis is important, as it improves the likelihood of treatment success. An eye care specialist can use dilating drops to examine the retina for signs of RP. Visual field testing measures side vision. An electroretinogram (ERG) measures the electrical response of the eye's light-sensitive cells in the retina. Optical coherence tomography may be helpful to assess macular cystic changes. Videonystagmography (VNG) measures involuntary eye movements that might signify a balance problem. Audiology testing determines hearing sensitivity at a range of frequencies.

Genetic testing may help diagnose Usher syndrome. So far, researchers have found nine genes that cause Usher syndrome. Genetic testing is available for all of them:

- Type 1 Usher syndrome: *MY07a, USH1C, CDH23, PCHD15, USH1G*

- Type 2 Usher syndrome: *USH2A, GPR98, DFNB31*

- Type 3 Usher syndrome: *CLRN1*

Genetic testing for Usher syndrome may be available through clinical research studies.

How Is Usher Syndrome Treated?

Presently, there is no cure for Usher syndrome. Treatment involves managing hearing, vision, and balance problems. Early diagnosis helps tailor educational programs that consider the severity of hearing and vision loss and a child's age and ability. Treatment may include hearing aids, assistive listening devices (ALDs), and cochlear implants. It may also include communication methods, such as American Sign Language (ASL), and orientation and mobility training for balance problems. Communication services and independent-living training may include braille instruction, low-vision services, or auditory (hearing) training.

Vitamin A may slow the progression of RP6, according to results from a long-term clinical trial supported by the National Eye Institute (NEI) and the Foundation Fighting Blindness. Based on the study, adults with a common form of RP may benefit from a daily supplement of 15,000 IU (international units) of the palmitate form of vitamin A. Patients should discuss this treatment option with their healthcare provider before proceeding. Because people with type 1 Usher syndrome did not take part in the study, high-dose vitamin A is not recommended for these patients.

General precautions for vitamin A supplementation:

- Do not substitute vitamin A palmitate with a beta carotene supplement.

- Do not take vitamin A supplements greater than the recommended dose of 15,000 IU or modify your diet to select foods with high levels of vitamin A.

- Pregnant women should not take high-dose vitamin A supplements due to the increased risk of birth defects. Women considering pregnancy should stop taking high-dose vitamin A supplements for six months before trying to conceive.

What Research Is Being Done?

Researchers are trying to identify additional genes that cause Usher syndrome. Efforts will lead to improved genetic counseling and earlier diagnosis, and may eventually expand treatment options.

Scientists are also developing mouse models with characteristics similar to Usher syndrome. Research using mouse models will help determine the function of Usher genes and will inform potential treatments.

137

Other areas of study include new methods for early identification of children with Usher syndrome, improving treatment strategies for children who use hearing aids and cochlear implants for hearing loss, and testing innovative intervention strategies to help slow or stop the progression of RP. Clinical researchers are also characterizing variability in balance among individuals with various types of Usher syndrome.

Section 12.4

Waardenburg Syndrome

This section includes text excerpted from "Waardenburg Syndrome," Genetics Home Reference (GHR), National Institutes of Health (NIH), March 19, 2019.

Waardenburg syndrome is a group of genetic conditions that can cause hearing loss and changes in coloring (pigmentation) of the hair, skin, and eyes. Although most people with Waardenburg syndrome have normal hearing, moderate to profound hearing loss can occur in one or both ears. The hearing loss is present from birth (congenital). People with this condition often have very pale blue eyes or different colored eyes, such as one blue eye and one brown eye. Sometimes, one eye has segments of two different colors. Distinctive hair coloring (such as a patch of white hair or hair that prematurely turns gray) is another common sign of the condition. The features of Waardenburg syndrome vary among affected individuals, even among people in the same family.

Types of Waardenburg Syndrome

There are four recognized types of Waardenburg syndrome, which are distinguished by their physical characteristics and sometimes by their genetic cause. Types I and II have very similar features, although people with type I almost always have eyes that appear widely spaced and people with type II do not. In addition, hearing loss occurs more often in people with type II than in those with type I.

Type III (sometimes called "Klein-Waardenburg syndrome") includes abnormalities of the arms and hands in addition to hearing loss and changes in pigmentation. Type IV (also known as "Waardenburg-Shah syndrome") has signs and symptoms of both Waardenburg syndrome and Hirschsprung disease, an intestinal disorder that causes severe constipation or blockage of the intestine.

Frequency

Waardenburg syndrome affects an estimated 1 in 40,000 people. It accounts for 2 to 5 percent of all cases of congenital hearing loss. Types I and II are the most common forms of Waardenburg syndrome, while types III and IV are rare.

Causes

Mutations in the *EDN3*, *EDNRB*, *MITF*, *PAX3*, *SNAI2*, and *SOX10* genes can cause Waardenburg syndrome. These genes are involved in the formation and development of several types of cells, including pigment-producing cells called "melanocytes." Melanocytes make a pigment called "melanin," which contributes to skin, hair, and eye color and plays an essential role in the normal function of the inner ear. Mutations in any of these genes disrupt the normal development of melanocytes, leading to abnormal pigmentation of the skin, hair, and eyes and problems with hearing.

Waardenburg syndrome types I and III are caused by mutations in the *PAX3* gene. Mutations in the *MITF* or *SNAI2* gene can cause Waardenburg syndrome type II.

Mutations in the *SOX10*, *EDN3*, or *EDNRB* gene can cause Waardenburg syndrome type IV. In addition to melanocyte development, these genes are important for the development of nerve cells in the large intestine. Mutations in one of these genes result in hearing loss, changes in pigmentation, and intestinal problems related to Hirschsprung disease.

In some cases, the genetic cause of Waardenburg syndrome has not been identified.

Inheritance Pattern

Waardenburg syndrome is usually inherited in an autosomal dominant pattern, which means one copy of the altered gene in each cell is sufficient to cause the disorder. In most cases, an affected person has one parent with the condition. A small percentage of cases result from new mutations in the gene; these cases occur in people with no history of the disorder in their family.

Some cases of Waardenburg syndrome type II and type IV appear to have an autosomal recessive pattern of inheritance, which means both copies of the gene in each cell have mutations. Most often, the parents of an individual with an autosomal recessive condition each carry one copy of the mutated gene, but do not show signs and symptoms of the condition.

Section 12.5

Other Types of Syndromic Deafness

This section contains text excerpted from the following sources: Text under the heading "Jervell Lange-Nielsen Syndrome" is excerpted from "Jervell Lange-Nielsen Syndrome," Genetic and Rare Diseases Information Center (GARD), National Center for Advancing Translational Sciences (NCATS), March 16, 2018; Text under the heading "Pendred Syndrome" is excerpted from "Pendred Syndrome," National Institute on Deafness and Other Communication Disorders (NIDCD), March 6, 2017; Text under the heading "Tietz Syndrome" is excerpted from "Tietz Syndrome," Genetic and Rare Diseases Information Center (GARD), National Center for Advancing Translational Sciences (NCATS), November 19, 2014. Reviewed April 2019; Text under the heading "Weissenbacher-Zweymüller Syndrome" is excerpted from "Weissenbacher-Zweymüller Syndrome," Genetics Home Reference (GHR), National Institutes of Health (NIH), March 19, 2019.

Jervell Lange-Nielsen Syndrome

Jervell Lange-Nielsen syndrome (JLNS) is an inherited disorder characterized by deafness present at birth and abnormalities of the electrical system of the heart. It is a form of long QT syndrome (LQTS). This refers to the QT interval measurement seen on the electrocardiogram. The severity of cardiac symptoms seen in individuals varies from no apparent symptoms to increasing heartbeat (tachycardia), fainting, and cardiac arrest. There are two different types of JLNS—type 1, caused by mutations in the *KCNQ1* gene, and type 2, caused by mutations in the *KCNE1* gene. Both types are inherited in an autosomal recessive manner. The treatment of individuals with JLNS focuses on treating hearing loss utilizing devices, such as cochlear implants, and preventing other symptoms, such as fainting and cardiac arrest.

Symptoms

Table 12.3 lists symptoms that people with this disease may have. For most diseases, symptoms will vary from person to person. People with the same disease may not have all the symptoms listed.

Table 12.3. Symptoms of Jervell Lange-Nielsen Syndrome

Medical Terms	Other Names
Percent of people who have these symptoms is not available through HPO	
Autosomal recessive inheritance	
Congenital sensorineural hearing impairment	
Prolonged QT interval	
Sudden cardiac death	Premature sudden cardiac death
Syncope	Fainting spell
Torsade de pointes	

Diagnosis

Making a diagnosis for a genetic or rare disease can often be challenging. Healthcare professionals typically look at a person's medical history, symptoms, physical exam, and laboratory test results in order to make a diagnosis. If you have questions about getting a diagnosis, you should contact a healthcare professional.

Pendred Syndrome

Pendred syndrome is a genetic disorder that causes early hearing loss in children. It also can affect the thyroid gland and sometimes creates problems with balance. The syndrome is named after Vaughan Pendred, the physician who first described people with the disorder.

Children who are born with Pendred syndrome may begin to lose their hearing at birth or by the time they are three years of age. Usually, their hearing will worsen over time. The loss of hearing often happens suddenly, although some individuals will later regain some hearing. Eventually, some children with Pendred syndrome become totally deaf.

Almost all children with Pendred syndrome have bilateral hearing loss, which means hearing loss in both ears, although one ear may have more hearing loss than the other.

Childhood hearing loss has many causes. Researchers believe that in the United States 50 to 60 percent of cases are due to genetic causes, and 40 to 50 percent of cases result from environmental causes. Healthcare professionals use different clues, such as when the hearing loss begins and whether there are anatomical differences in the ears, to help determine whether a child has Pendred syndrome or some other type of progressive deafness.

How Does Pendred Syndrome Affect Other Parts of the Body?

Pendred syndrome can make the thyroid gland grow larger. An enlarged thyroid gland is called a "goiter." The thyroid is a small, butterfly-shaped gland in the front of the neck, just above the collar-bones. The thyroid plays a major role in how the body uses energy from food. In children, the thyroid is important for normal growth and development. Children with Pendred syndrome, however, rarely have problems growing and developing properly, even if their thyroid is affected. Their levels of thyroid hormones are usually normal.

People with Pendred syndrome are significantly more likely than the general population to develop a goiter in their lifetime, although not everyone who has Pendred syndrome gets a goiter. The typical age for a goiter to develop is in adolescence or early adulthood. If a goiter becomes large, there may be problems with breathing and swallowing. In this case, a health professional should check the goiter and decide whether treatment is necessary. People with Pendred syndrome may need to visit an endocrinologist, who is a specially trained doctor familiar with diseases and disorders that involve the endocrine system, including the thyroid gland.

Pendred syndrome also can affect the vestibular system, which controls balance. Some people with Pendred syndrome will show vestibular weakness when their balance is tested. However, the brain is very good at making up for a weak vestibular system, and most children and adults with Pendred syndrome do not have a problem with their balance or have difficulty doing routine tasks. Some babies with Pendred syndrome may start walking later than other babies, however.

Scientists do not know why some people with Pendred syndrome develop a goiter or have balance problems and others do not.

What Causes Pendred Syndrome

Pendred syndrome can be caused by changes, or mutations, in a gene called "*SLC26A4*" (formerly known as the "*PDS* gene") on chromosome 7. Because it is a recessive trait, a child needs to inherit two mutated *SLC26A4* genes—one from each parent—to have Pendred syndrome. Since the child's parents are only carriers of a mutation in the *SLC26A4* gene, there are no health implications for them.

Couples who are concerned that they could pass Pendred syndrome to their children might want to seek genetic testing. A possible sign that someone might be a carrier of a mutated *SLC26A4* gene is a family history of early hearing loss. Another sign is a family member who has both a goiter and hearing loss. However, often there is no family history of Pendred syndrome in the families of children who have the disorder. A mutation in the *SLC26A4* gene can be determined by genetic testing of a blood sample.

The decision to have a genetic test is complicated. Most people talk with a genetic counselor trained to help them weigh the medical, emotional, and ethical considerations of testing. A genetic counselor is a health professional who provides information and support to people (and their families) who have a genetic disorder or who are at risk for a genetic disorder.

How Is Pendred Syndrome Diagnosed?

An otolaryngologist (a doctor who specializes in diseases of the ear, nose, throat, head, and neck) or a clinical geneticist will consider hearing loss, inner ear structures, and sometimes the thyroid in diagnosing Pendred syndrome. She or he will evaluate the timing, amount, and pattern of hearing loss and ask questions such as "When did the hearing loss start?," "Has it worsened over time?," and "Did it happen suddenly or in stages?" Early hearing loss is one of the most common characteristics of Pendred syndrome; however, this symptom alone does not mean a child has the condition.

The specialist will use inner ear imaging techniques, such as magnetic resonance imaging (MRI) or a computed tomography (CT scan), to look for two characteristics of Pendred syndrome. One characteristic might be a cochlea with too few turns. The cochlea is the spiral-shaped part of the inner ear that converts sound into electrical signals that are sent to the brain. A healthy cochlea has two-and-a-half turns, but the cochlea of a person with Pendred syndrome may have only one-and-a-half turns. Not everyone with Pendred syndrome, however, has an abnormal cochlea.

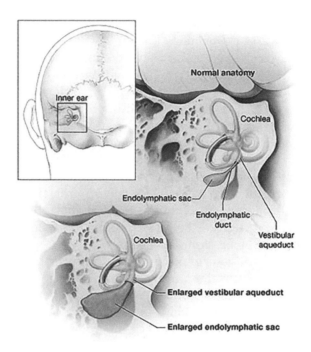

Figure 12.1. *The Inner Ear* (Source: National Institutes of Health (NIH) Medical Arts.)

The second characteristic of Pendred syndrome is an enlarged vestibular aqueduct. The vestibular aqueduct is a bony canal that runs from the vestibule (a part of the inner ear between the cochlea and the semicircular canals) to the inside of the skull. Inside the vestibular aqueduct is a fluid-filled tube called the "endolymphatic duct," which ends at the balloon-shaped endolymphatic sac. The endolymphatic duct and sac usually are also enlarged.

Experts do not recommend testing thyroid hormone levels in children with Pendred syndrome, since levels are usually normal. Some children might be given a "perchlorate washout test," a test that determines whether the thyroid is functioning properly. Although this test is probably the best test for determining thyroid function in Pendred syndrome, it is not used often and has largely been replaced by genetic testing. People who have developed a goiter may be referred to an endocrinologist, a doctor who specializes in glandular disorders, to determine whether the goiter is due to Pendred syndrome or to another cause. Goiter is a common feature of Pendred syndrome, but many individuals who develop a goiter do not have Pendred syndrome. Conversely, many people who have Pendred syndrome never develop a goiter.

How Common Is Pendred Syndrome?

The *SLC26A4* gene accounts for about 5 to 10 percent of hereditary hearing loss. As researchers gain more knowledge about the syndrome and its features, they hope to improve doctors' ability to detect and diagnose the disorder.

Can Pendred Syndrome Be Treated?

Treatment options for Pendred syndrome are available. Because the syndrome is inherited and can involve thyroid and balance problems, many specialists may be involved in treatment, including a primary care physician, an audiologist, an endocrinologist, a clinical geneticist, a genetic counselor, an otolaryngologist, and a speech-language pathologist.

To reduce the likelihood of hearing loss progression, children and adults with Pendred syndrome should avoid contact sports that might lead to head injury; wear head protection when engaged in activities, such as bicycle riding and skiing, that might lead to head injury; and avoid situations that can lead to barotrauma (extreme, rapid changes in pressure), such as scuba diving or hyperbaric oxygen treatment.

Pendred syndrome is not curable, but a medical team will work together to encourage informed choices about treatment options. They also can help people prepare for increased hearing loss and other possible long-term consequences of the syndrome.

Children with Pendred syndrome should start early treatment to gain communication skills, such as learning sign language or cued speech or learning to use a hearing aid. Most people with Pendred syndrome will have hearing loss significant enough to be considered eligible for a cochlear implant. A cochlear implant is an electronic device that is surgically inserted into the cochlea. While a cochlear implant does not restore or create normal hearing, it bypasses injured areas of the ear to provide a sense of hearing in the brain. Children, as well as adults, are eligible to receive an implant.

People with Pendred syndrome who develop a goiter need to have it checked regularly. The type of goiter found in Pendred syndrome is unusual because even though it grows in size, it still continues to make normal amounts of thyroid hormone. Such a goiter often is called a "euthyroid goiter."

What Research Is Being Conducted?

The National Institute on Deafness and Other Communication Disorders (NIDCD) is funding researchers who are working to understand hearing loss caused by inherited syndromes, such as Pendred syndrome, as well as from other causes. Researchers also are looking carefully at the characteristics of the disorder and how the syndrome might cause problems in different parts of the body such as the thyroid and inner ear.

Scientists continue to study the genetic basis of Pendred syndrome. The protein that the *SLC26A4* gene makes, called "pendrin," is found in the inner ear, kidney, and thyroid gland. Researchers have identified more than 150 deafness-causing mutations or alterations of this gene.

By studying mice, scientists are gaining a greater understanding of how an abnormal *SLC26A4* gene affects the form and function of different parts of the body. For example, by studying the inner ears of mice with *SLC26A4* mutations, scientists now realize that the enlarged vestibular aqueduct associated with Pendred syndrome is not caused by a sudden stop in the normal development of the ear. Studies such as this are important because they help scientists rule out some causes of a disorder while helping to identify areas needing more research. Researchers are hopeful these studies eventually will lead to therapies that can target the basic causes of the condition.

Tietz Syndrome

Tietz syndrome is a rare condition characterized by hearing loss, fair skin, and light-colored hair. The hearing loss in affected individuals is caused by abnormalities of the inner ear (sensorineural hearing loss) and is present from birth. People with Tietz syndrome are born with white hair and very pale skin but their hair color often darkens over time; The colored part of the eye (the iris) is blue. It is caused by changes (mutations) in the *MITF* gene which affects the development of melanocytes. The inheritance is autosomal dominant. The goal of treatment is to improve hearing; cochlear implantation may be considered.

Symptoms

The signs and symptoms of Tietz syndrome are usually present at birth and may include:

- Severe, bilateral (both ears) sensorineural hearing loss
- Fair skin
- Light-colored hair
- Blue eyes

Table 12.4 lists symptoms that people with this disease may have. For most diseases, symptoms will vary from person to person. People with the same disease may not have all the symptoms listed. This information comes from a database called the "Human Phenotype Ontology" (HPO). The HPO collects information on symptoms that have been described in medical resources. The HPO is updated regularly. Use the HPO ID to access more in-depth information about a symptom.

Table 12.4. Symptoms of Tietz Syndrome

Medical Terms	Other Names
80% to 99% of people have these symptoms	
Abnormal anterior chamber morphology	
Hearing impairment	Deafness Hearing defect
Hypopigmentation of hair	Loss of hair color
Hypopigmentation of the skin	Patchy lightened skin
White eyebrow	Pale eyebrow
Percent of people who have these symptoms is not available through HPO	
Autosomal dominant inheritance	
Bilateral sensorineural hearing impairment	
Blue irides	Blue eyes
Congenital sensorineural hearing impairment	
Generalized hypopigmentation	Fair skin Pale pigmentation
Hypopigmentation of the fundus	
White eyelashes	Blonde eyelashes Pale eyelashes

Diagnosis

A diagnosis of Tietz syndrome is suspected in people with severe, bilateral (both ears) sensorineural hearing loss; fair skin; and light-colored hair. Identification of a change (mutation) in the *MITF* gene also supports this diagnosis.

Diagnosing Tietz syndrome can be complicated since there are several different genetic conditions that can cause deafness and hypopigmentation, some of which are also caused by mutations in the *MITF* gene. It is, therefore, important for people with suspected Tietz syndrome to be evaluated by a healthcare provider who specializes in genetics.

The Genetic Testing Registry (GTR) provides information about the genetic tests for this condition. Patients and consumers with specific questions about a genetic test should contact a healthcare provider or a genetics professional.

Weissenbacher-Zweymüller Syndrome

Weissenbacher-Zweymüller syndrome is a condition that affects bone growth. It is characterized by skeletal abnormalities, hearing loss, and distinctive facial features. The features of this condition significantly overlap those of two similar conditions, otospondylomegaepiphyseal dysplasia (OSMED) and Stickler syndrome type III. All of these conditions are caused by mutations in the same gene, and in some cases, it can be difficult to tell them apart. Some researchers believe they represent a single disorder with a range of signs and symptoms.

Infants born with Weissenbacher-Zweymüller syndrome are smaller than average because the bones in their arms and legs are unusually short. The thigh and upper arm bones are wider than usual at the ends (described as dumbbell-shaped), and the bones of the spine (vertebrae) may also be abnormally shaped. High-frequency hearing loss occurs in some cases. Distinctive facial features include wide-set protruding eyes, a small and upturned nose with a flat bridge, and a small lower jaw. Some affected infants are born with an opening in the roof of the mouth (a cleft palate).

Most people with Weissenbacher-Zweymüller syndrome experience significant "catch-up" growth in the bones of the arms and legs during childhood. As a result, adults with this condition are not unusually short. However, affected adults still have other signs and symptoms of Weissenbacher-Zweymüller syndrome, including distinctive facial features and hearing loss.

Frequency

Weissenbacher-Zweymüller syndrome is very rare; only a few affected families worldwide have been described in the medical literature.

Causes

Weissenbacher-Zweymüller syndrome is caused by mutations in the *COL11A2* gene. This gene provides instructions for making one component of type XI collagen, which is a complex molecule that gives structure and strength to the connective tissues that support the body's joints and organs. Type XI collagen is found in cartilage, a tough but flexible tissue that makes up much of the skeleton during early development. Most cartilage is later converted to bone, except for the cartilage that continues to cover and protect the ends of bones and is present in the nose and external ears. Type XI collagen is also part of the inner ear and the nucleus pulposus, which is the center portion of the discs between vertebrae.

At least one mutation in the *COL11A2* gene can cause Weissenbacher-Zweymüller syndrome. This mutation disrupts the assembly of type XI collagen molecules. The defective collagen weakens connective tissues in many parts of the body, including the long bones, spine, and inner ears, which impairs bone development and underlies the other signs and symptoms of this condition. It is not well understood why "catch-up" bone growth occurs in childhood.

Inheritance Pattern

This condition is inherited in an autosomal dominant pattern, which means one copy of the altered gene in each cell is sufficient to cause the disorder.

Most cases of this condition result from a new mutation in the gene that occurs during the formation of reproductive cells (eggs or sperm) or in early embryonic development. These cases occur in people with no history of the disorder in their family.

Section 12.6

Otospondylomegaepiphyseal Dysplasia

This section includes text excerpted from
"Otospondylomegaepiphyseal Dysplasia," Genetics Home
Reference (GHR), National Institutes of
Health (NIH), March 19, 2019.

Otospondylomegaepiphyseal dysplasia (OSMED) is a condition characterized by skeletal abnormalities, distinctive facial features, and severe hearing loss. The term "otospondylomegaepiphyseal" refers to the parts of the body that this condition affects: the ears (oto-), the bones of the spine (spondylo-), and the ends (epiphyses) of long bones in the arms and legs. The features of this condition significantly overlap those of two similar conditions, Weissenbacher-Zweymüller syndrome and Stickler syndrome type III. All of these conditions are caused by mutations in the same gene, and in some cases, it can be difficult to tell the conditions apart. Some researchers believe they represent a single disorder with a range of signs and symptoms.

People with OSMED are often shorter than average because the long bones in their legs are unusually short. Other skeletal features include enlarged joints; short arms, hands, and fingers; and flattened bones of the spine (platyspondyly). People with the disorder often experience back and joint pain, limited joint movement, and arthritis that begins early in life.

Severe high-frequency hearing loss is common in people with OSMED. Typical facial features include protruding eyes; a flattened bridge of the nose; an upturned nose with a large, rounded tip; and a small lower jaw. Almost all affected infants are born with an opening in the roof of the mouth (a cleft palate).

Frequency

This condition is rare; its prevalence is unknown. Only a few families with OSMED worldwide have been described in the medical literature.

Causes

OSMED is caused by mutations in the *COL11A2* gene. This gene provides instructions for making one component of type XI collagen, which is a complex molecule that gives structure and strength to the connective tissues that support the body's joints and organs. Type XI collagen is found in cartilage, a tough but flexible tissue that makes up much of the skeleton during early development. Most cartilage is later converted to bone, except for the cartilage that continues to cover and protect the ends of bones and is present in the nose and external ears. Type XI collagen is also part of the inner ear and the nucleus pulposus, which is the center portion of the discs between vertebrae.

The *COL11A2* gene mutations that cause OSMED disrupt the production or assembly of type XI collagen molecules. The defective collagen weakens connective tissues in many parts of the body, including the long bones, spine, and inner ears, which impairs bone development and underlies the other signs and symptoms of this condition.

Inheritance Pattern

This condition is inherited in an autosomal recessive pattern, which means both copies of the gene in each cell have mutations. The parents of an individual with an autosomal recessive condition each carry one copy of the mutated gene, but they typically do not show signs and symptoms of the condition.

Section 12.7

Nonsyndromic Deafness

This section includes text excerpted from "Nonsyndromic Hearing Loss," Genetics Home Reference (GHR), National Institutes of Health (NIH), March 19, 2019.

Nonsyndromic hearing loss is a partial or total loss of hearing that is not associated with other signs and symptoms. In contrast, syndromic hearing loss occurs with signs and symptoms affecting other parts of the body.

Nonsyndromic hearing loss can be classified in several different ways. One common way is by the condition's pattern of inheritance: autosomal dominant (DFNA), autosomal recessive (DFNB),

X-linked (DFNX), or mitochondrial (which does not have a special designation). Each of these types of hearing loss includes multiple subtypes. DFNA, DFNB, and DFNX subtypes are numbered in the order in which they were first described. For example, DFNA1 was the first type of autosomal dominant nonsyndromic hearing loss to be identified.

The characteristics of nonsyndromic hearing loss vary among the different types. Hearing loss can affect one ear (unilateral) or both ears (bilateral). Degrees of hearing loss range from mild (difficulty understanding soft speech) to profound (inability to hear even very loud noises). The term "deafness" is often used to describe severe-to-profound hearing loss. Hearing loss can be stable, or it may be progressive, becoming more severe as a person gets older. Particular types of nonsyndromic hearing loss show distinctive patterns of hearing loss. For example, the loss may be more pronounced at high, middle, or low tones.

Most forms of nonsyndromic hearing loss are described as sensorineural, which means they are associated with a permanent loss of hearing caused by damage to structures in the inner ear. The inner ear processes sound and send the information to the brain in the form of electrical nerve impulses. Less commonly, nonsyndromic hearing loss is described as conductive, meaning it results from changes in the middle ear. The middle ear contains three tiny bones that help transfer sound from the eardrum to the inner ear. Some forms of nonsyndromic hearing loss, particularly a type called "DFNX2," involve changes in both the inner ear and the middle ear. This combination is called "mixed hearing loss."

Depending on the type, nonsyndromic hearing loss can become apparent at any time from infancy to old age. Hearing loss that is present before a child learns to speak is classified as prelingual or congenital. Hearing loss that occurs after the development of speech is classified as postlingual.

Frequency

Between 2 and 3 per 1,000 children in the United States are born with detectable hearing loss in one or both ears. The prevalence of hearing loss increases with age; the condition affects 1 in 8 people in the United States 12 years of age and older, or about 30 million people. By the age of 85, more than half of all people experience hearing loss.

Causes

The causes of nonsyndromic hearing loss are complex. Researchers have identified more than 90 genes that, when altered, are associated with nonsyndromic hearing loss. Many of these genes are involved in the development and function of the inner ear. Mutations in these genes contribute to hearing loss by interfering with critical steps in processing sound. Different mutations in the same gene can be associated with different types of hearing loss, and some genes are associated with both syndromic and nonsyndromic forms. In many affected families, the factors contributing to hearing loss have not been identified.

Most cases of nonsyndromic hearing loss are inherited in an autosomal recessive pattern. About half of all severe-to-profound autosomal recessive nonsyndromic hearing loss results from mutations in the *GJB2* gene; these cases are designated DFNB1. The *GJB2* gene provides instructions for making a protein called "connexin 26," which is a member of the connexin protein family. Mutations in another connexin gene, *GJB6*, can also cause DFNB1. The *GJB6* gene provides instructions for making a protein called "connexin 30." Connexin proteins form channels called "gap junctions," which allow communication between neighboring cells, including cells in the inner ear. Mutations in the *GJB2* or *GJB6* gene alter their respective connexin proteins, which changes the structure of gap junctions and may affect the function or survival of cells that are needed for hearing.

The most common cause of moderate autosomal recessive nonsyndromic hearing loss is mutations in the *STRC* gene. These mutations cause a form of the condition known as "DFNB16." Mutations in more than 60 other genes can also cause autosomal recessive nonsyndromic hearing loss. Many of these gene mutations have been found in one or a few families.

Nonsyndromic hearing loss can also be inherited in an autosomal dominant pattern. Mutations in at least 30 genes have been identified in people with autosomal dominant nonsyndromic hearing loss; mutations in some of these genes (including *GJB2* and *GJB6*) can also cause autosomal recessive forms of the condition. Although no single gene is associated with a majority of autosomal dominant nonsyndromic hearing loss cases, mutations in a few genes, such as *KCNQ4* and *TECTA*, are relatively common. Mutations in many of the other genes associated with autosomal dominant nonsyndromic hearing loss have been found in only one or a few families.

X-linked and mitochondrial forms of nonsyndromic hearing loss are rare. About half of all X-linked cases are caused by mutations in the *POU3F4* gene. This form of the condition is designated DFNX2. Mutations in at least three other genes have also been identified in people with X-linked nonsyndromic hearing loss.

Mitochondrial forms of hearing loss result from changes in mitochondrial DNA (mtDNA). Mitochondria are structures within cells that convert the energy from food into a form that cells can use. Although most DNA is packaged in chromosomes within the nucleus, mitochondria also have a small amount of their own DNA. Only a few mutations in mtDNA have been associated with hearing loss, and their role in the condition is still being studied.

Mutations in some of the genes associated with nonsyndromic hearing loss can also cause syndromic forms of hearing loss, such as Usher syndrome (*CDH23* and *MYO7A*, among others), Pendred syndrome (*SLC26A4*), Wolfram syndrome (*WFS1*), and Stickler syndrome (*COL11A2*). It is often unclear how mutations in the same gene can cause isolated hearing loss in some individuals and hearing loss with additional signs and symptoms in others.

In addition to genetic changes, hearing loss can result from environmental factors or a combination of genetic risk and a person's environmental exposures. Environmental causes of hearing loss include certain medications, specific infections before or after birth, and exposure to loud noise over an extended period. Age is also a major risk factor for hearing loss. Age-related hearing loss (presbycusis) is thought to have both genetic and environmental influences.

Inheritance Pattern

As discussed above, nonsyndromic hearing loss has different patterns of inheritance. Between 75 and 80 percent of cases are inherited in an autosomal recessive pattern, which means both copies of the gene in each cell have mutations. Usually, each parent of an individual with autosomal recessive hearing loss carries one copy of the mutated gene but does not have hearing loss.

Another 20 to 25 percent of nonsyndromic hearing loss has an autosomal dominant pattern of inheritance, which means one copy of the altered gene in each cell is sufficient to cause the condition. Most people with autosomal dominant hearing loss inherit an altered copy of the gene from a parent who also has hearing loss.

Between one and two percent of cases have an X-linked pattern of inheritance. A condition is considered X-linked if the mutated gene that causes the disorder is located on the X chromosome, one of the two sex chromosomes in each cell. Males with X-linked nonsyndromic hearing loss tend to develop more severe hearing loss earlier in life than females who inherit a copy of the same gene mutation. A characteristic of X-linked inheritance is that fathers cannot pass X-linked traits to their sons.

Mitochondrial forms of the condition, which result from changes to mtDNA, account for less than one percent of all nonsyndromic hearing loss in the United States. These cases are inherited in a mitochondrial pattern, which is also known as maternal inheritance. This pattern of inheritance applies to genes contained in mtDNA. Because egg cells, but not sperm cells, contribute mitochondria to the developing embryo, children can only inherit disorders resulting from mtDNA mutations from their mother. These disorders can appear in every generation of a family and can affect both males and females, but fathers do not pass traits associated with changes in mtDNA to their children.

In some cases, hearing loss occurs in people with no history of the condition in their family. These cases are described as sporadic, and the cause of the hearing loss is often unknown. When hearing loss results from environmental factors, it is not inherited.

Chapter 13

Sensorineural Hearing Disorders

Chapter Contents

Section 13.1

Auditory Neuropathy

This section includes text excerpted from "Auditory Neuropathy," National Institute on Deafness and Other Communication Disorders (NIDCD), January 26, 2018.

What Is Auditory Neuropathy?

Auditory neuropathy is a hearing disorder in which the inner ear successfully detects sound but has a problem with sending sound from the ear to the brain. It can affect people of all ages, from infancy through adulthood. The number of people affected by auditory neuropathy is not known, but current information suggests that auditory neuropathies play a substantial role in hearing impairments and deafness.

When their hearing sensitivity is tested, people with auditory neuropathy may have normal hearing or hearing loss ranging from mild to severe. They always have poor speech perception abilities, meaning that they have trouble understanding speech clearly. People with auditory neuropathy have greater impairment in speech perception than hearing health experts would predict based upon their degree of hearing loss on a hearing test. For example, a person with auditory neuropathy may be able to hear sounds but still has difficulty recognizing spoken words. Sounds may fade in and out or seem out of sync for these individuals.

What Causes Auditory Neuropathy

Researchers report several causes of auditory neuropathy. In some cases, the cause may involve damage to the inner hair cells—specialized sensory cells in the inner ear that transmit information about sounds through the nervous system to the brain. In other cases, the cause may involve damage to the auditory neurons that transmit sound information from the inner hair cells to the brain. Other possible causes may include inheriting genes with mutations or suffering damage to the auditory system, either of which may result in faulty connections between the inner hair cells and the auditory nerve (the nerve leading from the inner ear to the brain) or damage to the auditory nerve itself. A combination of these problems may occur in some cases.

What Are the Roles of the Outer and Inner Hair Cells?

Outer hair cells help amplify sound vibrations entering the inner ear from the middle ear. When hearing is working normally, the inner hair cells convert these vibrations into electrical signals that travel as nerve impulses to the brain, where the brain interprets the impulses as sound.

Although outer hair cells—hair cells next to and more numerous than inner hair cells—are generally more prone to damage than inner hair cells; outer hair cells seem to function normally in people with auditory neuropathy.

Are There Risk Factors for Auditory Neuropathy?

There are several ways that children may acquire auditory neuropathy. Some children diagnosed with auditory neuropathy experienced particular health problems before or during birth or as newborns. These problems include inadequate oxygen supply during or prior to birth, premature birth, jaundice, low birth weight (LBW), and dietary thiamine deficiency. In addition, some drugs used to treat pregnant women or newborns may damage the baby's inner hair cells, causing auditory neuropathy. Adults may also develop auditory neuropathy along with age-related hearing loss.

Auditory neuropathy runs in some families, and in some cases, scientists have identified genes with mutations that compromise the ear's ability to transmit sound information to the brain. Thus, inheritance of mutated genes is also a risk factor for auditory neuropathy.

Some people with auditory neuropathy have neurological disorders that also cause problems outside of the hearing system. Examples of such disorders are Charcot-Marie-Tooth syndrome and Friedreich ataxia.

How Is Auditory Neuropathy Diagnosed?

Health professionals—including otolaryngologists (ear, nose, and throat doctors), pediatricians, and audiologists—use a combination of methods to diagnose auditory neuropathy. These include tests of auditory brainstem response (ABR) and otoacoustic emissions (OAEs). The hallmark of auditory neuropathy is an absent or very abnormal ABR reading together with a normal OAE reading. A normal OAE reading is a sign that the outer hair cells are working normally.

An ABR test uses electrodes placed on a person's head and ears to monitor brain wave activity in response to sound. An OAE test uses a small, very sensitive microphone inserted into the ear canal to monitor the faint sounds produced by the outer hair cells in response to auditory stimulation. ABR and OAE testing are painless and can be used for newborn babies and infants, as well as older children and adults. Other tests may also be used as part of a comprehensive evaluation of an individual's hearing and speech perception abilities.

Does Auditory Neuropathy Ever Get Better or Worse?

Some newborn babies who have been diagnosed with auditory neuropathy improve and start to hear and speak within a year or two. Other infants stay the same, while some get worse and show signs that the outer hair cells no longer function (abnormal otoacoustic emissions). In people with auditory neuropathy, hearing sensitivity can remain stable, get better or worse, or gradually worsen, depending on the underlying cause.

What Treatments, Devices, and Other Approaches Can Help People with Auditory Neuropathy to Communicate?

Researchers are still seeking effective treatments for people with auditory neuropathy. Meanwhile, professionals in the hearing field differ in their opinions about the potential benefits of hearing aids, cochlear implants, and other technologies for people with auditory neuropathy. Some professionals report that hearing aids and personal listening devices, such as frequency modulation (FM) systems, are helpful for some children and adults with auditory neuropathy. Cochlear implants (electronic devices that compensate for damaged or nonworking parts of the inner ear) may also help some people with auditory neuropathy. No tests are currently available, however, to determine whether an individual with auditory neuropathy might benefit from a hearing aid or cochlear implant.

Debate also continues about the best ways to educate and improve communication skills in infants and children who have hearing impairments, such as auditory neuropathy. One approach favors sign language as the child's first language. A second approach encourages the use of listening skills—together with technologies, such as hearing aids and cochlear implants—and spoken language. A combination of these two approaches may also be used. Some health professionals believe it may be especially difficult for children with auditory neuropathy to learn to communicate only through spoken language because their ability to understand speech is often severely impaired. Adults with auditory neuropathy and older children who have already developed spoken language may benefit from learning how to speechread (also known as "lip reading").

What Research Is Being Done on Auditory Neuropathy?

Scientists have identified genes involved in causing some cases of auditory neuropathy, and they are working to identify what goes wrong in the auditory system when a person inherits a mutant gene. Researchers are also continuing to investigate the potential benefits of cochlear implants for children with auditory neuropathy and examining why cochlear implants may benefit some people with the condition but not others.

Section 13.2

Age-Related Hearing Loss (Presbycusis)

This section includes text excerpted from "Age-Related Hearing Loss," National Institute on Deafness and Other Communication Disorders (NIDCD), July 17, 2018.

What Is Age-Related Hearing Loss?

Age-related hearing loss (presbycusis) is the loss of hearing that gradually occurs in most of us as we grow older. It is one of the most common conditions affecting older and elderly adults.

Approximately 1 in 3 people in the United States between the ages of 65 and 74 has hearing loss, and nearly half of those older than 75 years of age have difficulty hearing. Having trouble hearing can make it hard to understand and follow doctor's advice; respond to warnings; and hear phones, doorbells, and smoke alarms. Hearing loss can also make it hard to enjoy talking with family and friends, leading to feelings of isolation.

Age-related hearing loss most often occurs in both ears, affecting them equally. Because the loss is gradual, if you have age-related hearing loss, you may not realize that you have lost some of your ability to hear.

There are many causes of age-related hearing loss. Most commonly, it arises from changes in the inner ear as we age, but it can also result from changes in the middle ear or from complex changes along the nerve pathways from the ear to the brain. Certain medical conditions and medications may also play a role.

How Do We Hear?

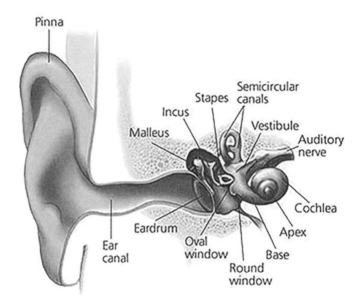

Figure 13.1. *The Auditory System* (Source: National Institutes of Health (NIH)/National Institute on Deafness and Other Communication Disorders (NIDCD))

Hearing depends on a series of events that change sound waves in the air into electrical signals. Your auditory nerve then carries these signals to your brain through a complex series of steps.

1. Sound waves enter the outer ear and travel through a narrow passageway called the "ear canal," which leads to the eardrum.

2. The eardrum vibrates from the incoming sound waves and sends these vibrations to three tiny bones in the middle ear. These bones are called the "malleus," "incus," and "stapes."

3. The bones in the middle ear couple the sound vibrations from the air to fluid vibrations in the cochlea of the inner ear, which is shaped like a snail and filled with fluid. An elastic partition runs from the beginning to the end of the cochlea, splitting it into an upper and lower part. This partition is called the "basilar membrane" because it serves as the base, or ground floor, on which key hearing structures sit.

4. Once the vibrations cause the fluid inside the cochlea to ripple, traveling waveforms along the basilar membrane. Hair cells— sensory cells sitting on top of the basilar membrane—ride the wave.

5. As the hair cells move up and down, microscopic hair-like projections (known as "stereocilia") that perch on top of the hair cells bump against an overlying structure and bend. Bending causes pore-like channels, which are at the tips of the stereocilia, to open up. When that happens, chemicals rush into the cells, creating an electrical signal.

6. The auditory nerve carries this electrical signal to the brain, which turns it into a sound that we recognize and understand.

Why Do We Lose Our Hearing as We Get Older?

Many factors can contribute to hearing loss as you get older. It can be difficult to distinguish age-related hearing loss from hearing loss that can occur for other reasons, such as long-term exposure to noise.

Noise-induced hearing loss is caused by long-term exposure to sounds that are either too loud or last too long. This kind of noise exposure can damage the sensory hair cells in your ear that allow you to hear. Once these hair cells are damaged, they do not grow back, and your ability to hear is diminished.

Conditions that are more common in older people, such as high blood pressure or diabetes, can contribute to hearing loss. Medications that are toxic to the sensory cells in your ears (for example, some chemotherapy drugs) can also cause hearing loss.

Rarely, age-related hearing loss can be caused by abnormalities of the outer ear or middle ear. Such abnormalities may include the reduced function of the tympanic membrane (the eardrum) or reduced function of the three tiny bones in the middle ear that carry sound waves from the tympanic membrane to the inner ear.

Most older people who experience hearing loss have a combination of both age-related hearing loss and noise-induced hearing loss.

Can I Prevent Age-Related Hearing Loss?

At this time, scientists do not know how to prevent age-related hearing loss. However, you can protect yourself from noise-induced hearing loss by protecting your ears from sounds that are too loud and last too long. It is important to be aware of potential sources of damaging noises, such as loud music, firearms, snowmobiles, lawn mowers, and leaf blowers. Avoiding loud noises, reducing the amount of time you are exposed to loud noise, and protecting your ears with ear plugs or earmuffs are easy things you can do to protect your hearing and limit the amount of hearing you might lose as you get older.

What Should I Do If I Have Trouble Hearing?

Hearing problems can be serious. The most important thing you can do if you think you have a hearing problem is to seek advice from a healthcare provider. There are several types of professionals who can help you. You might want to start with your primary care physician, an otolaryngologist, an audiologist, or a hearing aid specialist. Each has a different type of training and expertise. Each can be an important part of your hearing healthcare.

- An otolaryngologist is a doctor who specializes in diagnosing and treating diseases of the ear, nose, throat, and neck. An otolaryngologist, sometimes called an "ENT," will try to find out why you are having trouble hearing and offer treatment options. She or he may also refer you to another hearing professional, an audiologist.

- An audiologist has specialized training in identifying and measuring the type and degree of hearing loss. Some audiologists may be licensed to fit hearing aids.

- A hearing aid specialist is someone who is licensed by your state to conduct and evaluate basic hearing tests, offer counseling, and fit and test hearing aids.

What Treatments and Devices Can Help?

Your treatment will depend on the severity of your hearing loss, so some treatments will work better for you than others. There are a number of devices and aids that help you hear better when you have hearing loss. Here are the most common ones:

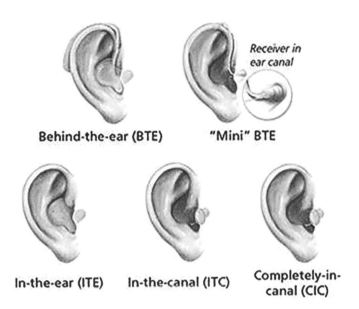

Figure 13.2. *Styles of Hearing Aids* (Source: National Institutes of Health (NIH)/National Institute on Deafness and Other Communication Disorders (NIDCD))

- **Hearing aids** are electronic instruments you wear in or behind your ear (see figure 13.2). They make sounds louder. To find the hearing aid that works best for you, you may have to try more than one. Be sure to ask for a trial period with your hearing aid, and understand the terms and conditions of the trial period. Work with your hearing aid provider until you are comfortable with putting on and removing the hearing aid, adjusting the volume level, and changing the batteries. Hearing aids are generally not covered by health insurance companies, although some are. Medicare does not cover hearing aids for adults; however, diagnostic evaluations are covered if they are ordered by a physician for the purpose of assisting the physician in developing a treatment plan.

- **Cochlear implants.** Cochlear implants are small electronic devices surgically implanted in the inner ear that help provide a sense of sound to people who are profoundly deaf or hard-of-hearing. If your hearing loss is severe, your doctor may recommend a cochlear implant in one or both ears.

- **Bone-anchored hearing systems** bypass the ear canal and middle ear, and are designed to use your body's natural ability to transfer sound through bone conduction. The sound processor picks up sound, converts it into vibrations, and then relays the vibrations through your skull bone to your inner ear.

- **Assistive listening devices** include telephone and cell phone amplifying devices, smartphone or tablet "apps," and closed-circuit systems (hearing loop systems) in places of worship, theaters, and auditoriums.

- **Lip reading or speech reading** is another option that helps people with hearing problems follow the conversational speech. People who use this method pay close attention to others when they talk by watching the speaker's mouth and body movements. Special trainers can help you learn how to lip read or speech read.

Can My Friends and Family Help Me?

You and your family can work together to make living with hearing loss easier. Here are some things you can do:

- Tell your friends and family about your hearing loss. The more friends and family you tell, the more people there will be to help you cope with your hearing loss.

- Ask your friends and family to face you when they talk so that you can see their faces. If you watch their faces move and see their expressions, it may help you to understand them better.

- Ask people to speak louder, but not shout. Tell them they do not have to talk slowly, just more clearly.

- Turn off the television or the radio when you are not actively listening to it.

- Be aware of the noise around you that can make hearing more difficult. When you go to a restaurant, for example, do not sit near the kitchen or near a band playing music. Background noise makes it hard to hear people talk.

Working together to hear better may be tough on everyone for a while. It will take time for you to get used to watching people as they talk and for people to get used to speaking louder and more clearly. Be patient and continue to work together. Hearing better is worth the effort.

What Research Is Being Done?

The National Institute on Deafness and Other Communication Disorders (NIDCD) is supporting research on the causes of age-related hearing loss, including genetic factors. Some NIDCD-supported scientists are exploring the potential to regrow new hair cells in the inner ear using drug or gene therapies. Other NIDCD-supported work is exploring medications that may reduce or prevent noise-induced and age-related hearing loss. Scientists supported by the NIDCD are also developing and refining devices that can be used to help people with age-related hearing loss.

Section 13.3

Hyperacusis

This section includes text excerpted from "Age-Related Hearing Loss," Genetic and Rare Diseases Information Center (GARD), National Center for Advancing Translational Sciences (NCATS), December 21, 2017.

Hyperacusis is a hearing disorder that results in difficulty tolerating sounds that would not bother most people. This condition may occur due to many different causes, such as head injury, viral infections, or neurological disorders. In some people with hyperacusis, sounds are perceived as being much louder than they would be by someone without this disorder. Some people may have emotional reactions to sounds, such as being annoyed or afraid. Others experience pain with low-level sounds. People with hyperacusis can have only one or different combinations of these symptoms. Another very common symptom is ringing in the ears (tinnitus).

Patients with hyperacusis typically first receive an otolaryngologic exam and hearing testing. These tests can be done by an audiologist or an otolaryngologist (ear, nose, and throat (ENT) doctor). Treatment may involve a program of sound therapy to train the brain to better process everyday sounds. This type of treatment involves listening to low-level white noise to gradually improve the ability to hear sounds.

Section 13.4

Sudden Deafness

This section includes text excerpted from "Sudden Deafness,"
National Institute on Deafness and Other Communication
Disorders (NIDCD), September 14, 2018.

What Is Sudden Deafness?

Sudden sensorineural (inner ear) hearing loss (SSHL), commonly known as "sudden deafness," is an unexplained, rapid loss of hearing either all at once or over a few days. SSHL happens because there is something wrong with the sensory organs of the inner ear. Sudden deafness frequently affects only one ear.

People with SSHL often discover the hearing loss upon waking up in the morning. Others first notice it when they try to use the deafened ear, such as when they use a phone. Still, others notice a loud, alarming "pop" just before their hearing disappears. People with sudden deafness may also notice one or more of these symptoms: a feeling of ear fullness, dizziness, and/or a ringing in their ears.

Sometimes, people with SSHL put off seeing a doctor because they think their hearing loss is due to allergies, a sinus infection, earwax plugging the ear canal, or other common conditions. However, you should consider sudden deafness symptoms a medical emergency and visit a doctor immediately. Although about half of people with SSHL recover some or all their hearing spontaneously, usually within one to two weeks from the onset, delaying SSHL diagnosis and treatment (when warranted) can decrease treatment effectiveness. Receiving timely treatment greatly increases the chance that you will recover at least some of your hearing.

Experts estimate that SSHL strikes between 1 and 6 people per 5,000 every year, but the actual number of new SSHL cases each year could be much higher because SSHL often goes undiagnosed. SSHL can happen to people at any age, but most often affects adults in their late forties and early fifties.

What Causes Sudden Deafness

A variety of disorders affecting the ear can cause SSHL, but only about 10 percent of people diagnosed with SSHL have an identifiable cause. Some of these conditions include:

- Infections
- Head trauma
- Autoimmune diseases
- Exposure to certain drugs that treat cancer or severe infections
- Blood circulation problems
- Neurological disorders, such as multiple sclerosis (MS)
- Disorders of the inner ear, such as Ménière disease

Most of these causes are accompanied by other medical conditions or symptoms that point to the correct diagnosis. Another factor to consider is whether hearing loss happens in one or both ears. For example, if sudden hearing loss occurs only in one ear, tumors on the auditory nerve should be ruled out as the cause. Autoimmune disease may cause SSHL in one or both ears.

How Is Sudden Deafness Diagnosed?

If you have sudden deafness symptoms, your doctor should rule out conductive hearing loss—hearing loss due to an obstruction in the ear, such as fluid or ear wax. For sudden deafness without an obvious, identifiable cause upon examination, your doctor should perform a test called "pure tone audiometry" within a few days of onset of symptoms to identify any sensorineural hearing loss.

With pure tone audiometry, your doctor can measure how loud different frequencies, or pitches, of sounds, need to be before you can hear them. One sign of SSHL could be the loss of at least 30 decibels (decibels are a measure of sound intensity) in 3 connected frequencies within 72 hours. This drop would, for example, make conversational speech sound as if it were a whisper. Patients may have more subtle, sudden changes in their hearing and may be diagnosed with other tests.

If you are diagnosed with sudden deafness, your doctor will probably order additional tests to try to determine an underlying cause for your SSHL. These tests may include blood tests, imaging (usually magnetic resonance imaging, or MRI), and balance tests.

How Is Sudden Deafness Treated?

The most common treatment for sudden deafness, especially when the cause is unknown, is corticosteroids. Steroids can treat many disorders and usually work by reducing inflammation, decreasing swelling, and helping the body fight illness. Previously, steroids were given in pill form. In 2011, a clinical trial supported by the National Institute on Deafness and Other Communication Disorders (NIDCD) showed that intratympanic (through the eardrum) injection of steroids was as effective as oral steroids. After this study, doctors started prescribing direct intratympanic injection of steroids into the middle ear; the medication then flows into the inner ear. The injections can be performed in the offices of many otolaryngologists, and are a good option for people who cannot take oral steroids or want to avoid their side effects.

Steroids should be used as soon as possible for the best effect and may even be recommended before all test results come back. Treatment that is delayed for more than two to four weeks is less likely to reverse or reduce permanent hearing loss.

Additional treatments may be needed if your doctor discovers an underlying cause of your SSHL. For example, if SSHL is caused by an infection, the doctor may prescribe antibiotics. If you took drugs that were toxic to the ear, you may be advised to switch to another drug. If an autoimmune condition caused your immune system to attack the inner ear, the doctor may prescribe drugs that suppress the immune system.

If your hearing loss is severe, does not respond to treatment, and/or happens in both ears, your doctor may recommend that you use hearing aids (to amplify sound) or even receive cochlear implants (to directly stimulate the auditory connections in the ear that go to the brain).

Chapter 14

Ototoxicity

What Is Ototoxicity?[1]

A change in hearing or balance caused by medications is called "ototoxicity." Many medications can harm the ear. For example, some medications used to treat cancer, and some antibiotics, can put you at risk for hearing and balance problems.

What Are Ototoxic Chemicals and Substances That Contain Ototoxicants?[2]

Ototoxic chemicals are classified as neurotoxicants, cochleotoxicants, or vestibulotoxicants based on the part of the ear they damage; these chemicals can reach the inner ear through the bloodstream and cause injury to inner parts of the ear and connected neural pathways. Neurotoxicants are ototoxic when they damage the nerve fibers that interfere with hearing and balance. Cochleotoxicants mainly affect the cochlear hair cells, which are the sensory receptors, and can impair the ability to hear. Vestibulotoxicants affect the hair cells on the spatial

This chapter includes text excerpted from documents published by two public domain sources. Text under the headings marked 1 are excerpted from "Ototoxicity: Medications and Hearing Loss," Office on Rehabilitation Research & Development Service (RR&D), U.S. Department of Veterans Affairs (VA), June 19, 2011. Reviewed Apirl 2019; Text under the headings marked 2 are excerpted from "Preventing Hearing Loss Caused by Chemical (Ototoxicity) and Noise Exposure," Centers for Disease Control and Prevention (CDC), March 8, 2018.

orientation and balance organs. The research on ototoxicants and their interactions with noise is limited. The dose-response, lowest observed effect level (LOEL) and no observed effect level (NOEL) has been identified in animal experiments for only a few substances.

The exposure threshold for ototoxicity varies for each chemical based on its compound family, properties, exposure route, exposure concentration and duration, synergy with noise, and noise exposure, along with an individual's risk factors.

Prevention[2]

The first step in preventing exposure to ototoxicants is to know if they are in the workplace. One way to identify ototoxicants in the workplace is by reviewing Safety Data Sheets (SDS) for ototoxic substances and/or chemicals, and ototoxic health hazards associated with ingredients in the product.

Employers must provide health and safety information, as well as training, to workers exposed to hazardous materials, including ototoxic chemicals. The training must be in a language and vocabulary that the worker understands. Additionally, complaints from workers about hearing loss should include investigating SDS for ototoxicants.

What Can I Do to Prevent Ototoxicity?[1]

You may not be able to prevent ototoxicity if you need an ototoxic drug to treat a life-threatening disease, but you can minimize it by working with your doctor to make good decisions about what treatment is best for you. One important action you can take is to have your hearing checked before and during treatment so that small changes in your hearing can be picked up early. Your doctor may then be able to adjust your medications to prevent more hearing loss.

Chapter 15

Tinnitus

What Is Tinnitus?

Tinnitus is commonly described as a ringing in the ears, but it also can sound like roaring, clicking, hissing, or buzzing. It may be soft or loud, high-pitched or low-pitched. You might hear it in either one or both ears. Roughly 10 percent of the adult population of the United States has experienced tinnitus lasting at least 5 minutes in the past year. This amounts to nearly 25 million Americans.

What Causes Tinnitus

Tinnitus is not a disease. It is a symptom that something is wrong in the auditory system, which includes the ear, the auditory nerve that connects the inner ear to the brain, and the parts of the brain that process sound. Something as simple as a piece of earwax blocking the ear canal can cause tinnitus. But, it can also be the result of a number of health conditions, such as:

- Noise-induced hearing loss

- Ear and sinus infections

- Diseases of the heart or blood vessels

This chapter includes text excerpted from "Tinnitus," National Institute on Deafness and Other Communication Disorders (NIDCD), March 6, 2017.

- Ménière disease

- Brain tumors

- Hormonal changes in women

- Thyroid abnormalities

Tinnitus is sometimes the first sign of hearing loss in older people. It also can be a side effect of medications. More than 200 drugs are known to cause tinnitus when you start or stop taking them.

People who work in noisy environments—such as factory or construction workers, road crews, or even musicians—can develop tinnitus over time when ongoing exposure to noise damages tiny sensory hair cells in the inner ear that help transmit sound to the brain. This is called "noise-induced hearing loss."

Service members exposed to bomb blasts can develop tinnitus if the shock wave of the explosion squeezes the skull and damages brain tissue in areas that help process sound. In fact, tinnitus is one of the most common service-related disabilities among veterans returning from Iraq and Afghanistan.

Pulsatile tinnitus is a rare type of tinnitus that sounds like a rhythmic pulsing in the ear, usually in time with your heartbeat. A doctor may be able to hear it by pressing a stethoscope against your neck or by placing a tiny microphone inside the ear canal. This kind of tinnitus is most often caused by problems with blood flow in the head or neck. Pulsatile tinnitus also may be caused by brain tumors or abnormalities in brain structure.

Even with all of these associated conditions and causes, some people develop tinnitus for no obvious reason. Most of the time, tinnitus is not a sign of a serious health problem; although, if it is loud or does not go away, it can cause fatigue, depression, anxiety, and problems with memory and concentration. For some, tinnitus can be a source of real mental and emotional anguish.

Why Do I Have This Noise in My Ears?

Although we hear tinnitus in our ears, its source is really in the networks of brain cells (what scientists call "neural circuits") that make sense of the sounds our ears hear. A way to think about tinnitus is that it often begins in the ear, but it continues in the brain.

Scientists still have not agreed upon what happens in the brain to create the illusion of sound when there is none. Some think that tinnitus is similar to chronic pain syndrome, in which the pain persists even after a wound or broken bone has healed.

Tinnitus could be the result of the brain's neural circuits trying to adapt to the loss of sensory hair cells by turning up the sensitivity to sound. This would explain why some people with tinnitus are over-sensitive to loud noise.

Tinnitus also could be the result of neural circuits thrown out of balance when damage in the inner ear changes, signaling activity in the auditory cortex—the part of the brain that processes sound. Or, it could be the result of abnormal interactions between neural circuits. The neural circuits involved in hearing are not solely dedicated to processing sound. They also communicate with other parts of the brain, such as the limbic region, which regulates mood and emotion.

What Should I Do If I Have Tinnitus?

The first thing is to see your primary care doctor, who will check if anything, such as ear wax, is blocking the ear canal. Your doctor will ask you about your current health, medical conditions, and medications to find out if an underlying condition is causing your tinnitus.

If your doctor cannot find any medical condition responsible for your tinnitus, you may be referred to an otolaryngologist (commonly called an "ear, nose, and throat doctor," or an "ENT"). The ENT will physically examine your head, neck, and ears and test your hearing to determine whether you have any hearing loss along with the tinnitus. You might also be referred to an audiologist who can also measure your hearing and evaluate your tinnitus.

What If the Sounds in My Ear Do Not Go Away?

Some people find their tinnitus does not go away or it gets worse. In some cases, it may become so severe that you find it difficult to hear, concentrate, or even sleep. Your doctor will work with you to help find ways to reduce the severity of the noise and its impact on your life.

Are There Treatments That Can Help Me?

Tinnitus does not have a cure yet, but treatments that help many people cope better with the condition are available. Most doctors will offer a combination of the treatments below, depending on the severity of your tinnitus and the areas of your life it affects the most.

- **Hearing aids** often are helpful for people who have hearing loss along with tinnitus. Using a hearing aid adjusted to carefully control outside sound levels may make it easier for you to hear. The better you hear, the less you may notice your tinnitus.

- **Counseling** helps you learn how to live with your tinnitus. Most counseling programs have an educational component to help you understand what goes on in the brain to cause tinnitus. Some counseling programs also will help you change the way you think about and react to your tinnitus. You might learn some things to do on your own to make the noise less noticeable, to help you relax during the day, or to fall asleep at night.

- **Wearable sound generators** are small electronic devices that fit in the ear and use a soft, pleasant sound to help mask the tinnitus. Some people want the masking sound to totally cover up their tinnitus, but most prefer a masking level that is just a bit louder than their tinnitus. The masking sound can be a soft "shhhhhhhhhhh," random tones, or music.

- **Tabletop sound generators** are used as an aid for relaxation or sleep. Placed near your bed, you can program a generator to play pleasant sounds, such as waves, waterfalls, rain, or the sounds of a summer night. If your tinnitus is mild, this might be all you need to help you fall asleep.

- **Acoustic neural stimulation** is a relatively new technique for people whose tinnitus is very loud or will not go away. It uses a palm-sized device and headphones to deliver a broadband acoustic signal embedded in music. The treatment helps stimulate change in the neural circuits in the brain, which eventually desensitizes you to the tinnitus. The device has been shown to be effective in reducing or eliminating tinnitus in a significant number of study volunteers.

- **Cochlear implants** are sometimes used in people who have tinnitus along with severe hearing loss. A cochlear implant bypasses the damaged portion of the inner ear and sends electrical signals that directly stimulate the auditory nerve. The device brings in outside sounds that help mask tinnitus and stimulate change in the neural circuits.

- **Antidepressants and antianxiety drugs** might be prescribed by your doctor to improve your mood and help you sleep.

- **Other medications** may be available at drugstores and on the Internet as an alternative remedy for tinnitus, but none of these preparations has been proved effective in clinical trials.

Can I Do Anything to Prevent Tinnitus or Keep It from Getting Worse?

Noise-induced hearing loss, the result of damage to the sensory hair cells of the inner ear, is one of the most common causes of tinnitus. Anything you can do to limit your exposure to loud noise—by moving away from the sound, turning down the volume, or wearing earplugs or earmuffs—will help prevent tinnitus or keep it from getting worse.

What Are Researchers Doing to Better Understand Tinnitus?

Along the path a hearing signal travels to get from the inner ear to the brain, there are many places where things can go wrong to cause tinnitus. If scientists can understand what goes on in the brain to start tinnitus and cause it to persist, they can look for those places in the system where a therapeutic intervention could stop tinnitus in its tracks.

In 2009, the National Institute on Deafness and Other Communication Disorders (NIDCD) sponsored a workshop that brought together tinnitus researchers to talk about the condition and develop fresh ideas for potential cures. During the course of the workshop, participants discussed a number of promising research directions, including:

- **Electrical or magnetic stimulation of brain areas involved in hearing.** Implantable devices that reduce the trembling of Parkinson disease and the anxieties of obsessive-compulsive disorder (OCD) already exist. Similar devices could be developed to normalize the neural circuits involved in tinnitus.

- **Repetitive transcranial magnetic stimulation (rTMS).** This technique, which uses a small device placed on the scalp to generate short magnetic pulses, is already being used to normalize electrical activity in the brains of people with epilepsy. Preliminary trials of rTMS in humans, funded by the NIDCD, are helping researchers pinpoint the best places in the brain to stimulate in order to suppress tinnitus. Researchers are also looking for ways to identify which people are most likely to respond well to stimulation devices.

- **Hyperactivity and deep brain stimulation.** Researchers have observed hyperactivity in neural networks after exposing the ear to intense noise. Understanding specifically where in the brain this hyperactivity begins and how it spreads to other areas could lead to treatments that use deep brain stimulation to calm the neural networks and reduce tinnitus.

• **Resetting the tonotopic map.** Researchers are exploring how to take advantage of the tonotopic map, which organizes neurons in the auditory cortex according to the frequency of the sound to which they respond. Previous research has shown a change in the organization of the tonotopic map after exposing the ear to intense noise. By understanding how these changes happen, researchers could develop techniques to bring the map back to normal and relieve tinnitus.

Chapter 16

Noise-Induced Hearing Loss

Chapter Contents

Section 16.1

Noise-Induced Hearing Loss: An Overview

This section includes text excerpted from "Noise-Induced Hearing Loss," National Institute on Deafness and Other Communication Disorders (NIDCD), January 23, 2018.

What Is Noise-Induced Hearing Loss?

Every day, we experience sound in our environment, such as the television, radio, washing machine, automobiles, buses, and trucks. But, when an individual is exposed to harmful sounds—sounds that are too loud or loud sounds over a long time—sensitive structures of the inner ear can be damaged, causing noise-induced hearing loss (NIHL).

How Do We Hear?

Hearing is a series of events in which the ear converts sound waves into electrical signals and causes nerve impulses to be sent to the brain, where they are interpreted as sound. The ear has three main parts: the outer, middle, and inner ear. Sound waves enter through the outer ear and reach the middle ear, where they cause the eardrum to vibrate. The vibrations are transmitted through three tiny bones in the middle ear called the "ossicles." These three bones are named the "malleus," "incus," and "stapes" (and are also known as the "hammer," "anvil," and "stirrup"). The eardrum and ossicles amplify

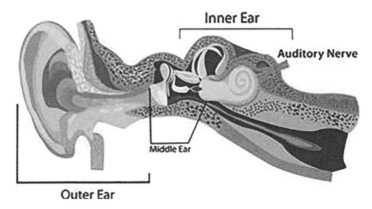

Figure 16.1. *Structure of Ear*

the vibrations and carry them to the inner ear. The stirrup transmits the amplified vibrations through the oval window and into the fluid that fills the inner ear. The vibrations move through fluid in the snail-shaped hearing part of the inner ear (cochlea) that contains the hair cells. The fluid in the cochlea moves the top portion of the hair cells, called the "hair bundle," which initiates the changes that lead to the production of the nerve impulses. These nerve impulses are carried to the brain, where they are interpreted as sound. Different sounds move the population of hair cells in different ways, thus allowing the brain to distinguish among various sounds, such as different vowel and consonant sounds.

What Sounds Cause Noise-Induced Hearing Loss?

NIHL can be caused by a one-time exposure to loud sound, as well as by repeated exposure to sounds at various loudness levels, over an extended period of time. The loudness of sound is measured in units called "decibels." For example, usual conversation is approximately 60 decibels, the humming of a refrigerator is 40 decibels, and city traffic noise can be 80 decibels. Examples of sources of loud noises that cause NIHL are motorcycles, firecrackers, and small arms fire, all emitting sounds from 120 to 140 decibels. Sounds of less than 75 decibels, even after long exposure, are unlikely to cause hearing loss.

Exposure to harmful sounds causes damage to the sensitive hair cells of the inner ear and to the nerve of hearing. These structures can be injured by noise in two different ways: from an intense brief impulse, such as an explosion, or from continuous exposure to noise, such as that in a woodworking shop.

What Are the Effects of Noise-Induced Hearing Loss?

The effect from impulse sound can be instantaneous and can result in an immediate hearing loss that may be permanent. The structures of the inner ear may be severely damaged. This kind of hearing loss may be accompanied by tinnitus, an experience of a sound such as ringing, buzzing, or roaring in the ears or head, which may subside over time. Hearing loss and tinnitus may be experienced in one or both ears, and tinnitus may continue constantly or intermittently throughout a lifetime.

The damage that occurs slowly over years of continuous exposure to loud noise is accompanied by various changes in the structure of the hair cells. It also results in hearing loss and tinnitus. Exposure to impulse and continuous noise may cause only a temporary hearing loss. If the hearing recovers, the temporary hearing loss is called a "temporary threshold shift." The temporary threshold shift largely disappears within 16 hours after exposure to loud noise.

Both forms of NIHL can be prevented by the regular use of hearing protectors, such as earplugs or earmuffs.

What Are the Symptoms of Noise-Induced Hearing Loss?

The symptoms of NIHL that occur over a period of continuous exposure increase gradually. Sounds may become distorted or muffled, and it may be difficult for the person to understand speech. The individual may not be aware of the loss, but it can be detected with a hearing test.

Who Is Affected by Noise-Induced Hearing Loss?

More than 30 million Americans are exposed to hazardous sound levels on a regular basis. 10 million Americans have suffered irreversible NIHL. Individuals of all ages, including children, adolescents, young adults, and older people, can develop NIHL. Exposure occurs in the workplace, in recreational settings, and at home. There is an increasing awareness of the harmful noises in recreational activities, such as target shooting or hunting, snowmobiles, go-carts, woodworking and other hobby equipment, power horns, cap guns, and model airplanes. Harmful noises at home may come from vacuum cleaners, garbage disposals, lawn mowers, leaf blowers, and shop tools. People who live in either urban or rural settings may be exposed to noisy devices on a daily basis.

Can Noise-Induced Hearing Loss Be Prevented?

NIHL is preventable. All individuals should understand the hazards of noise and how to practice good hearing health in everyday life.

- Know which noises can cause damage (those above 75 decibels).

- Wear earplugs or other hearing protective devices when involved in a loud activity. (Special earplugs and earmuffs are available at hardware stores and sporting good stores.)

- Be alert to hazardous noise in the environment.

- Protect children who are too young to protect themselves.

- Make family, friends, and colleagues aware of the hazards of noise.

- Have a medical examination by an otolaryngologist, a physician who specializes in diseases of the ears, nose, throat, head, and neck, and a hearing test by an audiologist, a health professional trained to identify and measure hearing loss and to rehabilitate persons with hearing impairments.

What Research Is Being Done for Noise-Induced Hearing Loss?

Scientists focusing their research on the mechanisms causing NIHL hope to understand more fully the internal workings of the ear, which will result in better prevention and treatment strategies. For example, scientists have discovered that damage to the structure of the hair bundle of the hair cell is related to temporary and permanent loss of hearing. They have found that when the hair bundle is exposed to prolonged periods of damaging sound, the basic structure of the hair bundle is destroyed, and the important connections among hair cells are disrupted, which directly leads to hearing loss.

Other studies are investigating potential drug therapies that may provide insight into the mechanisms of NIHL. For example, scientists studying altered blood flow in the cochlea are seeking the effect on the hair cells. They have shown reduced cochlear blood flow following exposure to noise. Further research has shown that a drug that promotes blood flow and is used for the treatment of peripheral vascular disease (any abnormal condition in blood vessels outside the heart) maintains circulation in the cochlea during exposure to noise. These findings may lead to the development of treatment strategies to reduce NIHL.

Continuing efforts will provide opportunities that can aid research on NIHL, as well as other diseases and disorders that cause hearing loss. Research is the way to develop new, more effective methods to prevent, diagnose, treat, and eventually eliminate these diseases and disorders and improve the health and quality of life (QOL) for all Americans.

Section 16.2

What Noises Cause Hearing Loss

This section includes text excerpted from "What Noises Cause Hearing Loss?" Centers for Disease Control and Prevention (CDC), December 11, 2018.

Loud Noise Can Cause Hearing Loss Quickly or over Time

Hearing loss can result from a single loud sound (such as firecrackers) near your ear. Or, more often, hearing loss can result over time from damage caused by repeated exposures to loud sounds. The louder the sound, the shorter the amount of time it takes for hearing loss to occur. The longer the exposure, the greater the risk for hearing loss (especially when hearing protection is not used or there is not enough time for the ears to rest between exposures).

Here are some sources of loud noise that you may be exposed to. If you are repeatedly exposed to them over time, they can cause hearing loss.

Everyday Activities

- Music from smartphones and personal listening devices, particularly when the volume is set close to the maximum
- Fitness classes
- Children's toys

Events

- Concerts, restaurants, and bars
- Sporting events, such as football, hockey, and soccer games
- Motorized sporting events, such as monster truck shows, stock car or road races, and snowmobiling
- Movie theaters

Tools and More

- Power tools
- Gas-powered lawn mowers and leaf blowers

- Sirens
- Firearms
- Firecrackers

Common Sources of Noise and Decibel Levels

Sound is measured in decibels (dB). A whisper is about 30 dB, normal conversation is about 60 dB, and a motorcycle engine running is about 95 dB. Noise above 85 dB over a prolonged period of time may start to damage your hearing. Loud noise above 120 dB can cause immediate harm to your ears.

The table below shows dB levels and how noise from everyday sources can affect your hearing.

Table 16.1. Noise and Their Decibel Levels

Everyday Sounds and Noises	Average Sound Level (Measured in Decibels)	Typical Response (after Routine or Repeated Exposure)
Softest sound that can be heard	0	
Normal breathing	10	
Ticking watch	20	
Soft whisper	30	
Refrigerator hum	40	Sounds at these dB levels typically don't cause any hearing damage.
Normal conversation, air conditioner	60	
Washing machine, dishwasher	70	You may feel annoyed by the noise
City traffic (inside the car)	80–85	You may feel very annoyed
Gas-powered lawnmowers and leaf blowers	90	Damage to hearing possible after 2 hours of exposure
Motorcycle	95	Damage to hearing possible after about 50 minutes of exposure
Approaching subway train, car horn at 16 feet (5 meters), and sporting events (such as hockey playoffs and football games)	100	Hearing loss possible after 15 minutes

Table 16.1. Continued

Everyday Sounds and Noises	Average Sound Level (Measured in Decibels)	Typical Response (after Routine or Repeated Exposure)
The maximum volume level for personal listening devices; a very loud radio, stereo, or television; and loud entertainment venues (such as nightclubs, bars, and rock concerts)	105–110	Hearing loss possible in less than 5 minutes
Shouting or barking in the ear	110	Hearing loss possible in less than 2 minutes
Standing beside or near sirens	120	Pain and ear injury
Firecrackers	140–150	Pain and ear injury

The time estimates listed in the "Typical Response" column are based on the National Institute of Occupational Safety and Health (NIOSH) exchange rate of 3 dB.

Sounds May Be Louder than What You Hear

How loud something sounds to you is not the same as the actual intensity of that sound. Sound intensity is the amount of sound energy in a confined space. It is measured in decibels (dB). The decibel scale is logarithmic, which means that loudness is not directly proportional to sound intensity. Instead, the intensity of a sound grows very fast. This means that a sound at 20 dB is 10 times more intense than a sound at 10 dB. Also, the intensity of a sound at 100 dB is one billion times more powerful compared to a sound at 10 dB.

Two sounds that have equal intensity are not necessarily equally loud. Loudness refers to how you perceive audible sounds. A sound that seems loud in a quiet room might not be noticeable when you are on a street corner with heavy traffic, even though the sound intensity is the same. In general, to measure loudness, a sound must be increased by 10 dB to be perceived as twice as loud. For example, 10 violins would sound only twice as loud as 1 violin.

The risk of damaging your hearing from noise increases with the sound intensity, not the loudness of the sound. If you need to raise your voice to be heard at an arm's length, the noise level in the environment is likely above 85 dB in sound intensity and could damage your hearing over time.

How Do I Know the Sound Level Is Safe?

You can use a sound level meter to measure noise around you. You can find free sound level meters developed as apps for smartphones. If the reading is higher than 85 dB, it might be okay if it is for a short time and followed by lower levels. The effect of lower volumes listened to over long periods is the same as that of louder sounds heard over a short period. For example, noise exposure at 85 dB for 8 hours is equivalent to exposure to 88 dB for 4 hours and 91 dB for 2 hours. At 100 dB, however, the safe duration of exposure would only be 15 minutes a day.

Section 16.3

How Do I Know If I Have Hearing Loss Caused by Loud Noise?

This section includes text excerpted from "How Do I Know If I Have Hearing Loss Caused by Loud Noise?" Centers for Disease Control and Prevention (CDC), December 11, 2018.

Prevention and early detection of hearing loss are important. If you have any signs of hearing loss or if you are at risk for hearing loss, get your hearing tested.

Signs of Hearing Loss

If you have any of these signs or symptoms, you may have hearing loss caused by noise:

- Speech and other sounds seem muffled
- Difficulty hearing high-pitched sounds (e.g., birds, doorbell, telephone, alarm clock)
- Difficulty understanding conversations when you are in a noisy place, such as a restaurant
- Difficulty understanding speech over the phone

- Trouble distinguishing speech consonants (e.g., difficulty distinguishing the difference between s and f, between p and t, or between sh and th in speech)

- Asking others to speak more slowly and clearly

- Asking someone to speak more loudly or repeat what they said

- Turning up the volume of the television or radio

- Ringing in the ears

- Hypersensitivity to certain sounds (certain sounds are very bothersome or create pain)

If you have any signs of hearing loss, get tested by a qualified healthcare provider.

Early Detection of Hearing Loss Are Important

Do not wait until you show signs of hearing loss. Have your hearing examined by your doctor during your regular checkup. A basic hearing evaluation usually includes a quick look in the ear with an special light for looking into the ear canal (otoscope) and other checks to assess the sounds you can hear.

Your doctor may refer you to a hearing specialist (audiologist) or other healthcare providers who is qualified to test hearing if you:

- Have a history of exposure to loud noise

- Feel your hearing has changed

- Have family or friends that say you have difficulty hearing and communicating with them. (Those around us can be the first to notice our hearing problems.)

The audiologist may have you listen to different sounds through headphones to determine the softest sounds you can hear, repeat lists of words, or complete other special tests.

Children Should Have Their Hearing Tested

Children should have their hearing tested before they enter school or any time there is a concern about the child's hearing. Children who do not pass the hearing screening need to get a full hearing test as soon as possible.

Are You at Risk for Loud Noise-Related Hearing Loss?

The following conditions and exposures can increase your risk for noise-induced hearing loss.

- Genetics and individual susceptibility to noise
- Long-standing (chronic) conditions, such as diabetes and high blood pressure
- Injuries to the ear
- Organic liquid chemicals, such as toluene
- Certain medicines

Medicines that damage the ear are called "ototoxic." The damage can result in hearing loss, ringing in the ears, or loss of balance. More than 200 medicines are ototoxic. They include certain antibiotics (for example, gentamicin), cancer treatment drugs (for example, cisplatin and carboplatin), pain relievers that contain salicylate (for example, aspirin, quinine, loop diuretics), and many other medicines.

Tips for People at Risk for Noise-Related Hearing Loss

- Avoid noisy places whenever possible.
- Use earplugs, protective earmuffs, or noise-canceling headphones when around loud noises.
- Keep the volume down when using earbuds or headphones.
- Ask your doctor for a hearing checkup if you suspect you have had hearing loss.

Regular Check-Ups Can Help Identify Early Hearing Loss

Regular check-ups are especially important if you are at risk for hearing loss, such as:

- If you have a family history of hearing loss not associated with noise exposure
- If you work in a noisy environment
- If you engage in noisy activities or hobbies

191

- If you take medicines that place you at greater risk for hearing loss (for example, certain antibiotics, cancer treatment drugs, pain relievers, and more)

Section 16.4

Preventing Hearing Loss from Loud Noise

This section includes text excerpted from "How Do I Prevent Hearing Loss from Loud Noise?" Centers for Disease Control and Prevention (CDC), December 11, 2018.

If You Need to Shout, the Sound Is Too Loud

Even without a device to measure sound, you can typically tell if the noise around you is too loud. If you or others need to shout in order to be heard or cannot understand each other even at arm's length away, the sound is too loud and may damage your hearing over time.

What about during Pregnancy and for Infants and Children

During pregnancy, use the same precautions specified above for at-home and public events. Also try to avoid your body touching the source of the noise (i.e., vibration).

For children and infants, also use the same precautions specified above. And keep children away from high noise levels, such as from very loud toys.

Use Hearing Protection

The best way to protect your hearing from noise is to avoid noisy activities. When you cannot avoid loud noise, use hearing protection. Hearing protection devices reduce the level of sound entering your ear. They do not block out sound completely. Hearing protection that does not fit properly will not protect your hearing.

Look for Noise Reduction Ratings

Hearing protection devices come with different noise reduction ratings. The noise reduction rating is usually labeled on the device container (it may say "NRR"), and it indicates the amount of potential protection the device provides.

Noise reduction ratings are measured in decibels (dB). Most hearing protection devices have ratings that range from 0 dB to 35 dB. A noise reduction rating is a "best case" rating measured in a laboratory; the actual sound reduction provided by the protector may be much less. It is best to choose a hearing protector that is comfortable and convenient, and that you are willing to wear consistently when exposed to noise. If you want to know exactly how much noise reduction you are getting, you can have the device "fit-tested" by a hearing professional.

More about Noise Reduction

The actual sound reduction may be lower than the number listed for the device even when worn correctly. As a basic guide, you can:

- Reduce the manufacturer's noise reduction rating by 25 percent for earmuffs

- Reduce the manufacturer's noise reduction rating by half (50%) for foam earplugs

- Reduce the manufacturer's noise reduction rating by 70 percent for all other earplugs

Choose the Right Hearing Protection

The choice of hearing protection device depends on your personal preferences of comfort and where you will wear it. How well the protection works depends on whether you wear it consistently and correctly. The most common types of hearing protection devices include earplugs, earmuffs, and specially made devices.

Insert-Type Earplugs

These devices provide an air-tight seal in the ear canal. They are generally cheap, effective, and easy to use. They can be any of the following types:

- Premolded (pliable devices of fixed proportions)

- Formable (usually made of expandable foam)

- Custom-molded (to fit precisely the size and shape of an individual's ear canal)

- Canal caps (earplugs on a flexible plastic or metal band) (During quiet times, when not needed, you can leave the canal caps hanging around your neck so they will be easy to find when needed.)

Earmuffs

Earmuffs come in many models designed to fit most people. They block out noise by completely covering the outer ear. Some earmuffs also include electronic parts to help users communicate or to block sound impulses or background noise. However, earmuffs might not work as well for people with heavy beards, sideburns, or glasses (which can create gaps between the earmuff cushion and your skull).

Wearing both earmuffs and earplugs can reduce the sound further. However, the noise reduction ratings for the two do not add together.

Specially Made Devices

You can also get specially made hearing protection devices. They can be styled and sized specifically for a person's individual ear. They can also have special features.

- Custom earplugs molded to fit your ear exactly

- Earmuffs with built-in radios or communication devices that allow you to listen at a safe level, while still protecting you from the loud noise outside (such as at sporting events)

- "Level-dependent" hearing protectors (such as earmuffs) that do not block sound when the environment is quiet, but block loud sounds. These can be very useful for hunters.

- Lightweight active noise cancellation headphones for reducing low-frequency noise (for example, in airplane cabins). Noise canceling devices work best for low-pitched droning sounds, such as from car and airplane engines and air conditioners. (These devices do not have a noise reduction rating.)

- Uniform-attenuation earplugs for musicians and concert attendees. These devices act just like turning down the volume on a stereo (in other words, the sound intensity is decreased).

Chapter 17

Hearing Protection

Chapter Contents

Section 17.1

How to Protect Your Hearing

This section includes text excerpted from documents
published by two public domain sources. Text under the
headings marked 1 are excerpted from "How Do You Protect
Your Hearing?" National Institute on Deafness and Other
Communication Disorders (NIDCD), January 10, 2018; Text
under the headings marked 2 are excerpted from "Protect Your
Child's Hearing," National Institute on Deafness and Other
Communication Disorders (NIDCD), July 22, 2016.

Protect Your Hearing[1]

Keep hearing the sounds you love. Earplugs and earmuffs help
protect your hearing from harmful noises. You will still be able to
hear the sounds you love, but your hearing will be protected from
damaging noise.

There are many types of hearing protectors, so you can wear the
ones that fit your style and are the most comfortable. Choose a great
color or design that matches what you are wearing.

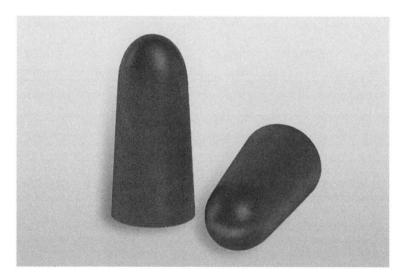

Figure 17.1. *Foam Earplugs*

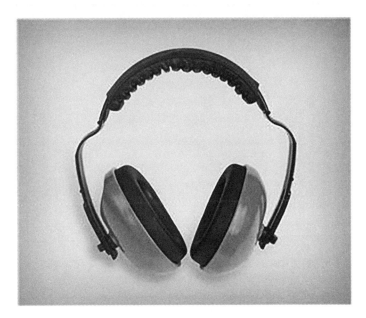

Figure 17.2. *Earmuffs*

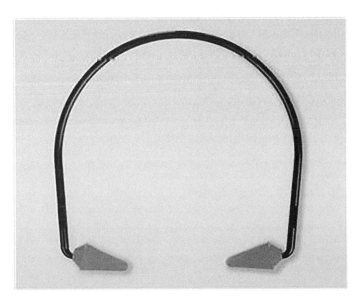

Figure 17.3. *Canal Caps*

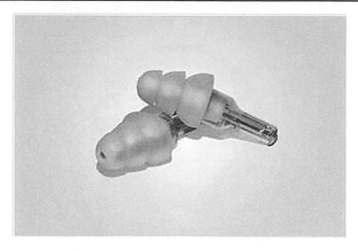

Figure 17.4. *High Fidelity Earplugs*

When to Use Hearing Protectors[2]

Hearing protectors limit the level of sound. They do not block out all noise—they just make noise softer. Use hearing protectors when you or your children are exposed to noise that is too loud or lasts too long. The louder the sound, the quicker hearing damage will occur.

For example, your children should use hearing protectors when:

- Attending loud events in stadiums, gymnasiums, amusement parks, theaters, auditoriums, and other entertainment facilities

- Attending auto races, sporting events, and music concerts of all types, including symphonies and rock concerts

- Riding a snowmobile, all-terrain vehicle, or farm tractor

- Participating in shooting sports. The sound of a gunshot can reach the same level as a jet engine at takeoff. At this decibel level, noise can damage your child's hearing immediately and permanently. Hearing protectors should be a standard part of shooting-safety gear.

Types of Hearing Protectors[2]

The amount of protection a hearing protector offers is measured by its noise reduction rating, or NRR. The higher the NRR, the better the device limits sound. Many companies now make hearing protectors in sizes to fit children. To find a list of companies on the Internet, search for "hearing protectors for children." Your local grocery, drug, and hardware stores may also carry some protectors.

Earplugs

Earplugs are either soft foam or hard plastic inserts that fit directly into the ear canal. They can be less expensive than earmuffs, and they come in both disposable and reusable options. Earplugs are also easy to carry around in a purse or pocket. Some even come with a neck strap so that your child would not lose one if it falls out.

Foam earplugs. These earplugs are rolled into a thin cylinder that is put halfway into the ear canal. Once in the ear, the earplug reshapes itself to fill the area snugly.

Get the right fit:

- Roll the earplug up into a small, thin "snake" with your fingers. You can use one or both hands.

- Pull the top of your ear up and back with your opposite arm to straighten out your ear canal. Use the other hand to slide the earplug in.

- Hold the earplug in with your finger. Count to 20 or 30 out loud while waiting for the plug to expand and fill the ear canal. Your voice will sound muffled when the plug has made a good seal.

- Check the fit when you are done. Most of the foam body of the earplug should be within the ear. Try cupping your hands tightly over your ears. If sounds are much more muffled with your hands in place, the earplug may not be sealing properly. Take the earplug out and try again.

Pre-molded earplugs. These earplugs are made from plastic, rubber, or silicone and are shaped like an ice cream cone. They are sold in different sizes. Your child will probably need a smaller size.

Earmuffs

Earmuffs often look like wireless headphones. The part that fits over the ear could be filled with fluid, foam, or both to make sure that the earmuff fits easily and closely. Earmuffs can often cost more than earplugs, but they are easier than earplugs for young children to put on correctly. You also will not have to worry about the earmuffs sliding out. Even if you buy earmuffs for your child, you might also want to have some spare earplugs on hand.

Get the right fit:

- Check to make sure the earmuffs are not too loose for your child's head.

- If your child wears glasses, check to make sure the earmuffs seal properly over them and are not uncomfortable.

Tips for Wearing Hearing Protectors[1]

- Practice wearing your hearing protectors around the house to get used to the fit.

- Bring an extra pair of earplugs or earmuffs when you go to a concert, game, or other noisy events. Share them with your friends so they can protect their hearing too.

Tips to Help Your Children Use Hearing Protectors[2]

- **Set clear rules for when hearing protectors should be worn.** Tell your children that you expect them to wear hearing protectors in noisy areas, even when you are not there to supervise. For example, is your child in the school band or going riding on a dirt bike? It is time for your child to put on hearing protectors.

- **Shop for hearing protectors with them.** Discuss with your children whether they would rather wear earplugs that can be hidden by hair or a hat, or make a fashion statement with more noticeable hearing protectors. Many colorful and comfortable styles of hearing protectors are available in stores and online.

- **Choose hearing protectors that fit in with your children's daily activities.** If your children play in a band or orchestra, earplugs can help protect their hearing. Special musicians' earplugs (often called "high fidelity earplugs") are available so that your children can hear instruments clearly, but at a softer level. You can also find hearing protectors designed specifically for hunting or shooting sports.

- **Make sure hearing protection is within reach.** Keep hearing protection devices in areas that are within easy reach of your children. Hearing protectors that are hidden in a drawer and are not worn will not do any good.

Section 17.2

Maintaining a Quiet Environment: At Home and Farm

This section contains text excerpted from the following sources: Text under the heading "Create a Quiet Home" is excerpted from "Quick Tips for a Quieter Home," National Institute on Deafness and Other Communication Disorders (NIDCD), July 22, 2016; Text under the heading "Keeping Noise down on the Farm" is excerpted from "Keeping Noise Down on the Farm," National Institute on Deafness and Other Communication Disorders (NIDCD), July 22, 2016.

Create a Quiet Home

Here are some helpful tips to maintain a quiet home:

Keep TV, Video Games, and Music at a Low Volume

Use the lowest volume that allows you to still hear clearly. If someone in the room has trouble hearing, try turning on the television (TV) captioning or subtitles rather than turning up the volume.

Create Ways to Reduce the Noise of Chores

Close the door between your kids and any appliances in use, such as the vacuum cleaner or equipment in a workshop or laundry room.

Buy Quiet Toys

Choose toys with volume controls, and use only the lowest volume setting.

Ask about Noise Ratings When Buying Appliances

When buying certain appliances, such as a fan, range hood, or dishwasher, ask about its noise rating. Some ratings are given in "sones." The lower the sone number, the quieter the unit.

Limit the Number of Noises Going on at One Time

Try to use just one noisy item at a time, such as the TV, hair dryer, vacuum, or power tools.

Keep Outdoor Noises Out

Close windows and doors when you hear outdoor sounds, such as leaf blowers, lawn mowers, power tools, and sirens.

Use Soft Furnishings to Soften Noise Indoors

Add cushions, curtains, and wall coverings to absorb noise. Placing carpets and area rugs (the thicker the better) over hard flooring can help reduce the noise too.

Put Earplugs or Earmuffs Where They Are Most Likely to Be Needed

Store them near a lawn mower, tractor, or all-terrain vehicle and in a woodworking shop and garage.

Put Red Stickers on Objects That Can Reach Unsafe Sound Levels

Remind your family members that a sticker means that they should use hearing protectors or limit the time that they are around these objects.

Keeping Noise Down on the Farm

Some people may think a farm is a quiet place, but if you live or work on one, you know that is not always the case. Combines, tractors, and even farm animals can create a noisy environment that puts your hearing at risk. The following tips can help parents teach children who live or work on a farm, how to prevent hearing loss from too much noise.

Be Alert to Potentially Damaging Sounds on the Farm

- A tractor with a closed cab, on average, can expose the operator to noise levels of about 85 decibels. Prolonged exposure to any noise at or above 85 decibels can cause gradual and permanent hearing loss.

- A tractor without a cab, a woodshop, or pig squeals can reach 100 decibels or higher—roughly the same noise level as a snowmobile. Try to limit your exposure to noises at or above 100 decibels to less than 15 minutes, if you do not have hearing protectors handy.

- Grain dryers and chain saws can reach 110 decibels or higher, about the same noise level as a rock concert. Regular unprotected exposure of more than one minute to sounds that are 110 decibels or higher risks permanent hearing damage.

Take Steps to Reduce Noise from Machinery

- Keep machinery running smoothly by replacing worn parts. Be sure engines are well lubricated and properly tuned to reduce noise from friction or vibrations.

- Put barriers between you and the noise, such as an acoustically designed cab on ride-on equipment or an insulated engine cover or barrier on stationary equipment.

- Install noise-reducing mufflers on engines.

Help Protect Your Family from Excessive Farm Noise

- Be aware of noise levels that put your hearing at risk. If you are running a piece of farm equipment and you have to shout to be heard over the noise, then you should likely be wearing hearing protectors. Any noise that leaves you or your child feeling stressed, or that leaves a ringing or buzzing sound in your ears, is too loud for any length of time without hearing protectors.

- Get hearing protectors and become comfortable using them. Hearing protectors reduce harmful levels of sound. Although carrying on a conversation may be more difficult in some situations, you will still be able to hear warning signals, which is very important for safety. Try out earmuffs before you buy them to ensure that the fit is right. Wear earplugs or earmuffs in and around the house so you become comfortable and familiar with how things sound when you are wearing them.

- Point out situations where family members should practice hearing safety. Remind your child to do chores or other activities away from noisy equipment or to wear hearing protectors when the chore involves noisy equipment.

- Post signs in potentially noisy areas. Use signs to identify work areas or equipment for which hearing protectors are essential.

- Keep hearing protectors on hand in potentially noisy areas. Ask family members to wear them whenever they are in these areas.

Equipment may start up without notice or emit a sudden blast of noise. Very loud noises, even if they last for only a short time, can cause immediate and permanent hearing damage.

Hearing Safety Is an Important Part of Farm Safety

The North American Guidelines for Children's Agricultural Tasks (NAGCAT) were developed by the National Children's Center for Rural and Agricultural Health and Safety (NCCRAHS) to help parents determine when children between 7 and 16 years of age can safely handle different farm chores. They advise the use of hearing protectors for certain chores that may put children's hearing at risk.

By taking some basic safety precautions and being a positive role model, you can teach your child how to have healthy hearing for life. At the same time, you will also be protecting your own hearing.

Decibel values for farm noises were obtained from the National Institute for Occupational Safety and Health (NIOSH), the National Agricultural Safety Database, and various state Cooperative Extension Service publications. Note that decibel values can vary widely according to many factors, including age, make, and model of the machinery; the operation being performed; and the amount of maintenance received. Furthermore, a person just inches away from the source is experiencing much higher decibel levels than someone standing 100 feet away.

Chapter 18

What If One Already Has Hearing Loss?

Chapter Contents

Section 18.1

Take Steps to Keep It from Getting Worse

This section includes text excerpted from "What If I
Already Have Hearing Loss?" Centers for Disease Control
and Prevention (CDC), December 11, 2018.

There is no medical or surgical treatment for hearing loss caused
by noise. Damaged hair cells do not grow back. As much as possible,
you should try to protect your hearing. If you do have hearing loss,
you should take steps to keep it from getting worse.

- Avoid noisy places whenever possible.
- Use earplugs, protective ear muffs, or noise-canceling
  headphones when around loud noises.
- Keep the volume down when listening through earbuds or
  headphones.
- Ask your doctor for a hearing check-up if you suspect you have
  hearing loss.

Many people with hearing loss can still hear some sounds. If you
already have a hearing loss, there are ways to help you make the most
out of the hearing you have. Read about the methods and devices below
that can help.

Things You Can Do to Help Compensate for Your Hearing Loss

- **Look at the speaker.** Your brain can pick up a lot of
  information from visual cues that can supplement what you hear
  to help you understand the message. Everyone reads lips more
  than they realize, and facial expressions and body language can
  provide helpful cues as well.
- **Find the best location for listening.** Placing yourself
  between the speaker and sources of background noise makes it
  much easier to hear and understand what is being said. Practice
  finding the best locations for different situations. For example,
  sit across from your host in a restaurant, or stay in a room apart
  from the music at a party.
- **Choose favorable listening environments whenever
  possible.** The physical characteristics of a room can make

it easier or harder to hear. For example, choose restaurants with better lighting or meeting rooms with carpeted floors and acoustic ceiling tiles that reduce the echo (or reverberation) in a room.

- **Pay attention to the conversation.** It is easier to understand a conversation context than to understand a statement that has no background to help you know what it is about.

- **Alert others to your hearing difficulty.** Speakers can use strategies to help you hear better as well, such as making sure they have your attention before they speak and giving you a clear view of their face.

- **Use closed captioning.** Use closed captioning (CC) when you watch TV, movies, and online videos. Closed captioning can enhance your ability to understand the program.

Consider Using a Device to Help You Hear

If you already have hearing loss, hearing devices can help you make the most out of the hearing you have.

- **Hearing aids.** Hearing aids make sounds louder. They can be adjusted to work best for your specific hearing loss. Making sounds louder can make them easier to understand. However, hearing aids may also make background sounds louder. If you have a hearing loss that distorts sounds, a hearing aid will not make sounds clearer.

- **Assistive listening devices (ALDs).** These devices help you hear sounds in specific everyday activities. Telephone amplifiers can make it easier to hear on the phone. A flashing or vibrating alarm clock can help you wake up in the morning. Loop, FM, and infrared systems can transmit sound to some types of earphones and certain hearing aids. They can help you hear television broadcasts, movies, and meetings in public places.

- **Cochlear implants.** These devices are for people who have very severe hearing loss. They stimulate the auditory nerve directly. Surgery is required to insert them.

- **Personal sound amplification products (PSAPs).** PSAPs allow people with normal hearing to hear better in specific situations. They might be used when hunting or bird-watching, for example, or to better hear a conversation or performance from a distance. PSAPs are not intended to compensate for hearing loss, and they are not individually programmed like hearing aids. However, they can be useful in some circumstances.

Section 18.2

Products and Devices to Improve Hearing

This section includes text excerpted from "Other Products and Devices to Improve Hearing," U.S. Food and Drug Administration (FDA), February 6, 2018.

Assistive Listening Devices

Assistive listening devices (ALDs), or assistive listening systems, include a large variety of devices designed to help you hear sounds in everyday activities. ALDs are available in some public places, such as auditoriums, movie theaters, houses of worship, and meeting rooms. They may be used by both normal-hearing and hearing-impaired people to improve listening in these settings.

ALDs can be used to overcome the negative effects of distance, poor room acoustics, and background noise. To achieve this purpose, many ALDs consist of a microphone near the source of the sound and a receiver near the listener. The listener can usually adjust the volume of the receiver as needed. Careful microphone placement allows the level of the speaker's voice to stay constant, regardless of the distance between the speaker and the audience. The speaker's voice is also heard clearly over room noises, such as chairs moving, fan motors running, and people talking.

ALDs can be used with or without hearing aids.

Cochlear Implants

A cochlear implant is an implanted electronic device that can produce useful hearing sensations by electrically stimulating nerves inside the inner ear. Cochlear implants currently consist of two main components:

- External component, comprised of an externally worn microphone, sound processor, and transmitter system

- Internal component, comprised of an implanted receiver and electrode system, which contains the electronic circuits that receive signals from the external system and send electrical signals to the inner ear

Cochlear implants are different from hearing aids in some aspects.

Table 18.1. Difference between Hearing Aids and Cochlear Implants

Hearing Aids	Cochlear Implants
Hearing aids are indicated for individuals with all degrees of hearing loss (from mild to profound).	Cochlear implants are indicated only for individuals with severe-profound hearing loss.
Most hearing aids are not implanted (although some bone-conduction hearing aids have an implanted component).	Cochlear implants are composed of both internal (implanted) and external components. A surgical procedure is needed to place the internal components.
In hearing aids, sound is amplified and conveyed through both the outer and middle ear and finally to the sensory receptor cells (hair cells) in the inner ear. The hair cells convert the sound energy into neural signals that are picked up by the auditory nerve.	Cochlear implants bypass the outer and middle ears, and the damaged hair cells and replace their functions by converting sound energy into electrical energy that directly stimulates the auditory nerve.

Implantable Middle Ear Hearing Devices

Implantable middle ear hearing devices (IMEHDs) help increase the transmission of sound to the inner ear. IMEHDs are small implantable devices that are typically attached to one of the tiny bones in the middle ear. When they receive sound waves, IMEHDs vibrate and directly move the middle ear bones. This creates sound vibrations in the inner ear, which helps you to detect the sound. This device is generally used for people with sensorineural hearing loss.

Bone-Anchored Hearing Aids

A bone-anchored hearing aid (BAHA), similar to a cochlear implant, has both implanted and external components. The implanted component is a small post that is surgically attached to the skull bone behind your ear. The external component is a speech processor which converts sound into vibrations; it connects to the implanted post and transmits sound vibrations directly to the inner ear through the skull, bypassing the middle ear. BAHAs are for people with middle ear problems (usually a mixed hearing loss) or who have no hearing in one ear.

Personal Sound Amplification Products

Personal sound amplification products (PSAPs), or sound amplifiers, increase environmental sounds for nonhearing impaired consumers. Examples of situations when these products would be used include hunting (listening for prey), bird watching, listening to a lecture with a distant speaker, and listening to soft sounds that would be difficult for normal hearing individuals to hear (e.g., distant conversations, performances). PSAPs are not intended to be used as hearing aids to compensate for hearing impairment.

Chapter 19

Electronic Hearing Devices

Chapter Contents

Section 19.1

Hearing Aids

This section contains text excerpted from the following
sources: Text beginning with the heading "What Are Hearing Aids?"
is excerpted from "Types of Hearing Aids," U.S. Food and Drug
Administration (FDA), January 16, 2018; Text beginning with the
heading "How Can Hearing Aids Help?" is excerpted from
"Hearing Aids," National Institute on Deafness and Other
Communication Disorders (NIDCD), March 6, 2017.

What Are Hearing Aids?

Hearing aids are sound-amplifying devices designed to aid people
who have a hearing impairment.

Most hearing aids share several similar electronic components,
including a microphone that picks up sound, amplifier circuitry that
makes the sound louder, a miniature loudspeaker (receiver) that delivers the amplified sound into the ear canal, and batteries that power
the electronic parts.

Hearing aids differ by:

- Design

- Technology used to achieve amplification (i.e., analog versus digital)

- Special features

Some hearing aids also have earmolds or earpieces to direct the
flow of sound into the ear and enhance sound quality. The selection of
hearing aids is based on the type and severity of hearing loss, listening
needs, and lifestyle.

What Are the Different Styles of Hearing Aids?

Behind-the-ear (BTE) aids: Most parts are contained in a small
plastic case that rests behind the ear; the case is connected to an earmold or an earpiece by a piece of clear tubing. This style is often chosen
for young children because it can accommodate various earmold types,
which need to be replaced as the child grows. Also, the BTE aids are
easily cleaned and handled and are relatively sturdy.

"Mini" BTE (or "on-the-ear") aids: A new type of BTE aid called
the "mini BTE" (or "on-the-ear") aid. It also fits behind/on the ear,

but it is smaller. A very thin, almost invisible, tube is used to connect the aid to the ear canal. Mini BTEs may have a comfortable earpiece for insertion ("open fit") but may also use a traditional earmold. Mini BTEs allow not only reduced occlusion or "plugged up" sensations in the ear canal, but also increase comfort, reduce feedback, and address cosmetic concerns for many users.

In-the-ear (ITE) aids: All parts of the hearing aid are contained in a shell that fills in the outer part of the ear. The ITE aids are larger than the in-the-canal and completely-in-the-canal aids (see below), and, for some people, may be easier to handle than smaller aids.

In-the-canal (ITC) aids and completely-in-the-canal (CIC) aids: These hearing aids are contained in tiny cases that fit partly or completely into the ear canal. They are the smallest hearing aids available and offer cosmetic and some listening advantages. However, their small size may make them difficult to handle and adjust for some people.

What Is the Difference between Analog and Digital Hearing Aids?

Analog hearing aids make continuous sound waves louder. These hearing aids essentially amplify all sounds (e.g., speech and noise) in the same way. Some analog hearing aids are programmable. They have a microchip which allows the aid to have settings programmed for different listening environments—for example, in a quiet place, such as at a library; in a noisy place, such as a restaurant; or in a large area, such as a soccer field. The analog programmable hearing aids can store multiple programs for various environments.

As the listening environment changes, hearing aid settings may be changed by pushing a button on the hearing aid. Analog hearing aids are becoming less and less common.

Digital hearing aids have all the features of analog programmable aids, but they convert sound waves into digital signals and produce an exact duplication of sound. Computer chips in digital hearing aids analyze speech and other environmental sounds. The digital hearing aids allow for more complex processing of sound during the amplification process, which may improve their performance in certain situations (for example, background noise and whistle reduction). They also have greater flexibility in hearing aid programming so that the sound they transmit can be matched to the needs for a specific pattern of hearing loss. Digital hearing aids also provide multiple program memories. Most individuals who seek hearing help are offered a choice of only digital technology these days.

What Are Some Features for Hearing Aids?

Hearing aids have optional features that can be built in to assist in different communication situations. For example:

- **Directional microphone** may help you converse in noisy environments. Specifically, it allows sound coming from a specific direction to be amplified to a greater level compared to sound from other directions. When the directional microphone is activated, sound coming from in front of you (as during a face-to-face conversation) is amplified to a greater level than sound from behind you.

- **T-coil (telephone switch)** allows you to switch from the normal microphone setting to a "T-coil" setting in order to hear better on the telephone. All wired telephones produced today must be hearing aid compatible. In the "T-coil" setting, environmental sounds are eliminated, and sound is picked up from the telephone. This also turns off the microphone on your hearing aid so you can talk without your hearing aid "whistling."

The T-coil works well in theaters, auditoriums, houses of worship, and other places that have an induction loop or frequency modulation (FM) installation. The voice of the speaker, who can be some distance away, is amplified significantly more than any background noise. Some hearing aids have a combination "M" (Microphone)/"T" (Telephone) switch, so that, while listening with an induction loop, you can still hear nearby conversation.

- **Direct audio input** allows you to plug in a remote microphone or an FM assistive listening system, connect directly to a TV, or connect to other devices, such as your computer, a CD player, tape player, radio, etc.

- **Feedback suppression** helps suppress squeals when a hearing aid gets too close to the phone or has a loose-fitting earmold.

The more complicated features may allow the hearing aids to best meet your particular pattern of hearing loss. They may improve their performance in specific listening situations; however, these sophisticated electronics may significantly add to the cost of the hearing aid as well.

How Can Hearing Aids Help?

Hearing aids are primarily useful in improving the hearing and speech comprehension of people who have hearing loss that results from damage to the small sensory cells in the inner ear, called "hair cells." This type of hearing loss is called "sensorineural hearing loss." The damage can occur as a result of disease, aging, or injury from noise or certain medicines.

A hearing aid magnifies sound vibrations entering the ear. Surviving hair cells detect the larger vibrations and convert them into neural signals that are passed along to the brain. The greater the damage to a person's hair cells, the more severe the hearing loss and the greater the hearing aid amplification needed to make up the difference. However, there are practical limits to the amount of amplification a hearing aid can provide. In addition, if the inner ear is too damaged, even large vibrations will not be converted into neural signals. In this situation, a hearing aid would be ineffective.

How Can I Find out If I Need a Hearing Aid?

If you think you might have hearing loss and could benefit from a hearing aid, visit your physician, who may refer you to an otolaryngologist or audiologist. An otolaryngologist is a physician who specializes in ear, nose, and throat (ENT) disorders and will investigate the cause of the hearing loss. An audiologist is a hearing health professional who identifies and measures hearing loss and will perform a hearing test to assess the type and degree of loss.

Which Hearing Aid Will Work Best for Me?

The hearing aid that will work best for you depends on the kind and severity of your hearing loss. If you have a hearing loss in both of your ears, two hearing aids are generally recommended because two aids provide a more natural signal to the brain. Hearing in both ears also will help you understand speech and locate where the sound is coming from.

You and your audiologist should select a hearing aid that best suits your needs and lifestyle. Price is also a key consideration because hearing aids range from hundreds to several thousand dollars. Similar to other equipment purchases, style and features affect cost. However, do not use price alone to determine the best hearing aid for you. Just because one hearing aid is more expensive than another does not necessarily mean that it will better suit your needs.

A hearing aid will not restore your normal hearing. With practice, however, a hearing aid will increase your awareness of sounds and their sources. You will want to wear your hearing aid regularly, so select one that is convenient and easy for you to use. Other features to consider include parts or services covered by the warranty, estimated schedule and costs for maintenance and repair, options and upgrade opportunities, and the hearing aid company's reputation for quality and customer service.

What Questions Should I Ask before Buying a Hearing Aid?

Before you buy a hearing aid, ask your audiologist these important questions:

- What features would be most useful to me?

- What is the total cost of the hearing aid? Do the benefits of newer technologies outweigh the higher costs?

- Is there a trial period to test the hearing aids? (Most manufacturers allow a 30- to 60-day trial period during which aids can be returned for a refund.) What fees are nonrefundable if the aids are returned after the trial period?

- How long is the warranty? Can it be extended? Does the warranty cover future maintenance and repairs?

- Can the audiologist make adjustments and provide servicing and minor repairs? Will loaner aids be provided when repairs are needed?

- What instruction does the audiologist provide?

How Can I Adjust to My Hearing Aid?

Hearing aids take time and patience to use successfully. Wearing your aids regularly will help you adjust to them.

Become familiar with your hearing aid's features. With your audiologist present, practice putting in and taking out the aid, cleaning it, identifying right and left aids, and replacing the batteries. Ask how to test it in listening environments where you have problems with hearing. Learn to adjust the aid's volume and to program it for sounds that are too loud or too soft. Work with your audiologist until you are comfortable and satisfied.

You may experience some of the following problems as you adjust to wearing your new aid.

- **My hearing aid feels uncomfortable.** Some individuals may find a hearing aid to be slightly uncomfortable at first. Ask your audiologist how long you should wear your hearing aid while you are adjusting to it.

- **My voice sounds too loud.** The "plugged-up" sensation that causes a hearing aid user's voice to sound louder inside the head is called the "occlusion effect," and it is very common for new hearing aid users. Check with your audiologist to see if a correction is possible. Most individuals get used to this effect over time.

- **I get feedback from my hearing aid.** A whistling sound can be caused by a hearing aid that does not fit or work well or is clogged by earwax or fluid. See your audiologist for adjustments.

- **I hear background noise.** A hearing aid does not completely separate the sounds you want to hear from the ones you do not want to hear. Sometimes, however, the hearing aid may need to be adjusted. Talk with your audiologist.

- **I hear a buzzing sound when I use my cell phone.** Some people who wear hearing aids or have implanted hearing devices experience problems with the radio frequency interference caused by digital cell phones. Both hearing aids and cell phones are improving, however, so these problems are occurring less often. When you are being fitted for a new hearing aid, take your cell phone with you to see if it will work well with the aid.

How Can I Care for My Hearing Aid?

Proper maintenance and care will extend the life of your hearing aid. Make it a habit to:

- Keep hearing aids away from heat and moisture

- Clean hearing aids as instructed. Earwax and ear drainage can damage a hearing aid.

- Avoid using hairspray or other hair care products while wearing hearing aids
- Turn off hearing aids when they are not in use
- Replace dead batteries immediately
- Keep replacement batteries and small aids away from children and pets

Are New Types of Aids Available?

Although they work differently than the hearing aids described above, implantable hearing aids are designed to help increase the transmission of sound vibrations entering the inner ear. A middle ear implant (MEI) is a small device attached to one of the bones of the middle ear. Rather than amplifying the sound traveling to the eardrum, an MEI moves these bones directly. Both techniques have the net result of strengthening sound vibrations entering the inner ear so that they can be detected by individuals with sensorineural hearing loss.

A bone-anchored hearing aid (BAHA) is a small device that attaches to the bone behind the ear. The device transmits sound vibrations directly to the inner ear through the skull, bypassing the middle ear. BAHAs are generally used by individuals with middle ear problems or deafness in one ear. Because surgery is required to implant either of these devices, many hearing specialists feel that the benefits may not outweigh the risks.

Can I Obtain Financial Assistance for a Hearing Aid?

Hearing aids are generally not covered by health insurance companies, although some are. For eligible children and young adults 21 years of age and younger, Medicaid will pay for the diagnosis and treatment of hearing loss, including hearing aids, under the Early and Periodic Screening, Diagnostic, and Treatment (EPSDT) service. Also, children may be covered by their state's early intervention program or state children's health insurance program.

Medicare does not cover hearing aids for adults; however, diagnostic evaluations are covered if they are ordered by a physician for the purpose of assisting the physician in developing a treatment plan. Since Medicare has declared the BAHA a prosthetic device and not a hearing aid, Medicare will cover the BAHA if other coverage policies are met.

Some nonprofit organizations provide financial assistance for hearing aids, while others may help provide used or refurbished aids.

Contact the National Institute on Deafness and Other Communication Disorders (NIDCD) with questions about organizations that offer financial assistance for hearing aids.

What Research Is Being Done on Hearing Aids?

Researchers are looking at ways to apply new signal processing strategies to the design of hearing aids. Signal processing is the method used to modify normal sound waves into amplified sound that is the best possible match to the remaining hearing for a hearing aid user. NIDCD-funded researchers also are studying how hearing aids can enhance speech signals to improve understanding.

In addition, researchers are investigating the use of computer-aided technology to design and manufacture better hearing aids. Researchers also are seeking ways to improve sound transmission and to reduce noise interference, feedback, and the occlusion effect. Additional studies focus on the best ways to select and fit hearing aids in children and other groups whose hearing ability is hard to test.

Another promising research focus is to use lessons learned from animal models to design better microphones for hearing aids. NIDCD-supported scientists are studying the tiny fly Ormia ochracea because its ear structure allows the fly to determine the source of a sound easily. Scientists are using the fly's ear structure as a model for designing miniature directional microphones for hearing aids. These microphones amplify the sound coming from a particular direction (usually the direction a person is facing) but not the sounds that arrive from other directions. Directional microphones hold great promise for making it easier for people to hear a single conversation, even when surrounded by other noises and voices.

Section 19.2

Cochlear Implants and Bone-Anchored Hearing Aids

This section contains text excerpted from the following sources:
Text beginning with the heading "What Is a Cochlear Implant?" is
excerpted from "Cochlear Implants—What Is a Cochlear Implant?"
U.S. Food and Drug Administration (FDA), February 4, 2018; Text
under the heading "Bone-Anchored Hearing Aids" is excerpted from
"Hearing Loss Treatment and Intervention Services," Centers for
Disease Control and Prevention (CDC), April 11, 2018.

What Is a Cochlear Implant?

A cochlear implant is an implanted electronic hearing device, designed to produce useful hearing sensations to a person with severe to profound nerve deafness by electrically stimulating nerves inside the inner ear.

These implants usually consist of two main components:

- The externally worn microphone, sound processor, and transmitter system

- The implanted receiver and electrode system, which contains the electronic circuits that receive signals from the external system and send electrical currents to the inner ear

Currently made devices have a magnet that holds the external system in place next to the implanted internal system. The external system may be worn entirely behind the ear or its parts may be worn in a pocket, belt pouch, or harness.

Who Uses Cochlear Implants

Cochlear implants are designed to help severely to profoundly deaf adults and children who get little or no benefit from hearing aids. Even individuals with severe or profound "nerve deafness" may be able to benefit from cochlear implants.

How Does a Cochlear Implant Work?

A cochlear implant receives sound from the outside environment, processes it, and sends small electric currents near the auditory nerve.

These electric currents activate the nerve, which then sends a signal to the brain. The brain learns to recognize this signal and the person experiences this as "hearing."

The cochlear implant somewhat simulates natural hearing, where sound creates an electric current that stimulates the auditory nerve. However, the result is not the same as normal hearing.

What Are the Benefits of Cochlear Implants?

For People with Implants

- Hearing ranges from near-normal ability to understand speech to no hearing benefit at all.

- Adults often benefit immediately and continue to improve for about three months after the initial tuning sessions. Then, although performance continues to improve, improvements are slower. Cochlear implant users' performances may continue to improve for several years.

- Children may improve at a slower pace. A lot of training is needed after implantation to help the child use the new "hearing" she or he now experiences.

- Most perceive loud, medium, and soft sounds. People report that they can perceive different types of sounds, such as footsteps, slamming of doors, sounds of engines, ringing of the telephone, barking of dogs, whistling of the tea kettle, rustling of leaves, the sound of a light switch being switched on and off, and so on.

- Many understand speech without lip-reading. However, even if this is not possible, using the implant helps lip-reading.

- Many can make telephone calls and understand familiar voices over the telephone. Some good performers can make normal telephone calls and even understand an unfamiliar speaker. However, not all people who have implants are able to use the phone.

- Many can watch TV more easily, especially when they can also see the speaker's face. However, listening to the radio is often more difficult as there are no visual cues available.

- Some can enjoy music. Some enjoy the sound of certain instruments (piano or guitar, for example) and certain voices. Others do not hear well enough to enjoy music.

What Are the Risks of Cochlear Implants?
General Anesthesia Risks

General anesthesia is drug-induced sleep. The drugs, such as anesthetic gases and injected drugs, may affect people differently. For most people, the risk of general anesthesia is very low. However, for some people with certain medical conditions, it is more risky.

Risks from the Surgical Implant Procedure

- Injury to the facial nerve—this nerve goes through the middle ear to give movement to the muscles of the face. It lies close to where the surgeon needs to place the implant, and, thus, it can be injured during the surgery. An injury can cause a temporary or permanent weakening or full paralysis on the same side of the face as the implant.

- Meningitis—this is an infection of the lining of the surface of the brain. People who have abnormally formed inner ear structures appear to be at greater risk of this rare, but serious complication.

- Cerebrospinal fluid leakage—the brain is surrounded by fluid that may leak from a hole created in the inner ear, or elsewhere from a hole, in the covering of the brain as a result of the surgical procedure.

- Perilymph fluid leak—the inner ear or cochlea contains fluid. This fluid can leak through the hole that was created to place the implant.

- Infection of the skin wound.

- Blood or fluid collection at the site of surgery.

- Attacks of dizziness or vertigo.

- Tinnitus, which is a ringing or buzzing sound in the ear.

- Taste disturbances—the nerve that gives taste sensation to the tongue also goes through the middle ear and might be injured during the surgery.

- Numbness around the ear.

- Reparative granuloma—this is the result of localized inflammation that can occur if the body rejects the implant.

- There may be other unforeseen complications that could occur with long-term implantation that we cannot now predict.

Other Risks Associated with the Use of Cochlear Implants

People with a cochlear implant:

- **May hear sounds differently.** Sound impressions from an implant differ from normal hearing, according to people who could hear before they became deaf. At first, users describe the sound as "mechanical," "technical," or "synthetic." This perception changes over time, and most users do not notice this artificial sound quality after a few weeks of cochlear implant use.

- **May lose residual hearing.** The implant may destroy any remaining hearing in the implanted ear.

- **May have unknown and uncertain effects.** The cochlear implant stimulates the nerves directly with electrical currents. Although this stimulation appears to be safe, the long-term effect of these electrical currents on the nerves is unknown.

- **May not hear as well as others** who have had successful outcomes with their implants.

- **May not be able to understand language well.** There is no test a person can take before surgery that will predict how well he or she will understand language after surgery.

- **May have to have it removed** temporarily or permanently if an infection develops after the implant surgery. However, this is a rare complication.

- **May have their implant fail.** In this situation, a person with an implant would need to have additional surgery to resolve this problem and would be exposed to the risks of surgery again.

- **May not be able to upgrade their implant** when new external components become available. Implanted parts are usually compatible with improved external parts. That way, as advances in technology development, one can upgrade her or his implant by changing only its external parts. In some cases, though, this would not work and the implant will need changing.

- **May not be able to have some medical examinations** and treatments. These treatments include:

  - Magnetic resonance (MRI) imaging. MRI is becoming a more routine diagnostic method for early detection of medical problems. Even being close to an MRI imaging unit will be dangerous because it may dislodge the implant or demagnetize its internal magnet. The U.S. Food and Drug Administration (FDA) has approved some implants, however, for some types of MRI studies done under controlled conditions.

  - Neurostimulation

  - Electrical surgery

  - Electroconvulsive therapy (ECT)

  - Ionic radiation therapy

- **Will depend on batteries** for hearing. For some devices, new or recharged batteries are needed every day.

- **May damage their implant.** Contact sports, automobile accidents, slips and falls, or other impacts near the ear can damage the implant. This may mean needing a new implant and more surgery. It is unknown whether a new implant would work as well as the old one.

- **May find them expensive.** Replacing damaged or lost parts may be expensive.

- **Will have to use it for the rest of life.** During a person's lifetime, the manufacturer of the cochlear implant could go out of business. Whether a person will be able to get replacement parts or other customer services in the future is uncertain.

- **May have lifestyle changes** because their implant will interact with the electronic environment. An implant may:

  - Set off theft detection systems

  - Set off metal detectors or other security systems

  - Be affected by cellular phone users or other radio transmitters

  - Have to be turned off during takeoffs and landings in aircraft

  - Interact in unpredictable ways with other computer systems

- **Will have to be careful of static electricity**. Static electricity may temporarily or permanently damage a cochlear implant. It may be good practice to remove the processor and headset before contact with static generating materials, such as children's plastic play equipment, TV screens, computer monitors, or synthetic fabric.

- **Have less ability to hear** both soft sounds and loud sounds without changing the sensitivity of the implant. The sensitivity of normal hearing is adjusted continuously by the brain, but the design of cochlear implants requires a person to manually change the sensitivity setting of the device as the sound environment changes.

- **May develop irritation** where the external part rubs on the skin and have to remove it for a while.

- **Cannot let the external parts get wet.** Damage from water may be expensive to repair, and the person may be without hearing until the implant is repaired. Thus, the person will need to remove the external parts of the device when bathing, showering, swimming, or participating in water sports.

- **May hear strange sounds** caused by its interaction with magnetic fields, such as those near airport passenger screening machines.

Can the Sound Processor Be Removed at Night?

Yes. But you should turn it off to save the battery. Some users wear the sound processor all night so they can hear.

Can I Use the Implant While Playing Sports?

Probably. Most implants are durable enough to allow playing sports. However, the external parts of most are not waterproof, so you would have to remove them before swimming or other water sports. Deep water diving may harm the internal implant due to high water pressure.

How Long Does It Take Me to Get Maximum Benefit from a Cochlear Implant?

It depends a lot on you and your rehabilitation group. It depends on how long you have been without hearing. It depends on whether you could speak well before you lost your hearing. Usually, there is a rapid rise in your ability to interpret the sounds after receiving an implant. This rapid rise slows after about three months but continues.

What Sounds Can Be Heard with a Cochlear Implant?

You will probably hear most sounds of medium-to-high loudness. Patients often report that they can hear footsteps, slamming of doors, ringing telephones, car engines, barking dogs, lawn mowers, and various other environmental sounds. You may hear some softer sounds too.

Will the Cochlear Implant Help Me Control the Loudness of My Voice?

Yes. The cochlear implant usually helps the wearer control the loudness because you can hear your voice in relation to background sounds.

Insurance Questions
Do Insurance Companies Pay for Cochlear Implants?

Because cochlear implants are recognized as a standard treatment for severe-to-profound nerve deafness, most insurance companies cover them. In 2004, Medicare, Medicaid, the Veteran's Administration, and other public healthcare plans covered cochlear implants. In 2004, more than 90 percent of all commercial health plans covered cochlear implants. Cochlear implant centers usually take the responsibility of obtaining prior authorization from the appropriate insurance company before proceeding with surgery.

Do I Pay for the Repairs?

Maybe. You will not have to pay for repairs if they are covered by a warranty or if you have insurance that covers repairs. Many health plans do not include specific benefits to cover repairs and replacement of parts for cochlear implants. However, the policy may have durable medical equipment (DME) benefits that can be applied. Read your benefits booklet for DME or prosthetic repair benefits, or check with the health plan.

My Health Plan Has Denied Coverage for a Cochlear Implant. How Can I Appeal?

First, determine specifically why the cochlear implant was denied. Make sure you have the denial in writing. If you do not receive a written denial, ask for one. An appeal is most effective when structured in response to the specific reason for denial of coverage. If a specific denial reason is not provided, contact the plan and ask for clarification. Second, contact your cochlear implant center and advocacy groups and ask for help.

My Health Plan Informs Me That I Have Exhausted My Rehabilitation Benefits. How Can I Appeal This Decision and Obtain Coverage for Additional Audiology or Speech Therapy Services?

Many health plans have limited rehabilitation services. They have a predetermined cut-off point for post-operative cochlear implant services. However, you may be able to get extended medical benefits based on your need for more services by having your clinician argue your case. You may have an easier case if your child is the implant user. The manufacturer of your implant may help your clinician develop the case.

How Can I Insure My External Parts against Theft, Damage or Loss?

External parts, if purchased new, probably carry a warranty from the manufacturer against defects and materials. Usually, under such warranties, equipment lost, damaged beyond repair, or stolen will be replaced one time at no cost.

After the warranty expires, you may have some options, such as:

- Buying a service contract from the implant manufacturer
- Getting repair and replacement coverage through your health plan
- Getting coverage through your personal home property and casualty or homeowner's policy

What Educators Need to Know

- Cochlear implants do not make hearing normal.
- The benefit of an implant depends, in part, on the:
  - Type of communication training (total communication, auditory-oral communication, cued speech, etc.) a student used before the implant
  - Type of communication the student uses after the implant

- To get maximum benefit from a cochlear implant, a student will need individual training, such as:
  - Speech training
  - Lipreading training
  - Auditory training
- To progress with their classmates, students with cochlear implants may still need:
  - Special accommodation in the classroom, such as:
    - Preferential seating
    - A note taker
    - A quiet environment, away from air handlers and other noisy equipment
    - A sign-language interpreter or a cued speech interpreter
- Students need time to adjust and accommodate to their cochlear implants. The amount of time they need varies. During the accommodation period, students need language input from all sources they used before their implants.
- Educators should treat their students with cochlear implants as individuals, each having particular communication needs. Students do not get equal benefits from cochlear implants.
- Students with cochlear implants may find it harder to:
  - Digest new and difficult subject matter
  - Interact in unfamiliar and complex social situations
- Educators should be aware that frequent changes to educational programs involving students with cochlear implants (program hopping) may impede learning.
- Educators can help their students in other ways to achieve full benefits from cochlear implants, such as:
  - Intervening early when there appears to be a problem
  - Promoting family counseling
  - Promoting specialized speech and language therapies
  - Explaining to families that speech and language are not the same thing, and that education is based on language development

- Getting more information and support from local and national organizations of teachers of those with impaired hearing

- To assure that students with cochlear implants do not fall behind their classmates, educators should frequently evaluate them and their educational settings.

- Particularly for their younger students, educators need to assure that external cochlear implant components are securely attached or removed during active school events. The components are expensive and are easily lost or damaged.

- Students will often need extra batteries, either new or recharged, for their implants to work.

- Students with cochlear implants are usually not able to interpret complex auditory signals, such as those in music.

Before, during, and after Implant Surgery
What Happens before Surgery

Primary care doctors usually refer patients to ear, nose and throat doctors (ENT doctors or otolaryngologists) to test them to see if they are candidates for cochlear implants.

Tests often done are:

- Examination of external, middle, and inner ear for signs of infection or abnormality

- Various tests of hearing, such as an audiogram

- A trial of hearing aid use to assess its potential benefit

- Exams to evaluate middle and inner ear structures, such as:

  - A computerized tomography (CT) scan. This type of X-ray helps the doctor see if the cochlea has a normal shape. This scan is especially important if the patient has a history of meningitis because it helps to see if there is new bone growth in the cochlea that could interfere with the insertion of the implant. This scan also may indicate which ear should be implanted.

  - A magnetic resonance imaging (MRI) scan

- Psychological examination to see if the patient can cope with the implant

- Physical exam to prepare for general anesthesia

229

What Happens during Surgery

The doctor or other hospital staff may:

- Insert some intravenous (IV) lines
- Shave or clean the scalp around the site of the implant
- Attach cables, monitors and patches to the patient's skin to monitor vital signs
- Put a mask on the patient's face to provide oxygen and anesthetic gas
- Administer drugs through the IV and the face mask to cause sleep and general anesthesia
- Awaken the patient in the operating room and take him or her to a recovery room until all the anesthesia is gone

What Happens after Surgery

Immediately after waking, a patient may feel:

- Pressure or discomfort over her or his implanted ear
- Dizziness
- Sick to the stomach (have nausea)
- Disoriented or confused for a while
- A sore throat for a while from the breathing tube used during general anesthesia

Then, a patient can expect to:

- Keep the bandages on for a while
- Have the bandages be stained with some blood or fluid
- Go home in about a day after surgery
- Have stitches for a while
- Get instructions about caring for the stitches, washing the head, showering, and general care and diet
- Have an appointment in about a week to have the stitches removed and have the implant site examined
- Have the implant "turned on" (activated) about three to six weeks later

Can a Patient Hear Immediately after the Operation?

No. Without the external transmitter part of the implant, a patient cannot hear. The clinic will give the patient the external components about a month after the implant surgery in the first programming session.

Why Is It Necessary to Wait Three to Six Weeks after the Operation before Receiving the External Transmitter and Sound Processor?

The waiting period provides time for the operative incision to heal completely. This usually takes three to six weeks. After the swelling is gone, your clinician can do the first fitting and programming.

What Happens during the Initial Programming Session

An audiologist adjusts the sound processor to fit the implanted patient, tests the patient to ensure that the adjustments are correct, determines what sounds the patient hears, and gives information on the proper care and use of the device.

Is It Beneficial If a Family Member Participates in the Training Program?

Yes. A family member should be included in the training program whenever possible to provide assistance. The family member should know how to manage the operations of the sound processor.

Do Patients Have More than One Implant?

Usually, patients have only one ear implanted, though a few patients have implants in both ears.

How Can I Help My Child Receive the Most Benefit from Their Cochlear Implant?

- Try to make hearing and listening as interesting and fun as possible
- Encourage your child to make noises
- Talk about things you do as you do them

- Show your child that he or she can consciously use and evaluate the sounds he or she receives from his or her cochlear implant

- Realize that the more committed you, your child's teachers, and your health professionals are to helping your child, the more successful she or he will be

What Can I Expect a Cochlear Implant to Achieve in My Child?

As a group, children are more adaptable and better able to learn than adults. Thus, they can benefit more from a cochlear implant. Significant hearing loss slows a child's ability to learn to talk and affects overall language development. The vocal quality and intelligibility of speech from children using cochlear implants seems to be better than from children who only have acoustic hearing aids.

How Important Is the Active Cooperation of the Patient?

Extremely important. The patient's willingness to experience new acoustic sounds and cooperate in an auditory training program are critical to the degree of success with the implant. The duration and complexity of the training varies from patient to patient.

Bone-Anchored Hearing Aids

This type of hearing aid can be considered when a child has either a conductive, mixed or unilateral hearing loss and is specifically suitable for children who cannot otherwise wear in-the-ear or behind-the-ear hearing aids.

Other Assistive Devices

Besides hearing aids, there are other devices that help people with hearing loss. The following are some examples of other assistive devices:

- Frequency modulation (FM) system

  An FM system is a kind of device that helps people with hearing loss hear in background noise. FM stands for frequency modulation. It is the same type of signal used for radios. FM systems send sound from a microphone used by someone speaking to a person wearing the receiver. This system is sometimes used with hearing aids. An extra piece is attached to the hearing aid that works with the FM system.

- Captioning

  Many television programs, videos, and DVDs are captioned. Television sets made after 1993 are made to show the captioning. You do not have to buy anything special. Captions show the conversation spoken in soundtrack of a program on the bottom of the television screen.

- Other devices

- There are many other devices available for children with hearing loss. Some of these include:

  - Text messaging

  - Telephone amplifiers

  - Flashing and vibrating alarms

  - Audio loop systems

  - Infrared (IR) listening devices

  - Portable sound amplifiers

  - TTY (text telephone or teletypewriter)

Chapter 20

Communicating with the Deaf and Hard of Hearing

Chapter Contents

Section 20.1

American Sign Language

This section includes text excerpted from "American Sign Language," National Institute on Deafness and Other Communication Disorders (NIDCD), April 25, 2017.

What Is American Sign Language?

American Sign Language (ASL) is a complete, complex language that employs signs made by moving the hands and is combined with facial expressions and postures of the body. It is the primary language of many North Americans who are deaf and is one of several communication options used by people who are deaf or hard-of-hearing.

Is Sign Language the Same in Other Countries?

No one form of sign language is universal. Different sign languages are used in different countries or regions. For example, British Sign Language (BSL) is a different language from ASL, and Americans who know ASL may not understand BSL.

Where Did American Sign Language Originate?

The exact beginnings of ASL are not clear, but some suggest that it arose more than 200 years ago from the intermixing of local sign languages and French Sign Language (LSF, or Langue des Signes Française). ASL includes some elements of LSF plus the original local sign languages, which, over the years, have melded and changed into a rich, complex, and mature language. Modern ASL and modern LSF are distinct languages and, while they still contain some similar signs, can no longer be understood by each other's users.

How Does American Sign Language Compare with Spoken Language?

The letters of the alphabet in American Sign Language. In spoken language, words are produced by using the mouth and voice to make sounds. But for people who are deaf (particularly those who are profoundly deaf), the sounds of speech are often not heard, and only a fraction of speech sounds can be seen on the lips. Sign languages are based on the idea that vision is the most useful tool a deaf person has to communicate and receive information.

ASL is a language completely separate and distinct from English. It contains all the fundamental features of language—it has its own rules for pronunciation, word order, and complex grammar. While every language has ways of signaling different functions, such as asking a question rather than making a statement, languages differ in how this is done. For example, English speakers ask a question by raising the pitch of their voice; ASL users ask a question by raising their eyebrows, widening their eyes, and tilting their bodies forward.

Just as with other languages, specific ways of expressing ideas in ASL vary as much as ASL users do. In addition to individual differences in expression, ASL has regional accents and dialects. Just as certain English words are spoken differently in different parts of the country, ASL has regional variations in the rhythm of signing, form, and pronunciation. Ethnicity and age are a few more factors that affect ASL usage and contribute to its variety.

How Do Most Children Learn?

Parents are often the source of a child's early acquisition of language, but for children who are deaf, additional people may be models for language acquisition. A deaf child born to parents who are deaf and who already use ASL will begin to acquire ASL as naturally as a hearing child picks up spoken language from hearing parents. However, for a deaf child with hearing parents who have no prior experience with ASL, language may be acquired differently. In fact, 9 out of 10 children who are born deaf are born to parents who hear. Some hearing parents choose to introduce sign language to their deaf children. Hearing parents who choose to learn sign language often learn it along with their child. Surprisingly, children who are deaf can learn to sign quite fluently from their parents, even when their parents might not be perfectly fluent themselves.

Why Emphasize Early Language Learning?

Parents should introduce a child who is deaf or hard-of-hearing to language as soon as possible. The earlier any child is exposed to and begins to acquire language, the better that child's communication skills will become. Research suggests that the first few years of life are the most crucial to a child's development of language skills, and even the early months of life can be important for establishing successful communication. Thanks to screening programs in place at almost all hospitals in the United States and its territories, newborn babies are tested for hearing before they leave the hospital. If a baby has hearing loss, this screening gives parents an opportunity to learn about communication options. Parents can then start their child's language learning process during this important early stage of development.

What Research Is Being Done on American Sign Language and Other Sign Languages?

The National Institute on Deafness and Other Communication Disorders (NIDCD) supports research looking at whether children with cochlear implants become bilingual in spoken language and sign language in the same way that (or in different ways from how) hearing children become bilingual in both languages. This research will tell us more about how language development in children with cochlear implants might differ between hearing and nonhearing families and could offer important insights to help guide educational decisions and parent counseling.

An NIDCD-funded researcher is studying Al-Sayyid Bedouin Sign Language (ABSL), a sign language used over the past 75 years by both hearing and nonhearing people in an isolated Bedouin village in Israel. Because it was developed among a small group of people with little to no outside influence and no direct linguistic input, ABSL offers researchers the opportunity to document a new language as it develops and evolves. It can also be used to model the essential elements and organization of natural language.

Another NIDCD-funded research team is also looking at sign language systems that develop in isolation. The research team is learning more about how grammar is built and expanded in situations where there is little linguistic input. In one setting, they are observing "home sign" systems used by deaf children who live in isolation. In another, they are studying a family sign language that has been used and handed down over several generations on a remote fishing island.

Section 20.2

Assistive Listening Devices

This section includes text excerpted from "Assistive Devices for
People with Hearing, Voice, Speech, or Language Disorders,"
National Institute on Deafness and Other Communication
Disorders (NIDCD), March 6, 2017.

What Are Assistive Devices?

The terms "assistive device" or "assistive technology" can refer to any device that helps a person with hearing loss or a voice, speech, or language disorder to communicate. These terms often refer to devices that help a person to hear and understand what is being said more clearly or to express thoughts more easily. With the development of digital and wireless technologies, more and more devices are becoming available to help people with hearing, voice, speech, and language disorders communicate more meaningfully and participate more fully in their daily lives.

What Types of Assistive Devices Are Available?

Health professionals use a variety of names to describe assistive devices.

- **Assistive listening devices** (ALDs) help amplify the sounds you want to hear, especially where there is a lot of background noise. ALDs can be used with a hearing aid or cochlear implant to help a wearer hear certain sounds better.

- **Augmentative and alternative communication (AAC) devices** help people with communication disorders to express themselves. These devices can range from a simple picture board to a computer program that synthesizes speech from text.

- **Alerting devices** connect to a doorbell, telephone, or alarm that emits a loud sound or blinking light to let someone with hearing loss know that an event is taking place.

What Types of Assistive Listening Devices Are Available?

Several types of ALDs are available to improve sound transmission for people with hearing loss. Some are designed for large facilities,

239

such as classrooms, theaters, places of worship, and airports. Other types are intended for personal use in small settings and for one-on-one conversations. All can be used with or without hearing aids or a cochlear implant. ALD systems for large facilities include hearing loop systems, frequency-modulated (FM) systems, and infrared systems.

- **Hearing loop (or induction loop) systems** use electromagnetic energy to transmit sound. A hearing loop system involves four parts:

  1. A sound source, such as a public address system, microphone, or home television (TV) or telephone

  2. An amplifier

  3. A thin loop of wire that encircles a room or branches out beneath carpeting

  4. A receiver worn in the ears or as a headset

  Amplified sound travels through the loop and creates an electromagnetic field that is picked up directly by a hearing loop receiver or a telecoil, a miniature wireless receiver that is built into many hearing aids and cochlear implants. To pick up the signal, a listener must be wearing the receiver and be within or near the loop. Because the sound is picked up directly by the receiver, the sound is much clearer, without as much of the competing background noise associated with many listening environments. Some loop systems are portable, making it possible for people with hearing loss to improve their listening environments, as needed, as they proceed with their daily activities. A hearing loop can be connected to a public address system, a television, or any other audio source. For those who do not have hearing aids with embedded telecoils, portable loop receivers are also available.

- **Frequency-modulated (FM) systems** use radio signals to transmit amplified sounds. They are often used in classrooms, where the instructor wears a small microphone connected to a transmitter and the student wears the receiver, which is tuned to a specific frequency, or channel. People who have a telecoil inside their hearing aid or cochlear implant may also wear a wire around the neck (called a "neckloop") or behind their aid or implant (called a "silhouette inductor") to convert the signal into magnetic signals that can be picked up directly by the telecoil. FM systems can transmit signals up to 300 feet and are able to be used in many public places. However, because radio signals are able to penetrate walls, listeners in one room may need to listen to a different channel than those in another room to avoid receiving mixed signals. Personal FM systems operate in the same way as larger scale systems and can be used to help people with hearing loss to follow one-on-one conversations.

- **Infrared (IR) systems** use infrared light to transmit sound. A transmitter converts sound into a light signal and beams it to a receiver that is worn by a listener. The receiver decodes the infrared signal back to sound. As with FM systems, people whose hearing aids or cochlear implants have a telecoil may also wear a neckloop or silhouette inductor to convert the infrared signal into a magnetic signal, which can be picked up through their telecoil. Unlike induction loop or FM systems, the infrared signal cannot pass through walls, making it particularly useful in courtrooms, where confidential information is often discussed, and in buildings where competing signals can be a problem, such as classrooms or movie theaters. However, infrared systems cannot be used in environments with too many competing light sources, such as outdoors or in strongly lit rooms.

- **Personal amplifiers** are useful in places in which the above systems are unavailable or when watching TV, being outdoors, or traveling in a car. About the size of a cell phone, these devices increase sound levels and reduce background noise for a listener. Some have directional microphones that can be angled toward a speaker or other source of sound. As with other ALDs, the amplified sound can be picked up by a receiver that the listener is wearing, either as a headset or as earbuds.

What Types of Augmentative and Alternative Communication Devices Are Available for Communicating Face-to-Face?

The simplest AAC device is a picture board or touch screen that uses pictures or symbols of typical items and activities that make up a person's daily life. For example, a person might touch the image of a glass to ask for a drink. Many picture boards can be customized and expanded based on a person's age, education, occupation, and interests.

Keyboards, touch screens, and sometimes a person's limited speech may be used to communicate desired words. Some devices employ a text display. The display panel typically faces outward so that two people can exchange information while facing each other. Spelling and word prediction software can make it faster and easier to enter information.

Speech-generating devices go one step further by translating words or pictures into speech. Some models allow users to choose from several different voices, such as male or female, child or adult, and even some regional accents. Some devices employ a vocabulary of prerecorded words, while others have an unlimited vocabulary, synthesizing speech as words are typed in. Software programs that convert personal computers into speaking devices are also available.

What Augmentative and Alternative Communication Devices Are Available for Communicating by Telephone?

For many years, people with hearing loss have used text telephone or telecommunications devices, called "TTY" or "TDD machines," to communicate by phone. This same technology also benefits people with speech difficulties. A TTY machine consists of a typewriter keyboard that displays typed conversations onto a readout panel or printed on paper. Callers will either type messages to each other over the system or, if a call recipient does not have a TTY machine, use the national toll-free telecommunications relay service at 711 to communicate. Through the relay service, a communications assistant serves as a bridge between two callers, reading typed messages aloud to the person with hearing while transcribing what is spoken into type for the person with hearing loss.

New electronic communication devices, however, TTY machines have almost become a thing of the past. People can place phone calls through the telecommunications relay service using almost any device with a keypad, including a laptop, personal digital assistant, and cell phone. Text messaging has also become a popular method of communication, skipping the relay service altogether.

Another system uses voice recognition software and an extensive library of video clips depicting American Sign Language (ASL) to translate a signer's words into text or computer-generated speech in real time. It is also able to translate spoken words back into sign language or text.

Finally, for people with mild to moderate hearing loss, captioned telephones allow you to carry on a spoken conversation, while providing a transcript of the other person's words on a readout panel or computer screen as back-up.

What Types of Alerting Devices Are Available?

Alerting or alarm devices use sound, light, vibrations, or a combination of these techniques to let someone know when a particular event is occurring. Clocks and wake-up alarm systems allow a person to choose to wake up to flashing lights, horns, or a gentle shaking.

Visual alert signalers monitor a variety of household devices and other sounds, such as doorbells and telephones. When the phone rings, the visual alert signaler will be activated and will vibrate or flash a light to let people know. In addition, remote receivers placed around the house can alert a person from any room. Portable vibrating pagers can let parents and caretakers know when a baby is crying. Some baby monitoring devices analyze a baby's cry and light up a picture to indicate if the baby sounds hungry, bored, or sleepy.

What Research Is Being Conducted on Assistive Technology?

The National Institute on Deafness and Other Communication Disorders (NIDCD) funds research into several areas of assistive technology, such as those described below.

Improved Devices for People with Hearing Loss

NIDCD-funded researchers are developing devices that help people with varying degrees of hearing loss communicate with others. One team has developed a portable device in which two or more users type messages to each other that can be displayed simultaneously in real time. Another team is designing an ALD that amplifies and enhances speech for a group of individuals who are conversing in a noisy environment.

Improved Devices for Nonspeaking People

- **More natural synthesized speech:** NIDCD-sponsored scientists are also developing a personalized text-to-speech synthesis system that synthesizes speech that is more intelligible and natural sounding to be incorporated in speech-generating devices. Individuals who are at risk of losing their speaking ability can pre-record their own speech, which is then converted into their personal synthetic voice.

- **Brain–computer interface research:** A relatively new and exciting area of study is called "brain–computer interface research." NIDCD-funded scientists are studying how neural signals in a person's brain can be translated by a computer to help someone communicate. For example, people with amyotrophic lateral sclerosis (ALS, or Lou Gehrig's disease) or brainstem stroke lose their ability to move their arms, legs, or body. They can also become locked-in, where they are not able to express words, even though they are able to think and reason normally. By implanting electrodes on the brain's motor cortex, some researchers are studying how a person who is locked-in can control communication software and type out words simply by imagining the movement of his or her hand. Other researchers are attempting to develop a prosthetic device that will be able to translate a person's thoughts into synthesized words and sentences. Another group is developing a wireless device that monitors brain activity that is triggered by visual stimulation. In this way, people who are locked-in can call for help during an emergency by staring at a designated spot on the device.

Section 20.3

Captions for Deaf and Hard-of-Hearing Viewers

This section includes text excerpted from "Captions for Deaf and Hard-of-Hearing Viewers," National Institute on Deafness and Other Communication Disorders (NIDCD), July 5, 2017.

What Are Captions?

Captions are words displayed on a television, computer, mobile device, or movie screen that describe the audio or sound portion of a program or video. Captions allow viewers who are deaf or hard-of-hearing to follow the dialogue and the action of a program simultaneously. For people with hearing loss who are not deaf, captions can even make the spoken words easier to hear—because hearing, similar to vision, is influenced by our expectations; when you have an idea of what someone might be about to say, her or his speech may seem more clear. Captions can also provide information about who is speaking or about sound effects that may be important to understanding a news story, a political event, or the plot of a program.

Captions are created from the program's transcript. A captioner separates the dialogue into captions and makes sure the words appear in sync with the audio they describe. Computer software encodes the captioning information and combines it with the audio and video to create a new master tape or digital file of the program. Ideally, the captions should appear near the bottom of the screen—not in the middle, where misplaced captions can cover the newscaster's face or the basketball hoop or quarterback.

Open and Closed Captions

Captions may be "open" or "closed." Open captions are always in view and cannot be turned off, whereas closed captions can be turned on and off by the viewer (using the menu settings on any television).

Closed captioning is available on digital television sets, including high-definition television sets, manufactured after July 1, 2002. Some digital captioning menus allow the viewer to control the caption display, including font style, text size and color, and background color.

Real-Time Captioning

Real-time captions, or communication access real-time translation, are created as an event takes place. A captioner (often trained as a court reporter or stenographer) uses a stenotype machine with a phonetic keyboard and special software. A computer translates the phonetic symbols into English captions almost instantaneously. The slight delay is based on the captioner's need to hear and code the word and on computer processing time. Real-time captioning can be used for programs that have no script; live events, including congressional proceedings; news programs; and nonbroadcast meetings, such as the national meetings of professional associations.

Although most real-time captioning is more than 98 percent accurate, the audience will see occasional errors. The captioner may mishear a word, hear an unfamiliar word, or have an error in the software dictionary.

Electronic Newsroom Captions

Electronic newsroom captions (ENR) are created from a news script computer or teleprompter and are commonly used for live newscasts. Only material that is scripted can be captioned using this technique. Therefore, spontaneous commentary, live field reports, breaking news, and sports and weather updates may not be captioned using ENR, and real-time captioning is needed.

Edited and Verbatim Captions

Captions can be produced as either edited or verbatim captions. Edited captions summarize ideas and shorten phrases. Verbatim captions include all of what is said. Although there are situations in which edited captions are preferred for ease in reading (such as for children's programs), most people who are deaf or hard-of-hearing prefer the full access provided by verbatim texts.

Rear-Window Captioning

Some movie theaters across the country offer this type of captioning system. An adjustable Lucite panel attaches to the viewer's seat and reflects the captions from a light-emitting diode (LED) panel at the back of the theater.

Captioned Telephone

A captioned telephone has a built-in screen to display in text (captions) whatever the other person on the call is saying. When an outgoing call is placed on a captioned telephone, the call is connected to a captioned telephone service (CTS). A specially trained CTS operator hears the person you want to talk to and repeats what that person says. Speech recognition technology automatically transcribes the CTS operator's voice into text that is displayed on the captioned telephone screen.

The Law

The Americans with Disabilities Act (ADA) of 1990 requires businesses and public accommodations to ensure that individuals with disabilities are not excluded from or denied services because of the absence of auxiliary aids. Captions are considered one type of auxiliary aid. Since the passage of the ADA, the use of captioning has expanded. Entertainment, educational, informational, and training materials are captioned for deaf and hard-of-hearing audiences at the time they are produced and distributed.

The Television Decoder Circuitry Act of 1990 requires that all televisions larger than 13 inches sold in the United States after July 1993 have a special built-in decoder that enables viewers to watch closed-captioned programming. The Telecommunications Act of 1996 directs the Federal Communications Commission (FCC) to adopt rules requiring closed captioning of most television programming.

Captions and the Federal Communications Commission

The FCC's rules on closed captioning became effective January 1, 1998. They require people or companies that distribute television programs directly to home viewers to caption those programs. The rules required all nonexempt programs to be closed-captioned by January 1, 2006; after that date, captioning was also required for all new nonexempt programs. As of January 1, 2010, all new nonexempt Spanish language video programming must also be provided with captions. Detailed guidelines and definitions of terms are available in the FCC's Electronic Code of Federal Regulations (e-CFR).

Who Is Required to Provide Closed Captions?

Congress requires video program distributors (cable operators, broadcasters, satellite distributors, and other multichannel video programming distributors) to close caption their TV programs. FCC rules ensure that viewers have full access to programming, address captioning quality, and provide guidance to video programming distributors and programmers. The rules require that captions be accurate, synchronous, complete, and properly placed. In addition, the rules distinguish between pre-recorded, live, and near-live programming, and explain how the standards apply to each type of programming, recognizing the greater challenges involved with captioning live or near-live programming.

What Programs Are Exempt?

Some advertisements, public service announcements, non-English-language programs (with the exception of Spanish programs), locally produced and distributed nonnews programming, textual programs, early-morning programs, and nonvocal musical programs are exempt from captioning.

To find out more about the FCC rules and captions, including information on the complaint process, call:

Toll-Free Voice: 888-CALL-FCC (888-225-5322)

Toll-Free TTY: 888-TELL-FCC (888-835-5322)

Section 20.4

Communication Problems in Hard-of-Hearing Individuals

This section includes text excerpted from "The Current State of Health Care for People with Disabilities," National Council on Disability (NCD), September 30, 2009. Reviewed April 2019.

Hard-of-Hearing Individuals

People who are deaf or hard-of-hearing experience extensive, largely unrecognized communication problems when they seek healthcare services. One researcher eloquently summarized these difficulties.

"Deaf or hard-of-hearing individuals in the United States must often cope with extraordinary communication barriers when working with their healthcare providers; receive healthcare services that are inadequate, inappropriate for their needs, and unethical due to the interplay of numerous complex individual, interpersonal, and systematic factors; and have a poorer self-reported health status than the general population. Within the subset of the U.S. population that uses English as a second language, Deaf individuals may be at greatest risk for poor physician-patient communication."

Health Status and Health Experiences

According to health experts, research about the health status, health behaviors, risk factors, and diseases experienced by people who are deaf or hard-of-hearing is limited because research is generally focused on hearing loss itself. Moreover, early studies may be misleading because they excluded certain important segments of the deaf population. Conflicting research and a relative lack of data, therefore, make it particularly challenging to identify the healthcare needs of this heterogeneous group. Further, few studies have examined deaf adults' experiences with the healthcare delivery system. Research has revealed, however, some important preliminary information about the health status of people who are deaf or hard-of-hearing, as well as some of the pressing problems this community encounters in the healthcare delivery system.

Distinct Cultural and Linguistic Group

Most researchers and most deaf individuals consider the Deaf Community a distinct cultural and linguistic group. As a distinct group, the Deaf Community is entitled to the same acknowledgment that society affords other groups with their own culture and language. The syntax and grammar of American Sign Language (ASL) is independent of English, and those who use it are a distinct linguistic group. People who use ASL as their primary language share experiences that parallel those of other cultural and linguistic minority groups. For example, the Deaf Community shares a cultural heritage that includes similar family and educational experiences and common social and community interests. Similarities to other minority groups include limited use of English in day-to-day communication; limited access to information from radio, television, and other forms of mass media; lack of access to information that is present in the ambient environment; and dependence on family members, friends, and others as interpreters.

People who use ASL frequently identify their linguistic identity by spelling "Deaf" with an uppercase "D," while "deaf" with a small "d" indicates hearing impairment as a physiological characteristic. However, not all people who are deaf identify with the cultural minority that uses ASL. The U.S. Census and other large population and health surveys do not inquire about ASL use, so the size of this community is not known; estimates range from 100,000 to 1,000,000 people. Among adults who are deaf, about 8 percent acquired their disability prelingually (i.e., before the age of three), and an estimated additional 11 percent became deaf between the ages of 3 and 19.

Health Disparities

The NCHS study reports that as hearing loss increases, people experience a higher prevalence of fair or poor health status; problems walking, bending, and reaching; and psychological distress. Adults in the study who were deaf or who experienced significant problems hearing were three times as likely to report fair or poor health compared with those who did not have hearing impairments. Hypertension and diabetes were more prevalent among adults who were deaf or had a lot of trouble hearing than among those who did not; they were highest among adults under the age of 65. People who were deaf or had a lot of trouble hearing were more likely to smoke (40 percent of those between the ages of 18 and 44, compared with 24 percent of people who were not deaf or hard-of-hearing). People who were deaf or had a lot of trouble hearing were also more likely to be overweight and less likely to participate in leisure time physical activity.

The NCHS study and other research have also shown that people who are deaf or have a lot of trouble hearing are more likely to drink alcohol at higher rates than adults with no hearing difficulties, and they have more difficulty finding appropriate accessible treatment services and programs. More than 40 percent of adults who are deaf, or have a lot of trouble hearing, smoke cigarettes, compared with 24 percent of people who do not have hearing problems. Deaf women of color appear to experience the greatest health disparities and difficulty accessing appropriate healthcare. They tend to have lower incomes and poorer health, and to be less educated compared with white women. Among women of color, African American deaf women experience the greatest health disadvantages.

Healthcare Experiences

People who are deaf or hard-of-hearing have a range of experiences with healthcare professionals, and these experiences may differ according to when they acquired hearing loss or became deaf. However, people who are deaf or hard-of-hearing have different healthcare experiences compared with people who do not have hearing loss. One study suggests that people who become deaf prelingually use healthcare at about the same rate as other minority language groups, while people who become deaf postlingually use healthcare services at about the same rate as individuals who have chronic illnesses. Medicare beneficiaries over the age of 65 who experience some hearing loss report lower satisfaction with healthcare access and quality of care than do other groups.

Barriers to Healthcare
Lack of Effective Communication

Communicating effectively in healthcare settings presents complex challenges for people who are deaf or hard-of-hearing. Research has revealed that people who are deaf or hard-of-hearing identify similar communication problems that compromise healthcare, including the following: medication errors and misdiagnosis, problems during surgery and anesthesia missed and delayed appointments, and less complete and accurate information than other patients receive.

Hearing loss varies from person to person, and communication styles and needs can be unique to the individual. As a result, diverse, individualized strategies are necessary to achieve effective communication. For example, while many people who are deaf communicate using ASL, others who are deaf or hard-of-hearing use speech-reading, speaking, writing, or a combination of these methods. Some people who are hard-of-hearing also use hearing aids or other devices, including assistive listening devices that are necessary to communicate effectively during medical visits. For others who are hard-of-hearing, effective communication may require that their healthcare provider modify the way he or she speaks. Because most hearing loss occurs in the higher frequencies, the provider's speech may be more accessible if he or she speaks in a lower voice. The patients may also need for the provider to be face to face and avoid turning away or covering his or her face. Some people may benefit if noise distractions are reduced.

Some people with hearing loss, including older people, may not acknowledge their hearing loss and may act as though they understand what is being communicated, while not in fact understanding. These individuals may require additional time and attention during healthcare provider visits to ensure that information has been communicated clearly and effectively.

Also, communications can be especially demanding physically and emotionally for patients who are deaf or hard-of-hearing, making fatigue a potential factor in determining effective communication. One study concluded that older adults with mild-to-moderate hearing loss may expend so much cognitive energy trying to hear accurately that their ability to remember spoken language suffers as a result. Thus, they may have difficulty retaining information presented during a healthcare visit.

Most healthcare practitioners have little understanding of how people with hearing loss communicate or how to communicate effectively with them. This lack of awareness directly affects the quality of health-care these practitioners can provide.

Focus group research has revealed widespread problems that affect health outcomes for many people; these problems often begin with provider assumptions about hearing loss. Most providers mistakenly assume that people who are deaf are fluent in both ASL and English. However, ASL is completely independent of English and does not have a written form. Attempts to write ASL using standard English words produces what appears to be broken English. This "broken" English leads some providers to assume that their deaf patients lack intelli-gence, an assumption they may not make about other people who are not fluent in English. If an immigrant from China with a Ph.D. in physics wrote in broken English, the healthcare provider would prob-ably assume that the immigrant's communication difficulties stemmed from the language barrier.

However, lack of awareness about ASL and assumptions about people who are deaf lead healthcare providers to incorrectly assume that a patient with limited English skills is cognitively impaired. As evidence of this, deaf patients often report that their physicians do not appear to respect their intelligence and think that they do not want to take responsibility for their health.

People who are deaf or hard-of-hearing report that healthcare providers rarely use appropriate and effective methods of commu-nication. Problems begin when an individual attempts to schedule an appointment with a healthcare provider and continue through office visits, diagnostic procedures, emergency room visits, hospital-izations, and even in hospice care. healthcare providers sometimes do not understand that providing appropriate methods of communication is medically necessary to ensure that healthcare is effective. Rather than asking the person what method of communication would be most effective, physicians and other healthcare practitioners frequently employ modes of communication that do not take into account specific individual needs. For example, they may rely on family members to interpret for patients who are deaf. Patients who are deaf can find it difficult to request an interpreter, because they are concerned that physicians might question the need or might expect the deaf individual to pay for the interpreter. In addition, some people who are deaf have reported that healthcare providers have denied requests for interpret-ers. Others have noted that interpreter services are not reimbursed by insurers, which presents a serious barrier to hiring them.

Many people who are deaf or significantly hard-of-hearing commu-nicate using Internet technologies, including videophone/video relay interpreting services (VP/VRS), facsimile (FAX), text messaging, and instant messaging. Others use older technologies, such as text telephones (TTYs), devices that allow the user to place a telephone call and then type a message to a person who also has such a device. Many people with hearing, speech, and language difficulties use the nationwide relay service established by the 1990 Americans with Disabilities Act (ADA). The relay service allows a caller using an Internet connection or TTY to contact a relay operator, who in turn places a call to the desired person and then "relays" the conversation between the two parties. Most healthcare practitioners, however, either are unaware that many people who are deaf and significantly hard-of-hearing people communicate using these technologies or are uncomfortable using them to communicate with patients. Moreover, some healthcare providers have raised the concern that these modes of communication do not preserve confidentiality and might violate the Health Insurance Portability and Accountability Act (HIPAA), even though they are the modes by which people who are deaf communicate most effectively.

Most practitioners have complex menu-driven voice message systems that make it difficult for relay operators to type the options to the caller before the connection times out. Thus, people who are deaf or hard-of-hearing are sometimes unable to make appointments with their healthcare providers or communicate directly with them. Regarding these basic communication barriers, one focus group participant said: "We just go right to the hospital. I wouldn't call my doctor at all. I just go right to the emergency room."

Typically, healthcare providers expect deaf patients to be able to read their handwriting or to lip-read as they speak. Deaf participants from several focus groups said they had significant problems with writing as a mode of communication, not only because it is slow and inefficient, but also because the vocabulary is unfamiliar and the handwriting often illegible. Because ASL is not English, medical terms are often interpreted using a vision description rather than a single corresponding word. This means that many deaf individuals never have the opportunity to learn medical terms.

For example, there is no sign for the word "cholesterol," so a certified interpreter would describe cholesterol as a type of fat buildup in the blood vessels. Another interpreter might simply fingerspell the word "cholesterol," but the patient might not know what the word means. Syntax differences between English and ASL can compound the communication problem when unfamiliar medical terms are used. Similarly, speech-reading is ineffective because only about 30 to 40 percent of spoken English can be understood using this technique. One focus group participant illustrated the problems with speech-reading: "I was so shocked when they had five people, doctors, and aides... All these people came towards me... I wondered what was going on. So I started writing notes to them... I could see they were talking... I had no idea why there were five people there looking at me."

Many deaf participants in focus groups said that they frequently relied on family members or friends to interpret for them during medical visits. This practice not only raises serious confidentiality issues for the person who is receiving care but also does not necessarily ensure effective communication between the patient and clinician. healthcare providers typically overestimate the sign language skills of friends or family members who are neither trained in medical interpretation nor certified as sign-language interpreters. Sometimes young children interpret for parents or family members. However, it can be quite difficult for children to accurately convey medical information. They may not fully understand the information or may find the information distressing. People who are deaf may have difficulty understanding their healthcare provider's instructions about therapeutic programs, prescription dosages, or side effects, which can lead to new health problems and reinforce stereotypes about the intellectual capacity of the person who is deaf. In one study, a deaf participant talked about having surgery without an interpreter available: "I needed a tonsillectomy. I went to the hospital, and I was scared. I was sedated and anesthetized, and I woke up afterward, scared and crying. I didn't know what to expect or what was going on with the swelling. There was no interpreter there."

Another deaf individual noted that the problems are a deterrent to seeking care. "There are a lot of deaf people who won't go to the doctor. [They think] I'll just bear with it until it goes away."

In several studies, deaf focus group participants indicated that communication is most effective when they have the opportunity to work with medically experienced, certified ASL interpreters. However, often, an interpreter is not available. One study revealed that even though physicians acknowledged that communication with deaf patients was most effective when ASL interpreters were available, they did not employ them frequently. This study also revealed that physicians overestimated the accuracy of speech-reading.

When people who are deaf or hard-of-hearing have access to deaf-friendly medical organizations (i.e., organizations in which methods for effective communication, such as ASL interpreters, and assistive listening devices are readily available and providers understand cultural aspects of deafness), screening rates for colorectal, cervical, and breast cancer are similar to rates for the general population.

Mental-Health System Concerns

For some people who are deaf or hard-of-hearing, longstanding concern over the lack of qualified interpreters is greater when seeking mental-health services, where inadequate communication has sometimes resulted in inappropriate institutionalization and loss of liberty. Research has shown that some people who are deaf or hard-of-hearing distrust mental-health providers in part because of concerns that communications will be ineffective in mental-health settings. Some focus group participants expressed fear that confidentiality might be violated and that the ASL skill levels of interpreters would not be adequate. Others said that in mental-health settings, people who were deaf were at the mercy of hearing authorities, who were likely to be prejudiced about deafness. Participants in several studies expressed the concern that people who were deaf would mistakenly be committed to mental-health facilities solely because of barriers to communication. People who are deaf or hard-of-hearing have expressed strong concern that mental-health professionals have misdiagnosed patients who are deaf and prescribed incorrect medication for them because of stigma, stereotypes, and ineffective communication.

Some healthcare providers who are deaf or hard-of-hearing have observed that standard psychological testing can be inappropriate for people who are deaf because testers are rarely fluent in ASL and rarely understand Deaf culture. Deaf patients who were willing to visit a therapist preferred to work with a deaf therapist. If that was not possible, they preferred to work with mental-health counselors and therapists who were fluent in sign language.

Perceptions of mental-health services can also depend on age. A study of senior, middle-aged, and young adults who were deaf asked the subjects what they would do if they needed mental-health services. Those in the senior group said they would seek help from a friend or family member, while younger people said they would probably seek a mental-health professional.

Lack of Insurance Coverage

According to unpublished data from the 2007 National Health Interview Survey (NHIS), among people in the United States, regarding the civilian population between the ages of 18 and 64 who identify as deaf or hard-of-hearing, 21.3 percent do not have any health insurance, while 34.2 percent are covered by private insurance, and 55.3 percent are covered by public insurance (30.1 percent by Medicare and 27.9 percent by Medicaid).

Disease Prevention and Health Promotion

Studies suggest that people who are deaf or hard-of-hearing experience specific barriers to participating in prevention programs, may have limited access to appropriate and accessible information about health promotion activities, and may not understand why such programs and activities are important. In particular, adults who are deaf tend to have less health literacy compared with the hearing population.

Lack of access to information in the media limits awareness of health-related information on the part of people who are deaf. Topics, such as the health studies, and information about prevention and health services, nutrition, alcohol and substance abuse, sex education, and domestic violence prevention are often discussed in popular media outlets, which are typically presented only in an audible format. It is not surprising, then, that adults who are deaf tend to have less health literacy compared with the hearing population. Some people who are deaf or hard-of-hearing are unaware of mental-health services available in the community and unfamiliar with terminology used by mental-health practitioners, suggesting a lack of information about these services as well.

For example, a comprehensive survey of 203 deaf patients in 2 healthcare systems that offer programs and services aimed at the Deaf community illustrated the respondents' lack of basic knowledge about health conditions. 40 percent of survey participants could not identify any of the 7 most common warning signs of a heart attack, while 62 percent could not identify any of the 7 most common warning signs of a stroke. In fact, 32 percent of study participants could not identify any risk factors for a heart attack or stroke, and 1 in 3 could not define the word "cancer." In another study, more than 70 percent of deaf participants said that people who were deaf could not get Human immunodeficiency virus (HIV), and more than 50 percent did not know the meaning of "HIV-positive." According to one survey, high-school students who are deaf or hard-of-hearing had some understanding about HIV and Acquired Immunodeficiency Syndrome (AIDs), but there were significant gaps in their awareness of how the infection is prevented and transmitted.

Focus group research has shown that women who are deaf have unique linguistic and cultural issues that affect their health and their healthcare experiences. Participants were unaware of the need to assess health risks through prevention and diagnostic screening procedures, including those for cardiovascular disease. Some participants also lacked knowledge and information about screening and diagnostic procedures for breast and cervical cancer and about the purpose and importance of treatments, such as surgery.

In general, women reported that they avoided visiting a healthcare provider because of the lack of effective communication, although they also reported positive experiences with some practitioners who use qualified interpreters. Studies comparing the prenatal healthcare of women who are deaf and women without hearing impairments reveal significant differences between the two groups. Women who were deaf were less satisfied with their prenatal care than hearing women, and they expressed less satisfaction with the quality of communication with their healthcare provider. When deaf patients had access to ASL interpreters and to providers who understand cultural aspects of deafness, screening rates for colorectal, cervical, and breast cancer were similar to rates for the general population.

A literature survey produced no information specifically aimed at men who are deaf regarding the benefits of early screening, detection, and treatment of prostate cancer. In response to this gap, a prostate cancer education program was adapted and tested on a small sample of men whose baseline knowledge about the disease increased, as shown in follow-up surveys. While this program evolved into an Internet ASL-accessible video on prostate health, research on the effectiveness of this strategy must still be conducted, and ensuring that all men who are deaf have access to such information remains a challenge.

Similarly, little research has been carried out on tobacco use by youth who are deaf or hard-of-hearing. However, a study reveals that middle- and high-school students generally smoke less than their hearing peers, and that students who attend integrated educational programs were more likely to have tried smoking than their peers in schools for deaf students. This study also shows that although healthcare providers are important sources of prevention information, few students reported that they had received anti-tobacco messages from their healthcare providers or in clinical settings—another missed opportunity to convey prevention guidance.

Conclusion

There is a tremendous need for increased attention to issues people who are deaf or hard-of-hearing have identified as deterrents to their health promotion and healthcare. The longstanding problems that arise from inequities in communication and poor access to culturally and linguistically appropriate healthcare and health information have failed to draw the level of institutional response from policymakers that is required to bring about systemic change.

At a minimum, additional public resources must be allocated to encourage and support ASL interpreter training and payment for interpreter services in medical settings. Congress should explicitly direct Medicare and Medicaid to pay for interpreter services, and states should require private health insurers to include payment for interpreters as a reimbursable expense to healthcare professionals or as an accepted cost to be negotiated in managed care provider payment schemes.

There is also an important role for medical educators, who must train young professionals, including people who are deaf or hard-of-hearing, about issues of concern to the deaf community and challenge negative stereotypes that currently influence practitioners' attitudes and methods for providing care. Accreditation organizations must include methods in their survey and monitoring mechanisms to evaluate the extent to which healthcare facilities have the capacity to provide interpreters for deaf or hard-of-hearing patients in a timely and effective manner. Patient education materials should also be assessed and modified to ensure that they are accessible.

Chapter 21

Frequently Asked Questions about Hearing Loss

Do We Lose Our Hearing as We Age?

It is true that most people's hearing gets worse as they get older. But, for the average person, aging does not cause impaired hearing before the age of 60. People who are not exposed to noise and are otherwise healthy, keep their hearing for many years. People who are exposed to noise and do not protect their hearing begin to lose their hearing at an early age. For example, by 25 years of age the average carpenter has "50-year-old" ears. That is, by the age of 25, the average carpenter has the same hearing as someone who is 50 years of age and has worked in a quiet job.

Can You Poke Out Your Eardrums with Earplugs?

That is unlikely for two reasons. First, the average ear canal is about 1 1/4 inches long. The typical ear plug is between 1/2 and 3/4 of an inch long. So, even if you inserted the entire earplug, it would still not touch the eardrum. Second, the path from the opening of the ear canal to the eardrum is not straight. In fact, it is quite irregular. This prevents you from poking objects into the eardrum.

This chapter includes text excerpted from "Noise and Hearing Loss Prevention—Frequently Asked Questions," Centers for Disease Control and Prevention (CDC), February 6, 2018.

I Work in a Dusty, Dirty Place. Should I Worry That Our Ears Will Get Infected by Using Earplugs?

Using earplugs will not cause an infection. But use common sense. Have clean hands when using earplugs that need to be rolled or formed with your fingers in order for you to insert them. If this is inconvenient, there are plenty of earplugs that are pre-molded or that have stems so that you can insert them without having to touch the part that goes into the ear canal.

Can You Hear Warning Sounds, Such as Backup Beeps, When Wearing Hearing Protectors?

The fact is that there are fatal injuries because people do not hear warning sounds. However, this is usually because the background noise was too high or because the person had severe hearing loss, not because someone was wearing hearing protectors. Using hearing protectors will bring both the noise and the warning sound down equally. So, if the warning sound is audible without the hearing protector, it will usually be audible when wearing the hearing protector. Also, many warning systems can be adjusted or changed so warning signals are easier to detect.

Won't Hearing Protectors Interfere with Our Ability to Hear Important Sounds Our Machinery and Equipment Make?

Hearing protectors will lower the noise level of your equipment; it will not eliminate it. However, some hearing protectors will reduce certain frequencies more than others; so wearing them can make noises sound different. In cases where it is important that the sound is quieter without any other changes, there are hearing protectors that can provide flat attenuation. There are also noise-activated hearing protectors that allow normal sounds to pass through the ear and only "turn-on" when the noise reaches hazardous levels. There are even protectors that professional concert musicians use that can lower the sound level while retaining sound fidelity.

Will We Be Able to Hear Each Other Talk When Wearing Hearing Protectors?

Some people find they can wear hearing protectors and still understand speech. Others will have trouble hearing speech while wearing hearing protectors. Being able to hear what other people say depends on many things: distance from the speaker, ability to see the speaker's face, general familiarity with the topic, level of background noise, and whether or not one has an existing hearing impairment. In some cases, wearing hearing protectors can make it easier to understand speech. In other instances, people may be using hearing protectors to keep out too much sound. You may need a protector that reduces the sound enough to be safe without reducing the sound too much to hear speech at a comfortably loud level. For those people who work in noise and must communicate, it may also be necessary to use communication headsets. Allow your employees to try different protectors. Some will work better than others at helping them to hear speech, and different protectors may work better for different people.

How Long Does It Take to Get Used to Hearing Protectors?

Think about getting a new pair of shoes. Some shoes take no time to get used to. Others—even though they are the right size—can take a while to get used to. Hearing protectors are no different from other safety equipment in terms of getting used to them. But if hearing protectors are the wrong size, or are worn out, they will not be comfortable. Also, workers may need more than one kind of protector in their job. For example, no one would wear golf shoes to go bowling. If hearing protectors are not suitable for the work being done, they probably will not feel comfortable.

How Do I Select and Use Hearing Protectors?

- Comfort—so you will wear them
- Consistency—use them every time, all the time, in hazardous noise
- Cleanliness—keep plugs and hands as clean as possible

How Do I Insert a Foam Earplug?

1. Roll the earplug
2. Pull up and away on the top of your ear with the opposite hand to open the ear
3. Hold the earplug after inserting it

How Long Can Someone Be in a Loud Noise before It Is Hazardous?

The degree of hearing hazard is related to both the level of the noise, as well as to the duration of the exposure. But, this question is similar to asking how long can people look at the sun without damaging their eyes. The safest thing to do is to ensure workers always protect their ears by wearing hearing protectors anytime they are around loud noise.

How Can I Tell If the Noise Is Too Loud?

There are two rules: First, if you have to raise your voice to talk to someone who is an arm's length away, then the noise is likely to be hazardous. Second, if your ears are ringing or sounds seem dull or flat after leaving a noisy place, then you probably were exposed to hazardous noise.

How Often Should My Hearing Be Tested?

Anyone regularly exposed to hazardous noise should have an annual hearing test. Also, anyone who notices a change in her or his hearing (or who develops tinnitus) should have her or his ears checked. People who have healthy ears and who are not exposed to hazardous noise should get a hearing test every three years.

Since I Already Have Hearing Loss and Wear a Hearing Aid, Hearing Prevention Programs Do Not Apply to Me, Right?

If you have hearing loss, it is important to protect the hearing that you have left. Loud noises can continue to damage your hearing making it even more difficult to communicate at work and with your family and friends.

Chapter 22

Novel Deafness and Hearing Loss Treatments

Chapter Contents

Section 22.1

Growing Hair Cells Might Lead to Hearing Loss Treatment

This section includes text excerpted from "New Way to Grow Hair Cells in the Lab Might Lead to Hearing Loss Treatment," National Institute on Deafness and Other Communication Disorders (NIDCD), July 6, 2018.

People who have lost their hearing may one day be able to get it back, thanks to recent research on the inner ear. Scientists funded by the National Institutes of Health (NIH) have discovered a way to replace the delicate cells in the inner ear that enable us to hear. Using inner ear tissue from mice, nonhuman primates (rhesus macaques), and humans, the scientists grew a large batch of the delicate sound-detecting cells, called "hair cells." The new study shows that the scientists can grow enough hair cells to test possible drug treatments for hearing loss in living cells.

Scientists on the team represented Harvard Medical School, Massachusetts Institute of Technology (MIT), Massachusetts Eye and Ear Infirmary (MEEI), and Brigham and Women's Hospital (BWH) and reported their findings in the February 21, 2017 issue of *Cell Reports*. Their big breakthrough came when they identified two small molecules that, when added to their earlier recipe for growing hair cells, helped them to increase the number of hair cells they could grow in the laboratory. A similar technique also helped them grow significantly more hair cells from nonhuman primate and human ear tissue. This is important because they now have enough cells to test potential drug treatments for hearing loss in living cells from both animal models and humans.

Hair cells detect sound and send sound information to the parts of our brain that interpret and respond to the sound. Our hair cells can be damaged or destroyed by exposure to loud noise, injury, and certain medications. Although fish and birds can replace damaged hair cells, mammals, including humans, cannot. Scientists have long sought to overcome this human inability to replace lost hair cells.

As their next step, the team will try to identify drugs that encourage lab-grown hair cells to multiply. They hope to use those drugs directly on damaged human inner ears to stimulate replacement of lost hair cells.

Hearing loss is a common problem. Approximately 15 percent of American adults (37.5 million) 18 years of age and older report some trouble hearing, and about 2 to 3 out of every 1,000 children in the United States are born with a detectable level of hearing loss in 1 or both ears. If scientists can help humans replace lost hair cells, we may one day be able to regain lost hearing.

Section 22.2

Drug Therapy Partially Restores Hearing

This section includes text excerpted from "Novel Drug Therapy Partially Restores Hearing in Mice," National Institutes of Health (NIH), June 28, 2018.

A small-molecule drug is one of the first to preserve hearing in a mouse model of an inherited form of progressive human deafness, report investigators at the University of Iowa (UI), Iowa City, and the National Institutes of Health's (NIH) National Institute on Deafness and Other Communication Disorders (NIDCD). The study sheds light on the molecular mechanism that underlies a form of deafness (DFNA27) and suggests a new treatment strategy.

"We were able to partially restore hearing, especially at lower frequencies, and save some sensory hair cells," said Thomas B. Friedman, Ph.D., chief of the Laboratory of Human Molecular Genetics at the NIDCD and a coauthor of the study. "If additional studies show that small-molecule-based drugs are effective in treating DFNA27 deafness in people, it's possible that using similar approaches might work for other inherited forms of progressive hearing loss."

The seed for the advance was planted a decade ago, when NIDCD researchers led by Friedman and Robert J. Morell, Ph.D., another co-author of the current study, analyzed the genomes of members of an extended family, dubbed LMG2. Deafness is genetically dominant in the LMG2 family, meaning that a child needs to inherit only one copy of the defective gene from a parent to have progressive hearing loss.

The investigators localized the deafness-causing mutation to a region on chromosome four called *"DFNA27,"* which includes a dozen or so genes. The precise location of the mutation eluded the NIDCD team, however.

A crucial clue to explain the DFNA27 form of progressive deafness arose from later studies of the mouse RE1 Silencing Transcription Factor, or *REST*, gene conducted by researchers at the University of Iowa. Botond Banfi, M.D., Ph.D. and Yoko Nakano, Ph.D., lead authors of the current study, discovered that mouse REST is regulated through an unusual mechanism in the sensory cells of the inner ear, and this regulation is critical for hearing in mice. Because the human counterpart of the mouse *REST* gene is located in the DFNA27 region, the Iowa and NIDCD researchers teamed up to reexamine the mystery of DFNA27 progressive deafness.

The coding sequence of a protein is generated from a gene by stitching together segments called "exons," while editing out the intervening segments. The resulting molecule serves as the template for a specific protein. Most previous studies had missed exon 4 in the *REST* gene because this small exon is not edited into the Rest mRNA in most cells. The normal function of the REST protein is to shut off genes that need to be active only in a very few cell types.

When Banfi's team deleted exon 4 of REST in mice, inner ear hair cells died, and mice became deaf. Many genes that should have been active were shut off in hair cells prior to their death. Working together, Friedman's and Banfi's groups pinpointed the deafness mutation in the LMG2 family. They discovered that the mutation lies near exon 4, altering the boundaries of exon 4, and interferes with the inactivation of REST in hair cells.

"We found that incorporating exon 4 into the REST messenger ribonucleic acid (mRNA) acts like a switch in sensory hair cells. It turns off REST and allows many genes to be turned on," said Banfi. "Some of these turned-on genes are important for hair cell survival and hearing."

The investigators used Banfi's exon 4-deficient mice as a model for DFNA27 deafness. Since REST suppresses gene expression through a process called histone deacetylation, they wanted to see if blocking this process could reduce hearing loss. Using small-molecule drugs that inhibit this process, the investigators were able to turn off REST and partially restore hearing.

"These results demonstrate the value of studying the molecular mechanisms that underlie inherited forms of deafness," said Andrew

J. Griffith, scientific director of the NIDCD. "By following these genetic leads, we find novel and unexpected pathways that can, in cases such as this one, uncover unexpected potential treatment strategies in humans."

Part Four

Vestibular Disorders

Chapter 23

Vestibular (Balance) Disorders: An Overview

Chapter Contents

Section 23.1

What Is a Vestibular (Balance) Disorder?

This section contains text excerpted from the following sources:
Text beginning with the heading "What Is a Balance Disorder?" is
excerpted from "Balance Disorders," National Institute on Deafness
and Other Communication Disorders (NIDCD), March 6, 2018; Text
under the heading "Balance or Vestibular Disorders in Adults" is
excerpted from "Science Capsule: Balance or Vestibular Disorders in
Adults," National Institute on Deafness and Other Communication
Disorders (NIDCD), January 27, 2017.

What Is a Balance Disorder?

A balance disorder is a condition that makes you feel unsteady or
dizzy. If you are standing, sitting, or lying down, you might feel as if
you are moving, spinning, or floating. If you are walking, you might
suddenly feel as if you are tipping over.

Everyone has a dizzy spell now and then, but the term "dizziness"
can mean different things to different people. For one person, dizziness
might mean a fleeting feeling of faintness, while for another it could
be an intense sensation of spinning (vertigo) that lasts a long time.

About 15 percent of American adults (33 million) had a balance or
dizziness problem in 2008. Balance disorders can be caused by certain
health conditions, medications, or a problem in the inner ear or the
brain. A balance disorder can profoundly affect daily activities and
cause psychological and emotional hardship.

What Are the Symptoms of a Balance Disorder?

If you have a balance disorder, your symptoms might include:

- Dizziness or vertigo (a spinning sensation)

- Falling or feeling as if you are going to fall

- Staggering when you try to walk

- Lightheadedness, faintness, or a floating sensation

- Blurred vision

- Confusion or disorientation

Other symptoms might include nausea and vomiting; diarrhea;
changes in heart rate and blood pressure; and fear, anxiety, or panic.

Symptoms may come and go over short time periods or last for a long time and can lead to fatigue and depression.

What Causes Balance Disorders

Causes of balance problems include medications, ear infection, a head injury, or anything else that affects the inner ear or brain. Low blood pressure can lead to dizziness when you stand up too quickly. Problems that affect the skeletal or visual systems, such as arthritis or eye muscle imbalance, can also cause balance disorders. Your risk of having balance problems increases as you get older.

Unfortunately, many balance disorders start suddenly and with no obvious cause.

How Does My Body Keep Its Balance?

Your sense of balance relies on a series of signals to your brain from several organs and structures in your body, specifically your eyes, ears, and the muscles and touch sensors in your legs. The part of the ear that assists in balance is known as the "vestibular system," or the "labyrinth," a maze-like structure in your inner ear made of bone and soft tissue.

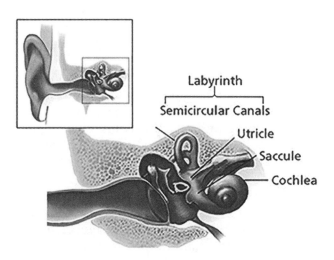

Figure 23.1. Structures of the Balance System inside the Inner Ear (Source: National Institutes of Health (NIH)/ National Institute on Deafness and Other Communication Disorders (NIDCD))

Within the labyrinth are structures known as "semicircular canals." The semicircular canals contain three fluid-filled ducts, which form loops arranged roughly at right angles to one another. They tell your brain when your head rotates. Inside each canal is a gelatin-like structure called the "cupula," stretched like a thick sail that blocks off one end of each canal. The cupula sits on a cluster of sensory hair cells. Each hair cell has tiny, thin extensions called "stereocilia" that protrude into the cupula.

When you turn your head, fluid inside the semicircular canals moves, causing the cupulae to flex or billow, similar to sails in the wind, which in turn bends the stereocilia. This bending creates a nerve signal that is sent to your brain to tell it which way your head has turned.

Between the semicircular canals and the cochlea (a snail-shaped, fluid-filled structure in the inner ear) lie two otolithic organs: fluid-filled pouches called the "utricle" and the "saccule." These organs tell your brain the position of your head with respect to gravity, such as whether you are sitting up, leaning back, or lying down, as well as any direction your head might be moving, such as side to side, up or down, forward or backward.

The utricle and the saccule also have sensory hair cells lining the floor or wall of each organ, with stereocilia extending into an overlying gel-like layer. Here, the gel contains tiny, dense grains of calcium carbonate called "otoconia." Whatever the position of your head, gravity pulls on these grains, which then move the stereocilia to signal your head's position to your brain. Any head movement creates a signal that tells your brain about the change in head position.

When you move, your vestibular system detects mechanical forces, including gravity, that stimulate the semicircular canals and the otolithic organs. These organs work with other sensory systems in your body, such as your vision and your musculoskeletal sensory system, to control the position of your body at rest or in motion. This helps you maintain stable posture and keep your balance when you are walking or running. It also helps you keep a stable visual focus on objects when your body changes position.

When the signals from any of these sensory systems malfunction, you can have problems with your sense of balance, including dizziness or vertigo. If you have additional problems with motor control, such as weakness, slowness, tremor, or rigidity, you can lose your ability to recover properly from imbalance. This raises the risk of falling and injury.

What Are Some Types of Balance Disorders?

There are more than a dozen different balance disorders. Some of the most common are:

- **Benign paroxysmal positional vertigo (BPPV) or positional vertigo:** A brief, intense episode of vertigo triggered by a specific change in the position of the head. You might feel as if you are spinning when you bend down to look under something, tilt your head to look up or over your shoulder, or roll over in bed. BPPV occurs when loose otoconia tumble into one of the semicircular canals and affect how the cupula works. This keeps the cupula from flexing properly, sending incorrect information about your head's position to your brain, and causing vertigo. BPPV can result from a head injury or can develop just from getting older.

- **Labyrinthitis:** An infection or inflammation of the inner ear that causes dizziness and loss of balance. It is often associated with an upper respiratory infection, such as the flu.

- **Ménière disease:** Episodes of vertigo, hearing loss, tinnitus (a ringing or buzzing in the ear), and a feeling of fullness in the ear. It may be associated with a change in fluid volume within parts of the labyrinth, but the cause or causes are still unknown.

- **Vestibular neuronitis:** An inflammation of the vestibular nerve that can be caused by a virus, and primarily causes vertigo.

- **Perilymph fistula:** A leakage of inner ear fluid into the middle ear. It causes unsteadiness that usually increases with activity, along with dizziness and nausea. Perilymph fistula can occur after a head injury, dramatic changes in air pressure (such as when scuba diving), physical exertion, ear surgery, or chronic ear infections. Some people are born with perilymph fistula.

- **Mal de Debarquement syndrome (MdDS):** A feeling of continuously rocking, swaying, or bobbing, typically after an ocean cruise or other sea travel, or even after prolonged running on a treadmill. Usually, the symptoms go away within a few hours or days after you reach land or stop using the treadmill. Severe cases, however, can last months or even years, and the cause remains unknown.

How Are Balance Disorders Diagnosed?

Diagnosis of a balance disorder is difficult. To find out if you have a balance problem, your primary doctor may suggest that you see an otolaryngologist and an audiologist. An otolaryngologist is a physician and surgeon who specializes in diseases and disorders of the ear, nose, neck, and throat. An audiologist is a clinician who specializes in the function of the hearing and vestibular systems.

You may be asked to participate in a hearing examination, blood tests, a video nystagmogram (a test that measures eye movements and the muscles that control them), or imaging studies of your head and brain. Another possible test is called "posturography." For this test, you stand on a special movable platform in front of a patterned screen.

Posturography measures how well you can maintain steady balance during different platform conditions, such as standing on an unfixed, movable surface. Other tests, such as rotational chair testing, brisk head-shaking testing, or even tests that measure eye or neck muscle responses to brief clicks of sound, may also be performed. The vestibular system is complex, so multiple tests may be needed to best evaluate the cause of your balance problem.

How Are Balance Disorders Treated?

The first thing an otolaryngologist will do if you have a balance problem is determine if another health condition or a medication is to blame. If so, your doctor will treat the condition, suggest a different medication, or refer you to a specialist if the condition is outside his or her expertise.

If you have BPPV, your otolaryngologist or audiologist might perform a series of simple movements, such as the Epley maneuver, to help dislodge the otoconia from the semicircular canal. In many cases, one session works; other people need the procedure several times to relieve their dizziness.

If you are diagnosed with Ménière disease, your otolaryngologist may recommend that you make some changes to your diet and, if you are a smoker, that you stop smoking. Antivertigo or antinausea medications may relieve your symptoms, but they can also make you drowsy. Other medications, such as gentamicin (an antibiotic) or corticosteroids, may be used. Although gentamicin may reduce dizziness better than corticosteroids, it occasionally causes permanent hearing loss. In some severe cases of Ménière disease, surgery on the vestibular organs may be needed.

Some people with a balance disorder may not be able to fully relieve their dizziness and will need to find ways to cope with it. A vestibular rehabilitation therapist can help you develop an individualized treatment plan.

Talk to your doctor about whether it is safe to drive and about ways to lower your risk of falling and getting hurt during daily activities, such as when you walk up or down stairs, use the bathroom, or exercise. To reduce your risk of injury from dizziness, avoid walking in the dark. Wear low-heeled shoes or walking shoes outdoors. If necessary, use a cane or walker, and modify conditions at your home and workplace, such as adding handrails.

When Should I Seek Help If I Think I Have a Balance Disorder?

To help you decide whether to seek medical help for dizziness or balance problems, ask yourself the following questions. If you answer "yes" to any of these questions, talk to your doctor:

- Do I feel unsteady?
- Do I feel as if the room is spinning around me, even for a very brief time?
- Do I feel as if I am moving when I know I am sitting or standing still?
- Do I lose my balance and fall?
- Do I feel as if I am falling?
- Do I feel lightheaded or as if I might faint?
- Do I have blurred vision?
- Do I ever feel disoriented—losing my sense of time or location?

How Can I Help My Doctor Make a Diagnosis?

You can help your doctor make a diagnosis and determine a treatment plan by answering the questions below. Be prepared to discuss this information during your appointment.

- The best way I can describe my dizziness or balance problem is:
  - Is there a spinning sensation, and if so, which way does the room spin?

277

- Is the dizziness/spinning caused by any specific motion, or does it occur even when sitting or lying still?

- Are there any other symptoms that occur at the same time as the dizziness/spinning, such as hearing loss, tinnitus, a feeling of pressure in one or both ears, or a headache?

- Does anything seem to help the dizziness/spinning?

- How often do I feel dizzy or have trouble keeping my balance? How long do the dizziness or spinning episodes last (seconds, minutes, hours, days)?

- Have I ever fallen?

  - When did I fall?

  - Where did I fall?

  - Under what conditions did I fall?

  - How often have I fallen?

- These are the medicines I take. Include all prescription medications; all over-the-counter (OTC) medicine, such as aspirin, antihistamines, or sleep aids; and all vitamin supplements and alternative or homeopathic remedies.

Section 23.2

Dizziness and Balance Problems in Children

This section includes text excerpted from "Dizziness and Balance Problems in Kids," *NIH News in Health*, National Institutes of Health (NIH), March 2016.

Most people feel dizzy now and then. Kids may occasionally feel lightheaded or unsteady. But, if such feelings repeat or interfere with everyday life, it could be a sign of a balance disorder.

Most balance problems are temporary and easy to treat. But, these problems may also signal a more serious condition that could have a lasting impact. Learn to recognize the signs of dizziness or balance problems that may warrant a trip to a doctor.

Experts have long suspected that dizziness and balance problems are often overlooked and untreated, but the scope of the problem was not fully understood. That is why the National Institutes of Health (NIH) supported the largest national survey to date to uncover information about these disorders in children. The study included data on nearly 11,000 kids between the ages of 3 and 17.

The researchers found that more than 1 in 20 kids in the U.S. had a dizziness or balance problem, and only one-third of them received treatment in the previous year. "The findings suggest that dizziness and balance problems are fairly common among children," says Dr. James F. Battey, Jr., a pediatrician, and director of NIH's National Institute on Deafness and Other Communication Disorders (NIDCD).

Our sense of balance is a complex process. It is managed by signals between the brain, ears, eyes, and sensors in the joints and other body parts. This intricate system helps your body monitor and maintain its position as you move throughout the day, without you even having to think about it. But, if any of these many sensory signals go wrong, it can weaken your sense of balance.

Balance disorders can make you stagger when walking. You might teeter or fall when trying to stand. Affected people might feel as if they themselves or the world around them is spinning or moving—a condition known as "vertigo." Other symptoms can include blurred vision, vomiting, diarrhea, confusion, and anxiety.

Common causes of balance problems in children range from ear infections, severe headaches, and certain medications to more serious neurological disorders, head or neck injuries, and genetic conditions. In many cases, the study's researchers found, an underlying cause was not reported.

Balance disorders can be difficult to recognize and understand. They can be especially hard to diagnose in young children. Kids may not know the right words to describe their symptoms. Affected children may talk about a "spinning feeling." They may say their tummy or head feels bad or weird. They may walk unsteadily or seem clumsy.

"Parents who notice dizziness and balance problems in their children should consult a healthcare provider to rule out a serious underlying condition," Battey says.

Your child's pediatrician will likely ask questions about when the symptoms first appeared, how long they last, how often they occur, and what medications the child is taking. Your child's eyes and ears will be examined, and hearing and balance may be tested. You may be referred to a specialist, such as an otolaryngologist—a doctor with expertise in the ear, nose, and throat.

Treatment will depend on the underlying cause. The good news is that most dizziness and balance problems in children are temporary and treatable. Still, it is important to check with a health professional if you notice any problems.

Tell Your Doctor

Dizziness and balance problems may be hard to spot in children. Younger kids may lack the vocabulary to describe their symptoms. Talk with a healthcare provider if your child:

- Falls frequently

- Seems unsteady upon standing or walking

- Feels as if the room is spinning around her or him.

- Feels as if moving when standing or sitting still.

- Feels as if she or he is falling

- Feels lightheaded, or as if she or he might faint

- Says that vision becomes blurred

Section 23.3

Vestibular (Balance) Disorders in Adults

This section includes text excerpted from "Science Capsule: Balance or Vestibular Disorders in Adults," National Institute on Deafness and Other Communication Disorders (NIDCD), January 27, 2017.

Balance disorders can result from trauma, disease, or the effects of aging on all the balance-related systems. Vestibular dysfunction can lead to dizziness, vertigo, nausea, migraines, blurred vision, and various forms of postural instability. Episodes of vestibular dizziness or nausea may be relatively brief but, when present, can be profoundly disturbing, including disorientation, falling, or even complete incapacitation from physical activity. About 15 percent of American adults (33 million) had a balance or dizziness problem during the past year. National Institute on Deafness and Other Communication Disorders (NIDCD) research is supporting the development of more efficient vestibular testing for improved clinical diagnoses and effective pharmacological treatments for vertigo.

A common balance disorder affecting more than one-half million Americans is Ménière disease. It can develop at any age, but most often occurs in adults between the ages of 40 and 60. Characteristic symptoms include a combination of vertigo, hearing loss, nausea, tinnitus, and a feeling of fullness in the ear. Ménière disease usually affects only one ear. At worst, intense vertigo causes a fall, called a "drop attack," with possible injury. Because episodes can be repetitive (recurring several times a day, coming and receding over weeks or months) and intense, it can be very debilitating.

Dysfunctions of the vestibular system can occur independently or with a hearing loss, from causes such as pharmacotoxicity or head trauma. NIDCD Intramural scientists, at the NIH Clinical Center, evaluate both hearing and vestibular function by testing individuals with and without balance disorders. The goal of the studies is to determine the best way to perform the testing and understand the variations among the test and different individuals. Examples of ongoing research include examining auditory or vestibular function in individuals with neurofibromatosis type 2, Usher syndrome, enlarged vestibular aqueducts, Niemann-Pick type C, xeroderma pigmentosum, and Moebius syndrome.

Balance disorders are associated, as mentioned, with falling, which is the leading cause of injury deaths among older adults. 1 in 3 Americans 65 years of age and older falls each year, and falls can result in severe trauma and even loss of life. Each year, more than 4 million older U.S. adults go to emergency departments for fall-related injuries at a cost of $4 billion. The NIDCD supports a longitudinal study that measures vestibular function in older adults. The NIDCD is also sponsoring the AVERT (Acute video-oculography for Vertigo in Emergency Rooms for rapid Triage) clinical trial to help diagnose vertigo, dizziness, and other balance problems. The team of researchers is using a diagnostic medical device (video-oculography or VOG) in the triage of patients who go to emergency room with complaints of vertigo and/or dizziness. The device measures abnormal eye movements to differentiate benign causes of the dizziness or imbalance from dangerous causes (such as stroke). This study offers the potential for improving standard of care in the diagnosis and treatment of patients with vertigo or dizziness, leading to better outcomes at lower cost.

Section 23.4

Coping with Balance Disorders

This section includes text excerpted from "Dizziness Can Be a Drag," *NIH News in Health*, National Institutes of Health (NIH), August 2012. Reviewed April 2019.

Imagine reaching for something on a grocery shelf and suddenly feeling unsteady, or looking over your shoulder to back up the car and having things start whirling around you. Most people feel dizzy now and then. But, if that feeling persists or interferes with your daily life, it could be a sign of a balance disorder.

A balance disorder makes you feel as if you are moving, spinning or floating, even though you are quite still. More than 4 in 10 Americans will experience an episode of dizziness sometime during their lives that is significant enough to send them to a doctor.

Dizziness can range from feeling lightheaded to woozy to disoriented. Feeling that you or your surroundings are spinning is called "vertigo." Any of these sensations can be extremely distressing.

"Balance is a multisystem function," explains National Institutes of Health (NIH) hearing and balance expert Dr. Daniel Sklare. It begins with a series of signals within the tiny balance organs of the inner ear. These organs work with your brain's visual system to give you a sense of your body's position. They also keep objects from blurring when your head moves. Sense receptors in skin, joints, and muscles also send balance-related signals to the brain. The brain receives and coordinates information from all these different body systems. Balance disorders can arise when any of these signals malfunction.

Because balance is so complex, it can be hard to figure out the underlying cause of certain problems. Some balance disorders can begin suddenly. They might arise from an ear infection, a head injury or certain medications. Low blood pressure can lead to dizziness when you stand up quickly. Disorders related to vision, muscles, bones, or joints can also contribute to balance problems.

"As America gets older, many people with imbalance have a collection of these problems," says Dr. Gordon Hughes, NIH clinical trials director for hearing and balance. "They might have aging of the ear, aging of vision, cataracts, muscle weakness from losing some muscle mass or arthritis in the hips, plus other problems like diabetes."

Researchers have identified more than a dozen different balance disorders. The most common is a sudden, often harmless burst of vertigo that might arise with an abrupt change in the position of the head, such as when you bend over to tie your shoes. Technically known as "benign paroxysmal positional vertigo" (BPPV), this condition can result from a head injury or simply from getting older. BPPV sometimes occurs when tiny calcium crystals in the inner ear become displaced. In that case, your doctor can treat BPPV by carefully moving the head and body to reposition these particles. An NIH-supported clinical trial showed that this treatment works well for BPPV.

Another common balance disorder is known as "Ménière disease." It can develop at any age, but most often strikes adults between 40 and 60 years of age. Symptoms include intense vertigo, hearing loss, nausea, tinnitus (a ringing or buzzing in the ear) and a feeling of fullness in the ear. Ménière disease usually affects only one ear.

Some people with Ménière disease have single attacks of dizziness separated by long periods of time. Others may experience many attacks closer together over a number of days. Some affected people have vertigo so extreme that they lose their balance and fall. These episodes are called "drop attacks."

An attack of Ménière's symptoms, while not life-threatening, can feel completely overwhelming. The symptoms arise because of a change in fluid volume within the inner ear. But, its underlying cause remains unknown. Scientists estimate that 6 in 10 people either get better on their own or can control their vertigo with diet, drugs, or devices. In severe cases, surgical therapies can end the dizziness but might affect hearing.

NIH-funded researchers at the University of Washington are now exploring a new treatment option to stop a Ménière's attack. An implant behind the ear is designed to control abnormal electrical activity in the nerve that sends balance information to the brain, bringing the sensation of spinning to a halt. The device is now being tested in clinical trials.

If you think you may have a balance disorder, talk with your healthcare provider. Your doctor can assess whether your symptoms might be caused by a serious disorder, such as a heart or blood condition. If an inner ear balance disorder is likely, you may be referred to a specialist, such as an otolaryngologist, a doctor with expertise in the ear, nose, and throat. You might receive a hearing test, a balance test, and possibly an imaging study of the brain.

Work with your doctor to figure out how to cope with your dizziness on a daily basis and reduce your risk of injury. For example, wear low-heeled shoes or walking shoes outdoors. You might decide to try using a cane or a walker. Safe, secure handrails in stairwells and grip handles in bathrooms can help make your home safer. Driving a car may be especially hazardous, so ask your doctor if it is safe for you to drive.

A specialized rehabilitation therapist can give you a set of head, body and eye exercises to help reduce dizziness and nausea.

Meanwhile, researchers continue to work to develop new, more effective approaches. In one experimental rehabilitation strategy, now in clinical trials, scientists have created a "virtual reality" grocery store. It allows people with balance disorders to walk safely on a treadmill through computer-generated store aisles. While holding onto a grocery cart, they can look up and down, turn their heads and reach for items on virtual shelves. By doing this, they safely learn how to navigate an environment that can be challenging for someone with a balance problem.

"The key for people looking for treatment is to go to the best team of clinical experts that they can gain access to," says Dr. Sklare. "It's very important to get that level of assessment."

Tell Your Doctor

Discuss your symptoms with a healthcare provider if:

- You often feel unsteady
- You feel as if the room is spinning around you
- You feel as if you are moving when you know you are standing or sitting still
- You lose your balance and fall
- You feel as if you are falling
- You feel lightheaded, or as if you might faint
- Your vision becomes blurred
- You sometimes feel disoriented, losing your sense of time, place or identity

Section 23.5

Presbyastasis

This section contains text excerpted from the following sources: Text
in this section begins with excerpts from "Older Consumer Safety:
Phase I—A Review and Summary of the Literature on Age-Related
Differences in the Adult Consumer Population, and Product Related
Interventions to Compensate for those Differences," U.S. Consumer
Product Safety Commission (CPSC), December 2005. Reviewed April
2019; Text under the heading "Balance Problems and Disorders" is
excerpted from "Balance Problems and Disorders," National Institute
on Aging (NIA), National Institutes of Health (NIH), May 1, 2017;
Text under the heading "Four Things You Can Do to Prevent Falls"
is excerpted from "What You Can Do to Prevent Falls," Centers for
Disease Control and Prevention (CDC), September 22, 2017.

Presbyastasis is the age-related impairment of vestibular functions that results in balance and equilibrium issues. As the condition progresses, it becomes intertwined with other sensory systems,
making it a complex condition that requires a holistic evaluation
and treatment.

The vestibular system contributes information regarding the position and movement of the head in space and is critical for maintaining
balance when visual or somatosensory information is absent or distorted; it also assists in resolving sensory conflict that arises in complex
visual environments. Changes in the vestibular system begin as early
as 30 years of age, with a gradual decline that continues progressively
through adulthood and results in reduced sensitivity to head movements. By the age of 70, the number of vestibular hair and nerve cells
declines by as much as 40 percent. With advancing age, there appears
to be a moderate reduction in the speed with which one can stabilize
vision when the head moves quickly through space. This reduction
adversely affects an older adult's ability to determine whether it is
the world or her- or himself that is moving in certain situations. Older
adults feel increasingly unsteady in complex visual environments and
may report sensations of dizziness or vertigo (spinning sensation) that
add to their perception of instability.

Balance and Falls

Balance can be defined as the process of controlling the body's center of mass or gravity relative to the base of support, typically one's

feet. Failing to maintain balance ultimately leads to a fall. Balance is often separated into two types: static balance, which involves the maintenance of balance while in a stationary position, and dynamic balance, which involves the maintenance of balance during locomotion or while moving.

Static Balance and Postural Stability

Static balance is commonly measured in two ways: postural sway during quiet standing and response to an outside perturbation of balance. Testing consistently finds that older adults (i.e., those over the age of 60) have poorer static balance than younger adults. For example, older adults show more body sway, in terms of both speed and range, than younger adults.

In response to postural sway and outside perturbations, people maintain balance through the use of ankle, hip, and step postural strategies. The ankle strategy is typically used for small perturbations and is also used to control body sway during quiet standing. When employing the ankle strategy, the upper and lower body moves as a single unit around the ankles as the muscles surrounding the ankles apply force to the standing surface and bring one's center of gravity back over the base of support. The hip strategy is employed after a larger or faster perturbation in which the center of gravity must be brought over the base of support more quickly to avoid a loss of balance, and it involves the use of the muscles surrounding the knee and hip as the upper and lower body move in directions opposite one another. The step strategy involves taking one or more steps to establish a new base of support. Although this strategy is used when the perturbation is so large that the hip strategy would likely be ineffective, it also appears to be a naturally preferred balance strategy.

The ability to maintain balance depends on the sensory, cognitive, and motor control systems. The visual, prioreceptive or somatosensory, and vestibular sensory systems provide a visual layout of the surrounding environment, information about body position with respect to the environment, body limb positions with respect to each other, and head position and movement. The cognitive system then processes and integrates this sensory information and may plan the appropriate response. Finally, the motor control system makes the necessary adjustments to maintain balance.

Age-related declines in some or all of these systems are likely to be responsible for observed age-related deficits in balance. For example, age-related declines in the visual, proprioceptive/somatosensory, and vestibular senses can result in reduced or distorted sensory information and in the slower integration of this information, which may limit one's ability to quickly and accurately perceive where the body is in space. Furthermore, the evidence indicates that older adults rely more on vision and visual feedback than younger adults, even when that information may be inaccurate or when vision is declining. Age-related cognitive impairments associated with working memory and attention are also likely to affect balance, since older adults tend to allocate more attention to maintaining balance than younger adults but are less capable of dividing attention. Thus, older adults are likely to have greater difficulty maintaining balance while simultaneously focusing on another task. Lastly, declines in muscular strength, power, and coordination are likely to limit the extent to which older adults can produce rapid and accurate adjustment forces or steps to maintain balance after an unexpected perturbation.

Advancing age is associated with deteriorations in the integration of movement senses and vestibular cues. Losses in these senses reduce the ability to control body positions and movements, which leaves older adults vulnerable to instability and falls. The senses of movement, touch, and position are due to receptors in the joints, muscles, and skin, and are more variable in old age.

Balance Problems and Disorders

Balance problems are among the most common reasons that older adults seek help from a doctor. They are often caused by disturbances of the inner ear. Vertigo, the feeling that you or the things around you are spinning, is a common symptom.

Having good balance means being able to control and maintain your body's position, whether you are moving or remaining still. Good balance helps you walk without staggering, get up from a chair without falling, climb stairs without tripping, and bend over without falling. Good balance is important to help you get around, stay independent, and carry out daily activities.

Balance disorders are one reason older people fall.

Causes of Balance Problems

People are more likely to have problems with balance as they get older. But age is not the only reason these problems occur. In some cases, you can help reduce your risk for certain balance problems.

287

Some balance disorders are caused by problems in the inner ear. The part of the inner ear that is responsible for balance is the vestibular system, also known as the "labyrinth." A condition called "labyrinthitis" occurs when the labyrinth becomes infected or swollen. It is typically accompanied by vertigo and imbalance. Upper respiratory infections, other viral infections, and, less commonly, bacterial infections can also lead to labyrinthitis.

Some diseases of the circulatory system, such as stroke, can cause dizziness and other balance problems. Low blood pressure can also cause dizziness. Head injury and many medicines may also lead to balance problems.

Check with your doctor if you notice a problem while taking a medication. Ask if other medications can be used instead. If not, ask if the dosage can be safely reduced. Sometimes it cannot. However, your doctor will help you get the medication you need while trying to reduce unwanted side effects.

Symptoms of Balance Disorders

If you have a balance disorder, you may stagger when you try to walk, or teeter or fall when you try to stand up. You might experience other symptoms such as:

- Dizziness or vertigo (a spinning sensation)

- Falling or feeling as if you are going to fall

- Lightheadedness, faintness, or a floating sensation

- Blurred vision

- Confusion or disorientation

Other symptoms might include nausea and vomiting; diarrhea; changes in heart rate and blood pressure; and fear, anxiety, or panic. Symptoms may come and go over short time periods or last for a long time, and they can lead to fatigue and depression.

Balance disorders can be signs of other health problems, such as an ear infection, stroke, or multiple sclerosis. In some cases, you can help treat a balance disorder by seeking medical treatment for the illness that is causing the disorder.

Some exercises help make up for a balance disorder by moving the head and body in certain ways. The exercises are developed specifically for a patient by a professional (often a physical therapist) who understands the balance system and its relationship with other systems in the body.

Balance problems due to high blood pressure can be managed by eating less salt (sodium), maintaining a healthy weight, and exercising. Balance problems due to low blood pressure may be managed by drinking plenty of fluids, such as water; avoiding alcohol; and being cautious regarding your body's posture and movement, such as standing up slowly and avoiding crossing your legs when you are seated.

Coping with a Balance Disorder

Some people with a balance disorder may not be able to fully relieve their dizziness and will need to find ways to cope with it. A vestibular rehabilitation therapist can help you develop an individualized treatment plan.

If you have trouble with your balance, talk to your doctor about whether it is safe to drive and about ways to lower your risk of falling during daily activities, such as walking up or down stairs, using the bathroom, or exercising. To reduce your risk of injury from dizziness, avoid walking in the dark. You should also wear low-heeled shoes or walking shoes outdoors. If necessary, use a cane or walker, and modify conditions at your home and workplace, such as by adding handrails.

Four Things You Can Do to Prevent Falls
Talk Openly with Your Healthcare Provider about Fall Risks and Prevention

Tell a provider right away if you fall, worry about falling, or feel unsteady. Have your doctor or pharmacist review all the medicines you take, even over-the-counter (OTC) medicines. As you get older, the way medicines work in your body can change. Some medicines, or combinations of medicines, can make you sleepy or dizzy and can cause you to fall. Ask your provider about taking vitamin D supplements to improve bone, muscle, and nerve health.

Exercise to Improve Your Balance and Strength

Exercises that improve balance and make your legs stronger lower your chances of falling. It also helps you feel better and more confident. An example of this kind of exercise is Tai Chi.

Lack of exercise leads to weakness and increases your chances of falling.

Ask your doctor or healthcare provider about the best type of exercise program for you.

Have Your Eyes and Feet Checked

Once a year, check with your eye doctor and update your eyeglasses if needed. You may have a condition, such as glaucoma or cataracts, that limits your vision. Poor vision can increase your chances of falling. Also, have your healthcare provider check your feet once a year. Discuss proper footwear, and ask whether seeing a foot specialist is advised.

Make Your Home Safer

- Remove things you can trip over (such as papers, books, clothes, and shoes) from stairs and places where you walk.

- Remove small throw rugs or use double-sided tape to keep the rugs from slipping.

- Keep items you use often in cabinets you can reach easily without using a step stool.

- Have grab bars put in next to and inside the tub and next to the toilet.

- Use nonslip mats in the bathtub and on shower floors.

- Improve the lighting in your home. As you get older, you need brighter lights to see well. Hang light-weight curtains or shades to reduce glare.

- Have handrails and lights installed on all staircases.

- Wear well-fitting shoes with good support inside and outside the house.

Section 23.6

Vestibular Rehabilitation

This section includes text excerpted from "William S. Middleton Memorial Veterans Hospital—Vestibular Rehabilitation," U.S. Department of Veterans Affairs (VA), June 9, 2015. Reviewed April 2019.

What Is Vestibular Rehabilitation and Balance Retraining?

A movement/exercise approach with the goals of:

- Decreasing/eliminating dizziness/vertigo (room spinning)
- Improving balance, function, and safety
- Reducing falls or risk for falls

What Are the Symptoms of a Vestibular Problem?

- Dizziness/vertigo (room spinning)
- Imbalance/unsteadiness
- Motion sensitivity/nausea

You may also experience muscular stiffness, imbalance, weakness, fatigue, headaches, anxiety, and memory problems.

What Will the Patient Need to Do?

One of the most important parts of treating vestibular problems is a home exercise program. These exercises need to be done consistently and daily in order to improve symptoms. Patients will be expected to complete the given exercises every day often multiple times per day.

A physical therapist will individually customize a program for your specific needs aimed at eliminating or decreasing your imbalance and dizziness.

Chapter 24

Vestibular Schwannoma

What Is a Vestibular Schwannoma (Acoustic Neuroma)?

A vestibular schwannoma (VS) (also known as "acoustic neuroma," "acoustic neurinoma," or "acoustic neurilemoma") is a benign, usually slow-growing tumor that develops from the balance and hearing nerves supplying the inner ear. The tumor comes from an overproduction of Schwann cells—the cells that normally wrap around nerve fibers like onion skin to help support and insulate nerves. As the vestibular schwannoma grows, it affects the hearing and balance nerves, usually causing unilateral (one-sided) or asymmetric hearing loss, tinnitus (ringing in the ear), and dizziness or loss of balance. As the tumor grows, it can interfere with the face sensation nerve (the trigeminal nerve), causing facial numbness. Vestibular schwannomas can also affect the facial nerve (for the muscles of the face), causing facial weakness or paralysis on the side of the tumor. If the tumor becomes large, it will eventually press against nearby brain structures (such as the brainstem and the cerebellum), becoming life-threatening.

This chapter includes text excerpted from "Vestibular Schwannoma (Acoustic Neuroma) and Neurofibromatosis," National Institute on Deafness and Other Communication Disorders (NIDCD), March 6, 2017.

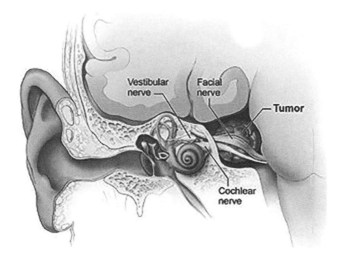

Figure 24.1. *Inner Ear with Vestibular Schwannoma (Tumor)*

A vestibular schwannoma (also known as acoustic neuroma, acoustic neurinoma, or acoustic neurilemoma) is a benign, usually slow-growing tumor that develops from the balance and hearing nerves supplying the inner ear.

How Is a Vestibular Schwannoma Diagnosed?

Unilateral or asymmetric hearing loss and/or tinnitus and loss of balance or dizziness are early signs of a vestibular schwannoma. Unfortunately, early detection of the tumor is sometimes difficult because the symptoms may be subtle and may not appear in the beginning stages of growth. Also, hearing loss, dizziness, and tinnitus are common symptoms of many middle and inner ear problems (the important point here is that unilateral or asymmetric symptoms are the worrisome ones). Once the symptoms appear, a thorough ear examination and hearing and balance testing (audiogram, electronystagmography, auditory brainstem responses) are essential for proper diagnosis. Magnetic resonance imaging (MRI) scans are critical in the early detection of a vestibular schwannoma and are helpful in determining the location and size of a tumor and in planning its microsurgical removal.

How Is a Vestibular Schwannoma Treated?

Early diagnosis of a vestibular schwannoma is key to preventing its serious consequences. There are three options for managing a vestibular schwannoma: surgical removal, radiation, and observation. Sometimes, the tumor is surgically removed (excised). The exact type of operation done depends on the size of the tumor and the level of hearing in the affected ear. If the tumor is small, hearing may be saved and accompanying symptoms may improve by removing it to prevent its eventual effect on the hearing nerve. As the tumor grows larger, surgical removal is more complicated because the tumor may have damaged the nerves that control facial movement, hearing, and balance and may also have affected other nerves and structures of the brain.

The removal of tumors affecting the hearing, balance, or facial nerves can sometimes make the patient's symptoms worse because these nerves may be injured during tumor removal.

As an alternative to conventional surgical techniques, radiosurgery (that is, radiation therapy, the "gamma knife," or linear accelerator (LINAC)) may be used to reduce the size or limit the growth of the tumor. Radiation therapy is sometimes the preferred option for elderly patients, patients in poor medical health, patients with bilateral vestibular schwannoma (tumor affecting both ears), or patients whose tumor is affecting their only hearing ear. When the tumor is small and not growing, it may be reasonable to "watch" the tumor for growth. MRI scans are used to carefully monitor the tumor for any growth.

What Is the Difference between Unilateral and Bilateral Vestibular Schwannomas?

Unilateral vestibular schwannomas affect only one ear. They account for approximately 8 percent of all tumors inside the skull; approximately 1 out of every 100,000 individuals per year develops a vestibular schwannoma. Symptoms may develop at any age but usually occur between the ages of 30 and 60. Most unilateral vestibular schwannomas are not hereditary and occur sporadically.

Bilateral vestibular schwannomas affect both hearing nerves and are usually associated with a genetic disorder called "neurofibromatosis type 2" (NF2). Half of the affected individuals have inherited the disorder from an affected parent, and half seem to have a mutation for the first time in their family. Each child of an affected parent has a 50 percent chance of inheriting the disorder. Unlike those with a unilateral vestibular schwannoma, individuals with NF2 usually develop symptoms in their teens or early adulthood. In addition, patients with NF2 usually develop multiple brain and spinal cord related tumors. They also can develop tumors of the nerves important for swallowing, speech, eye and facial movement, and facial sensation. Determining the best management of the vestibular schwannomas, as well as the additional nerve, brain, and spinal cord tumors, are more complicated than deciding how to treat a unilateral vestibular schwannoma. Further research is needed to determine the best treatment for individuals with NF2.

Scientists believe that both unilateral and bilateral vestibular schwannomas form following the loss of the function of a gene on chromosome 22. (A gene is a small section of deoxyribonucleic acid (DNA) responsible for a particular characteristic, such as hair color or skin tone.) Scientists believe that this particular gene on chromosome 22 produces a protein that controls the growth of Schwann cells. When this gene malfunctions, Schwann cell growth is uncontrolled, resulting in a tumor. Scientists also think that this gene may help control the growth of other types of tumors. In NF2 patients, the faulty gene on chromosome 22 is inherited. For individuals with unilateral vestibular schwannoma, however, some scientists hypothesize that this gene somehow loses its ability to function properly.

What Is Being Done about Vestibular Schwannoma?

Scientists continue studying the molecular pathways that control normal Schwann cell development to better identify gene mutations that result in vestibular schwannomas. Scientists are working to better understand how the gene works so they can begin to develop new therapies to control the overproduction of Schwann cells in individuals with vestibular schwannoma. Learning more about the way genes help control Schwann cell growth may help prevent other brain tumors. In addition, scientists are developing robotic technology to assist physicians with acoustic neuroma surgery.

Chapter 25

Enlarged Vestibular Aqueducts

What Are Vestibular Aqueducts?

Vestibular aqueducts are narrow, bony canals that travel from the inner ear to deep inside the skull (see Figure 25.1). The aqueducts begin inside the temporal bone, the part of the skull just above the ear. The temporal bone also contains two sensory organs that are part of the inner ear. These organs are the cochlea, which detects sound waves and turns them into nerve signals, and the vestibular labyrinth, which detects movement and gravity. These organs, together with the nerves that send their signals to the brain, work to create normal hearing and balance. Running through each vestibular aqueduct is a fluid-filled tube called the "endolymphatic duct," which connects the inner ear to a balloon-shaped structure called the "endolymphatic sac."

Recent studies indicate that a vestibular aqueduct is abnormally enlarged if it is larger than one millimeter, roughly the size of the head of a pin. This is called an "enlarged vestibular aqueduct" or "EVA"; the condition is also known as a "dilated vestibular aqueduct" or a "large vestibular aqueduct." If a vestibular aqueduct is

This chapter includes text excerpted from "Enlarged Vestibular Aqueducts and Childhood Hearing Loss," National Institute on Deafness and Other Communication Disorders (NIDCD), February 13, 2017.

enlarged, the endolymphatic duct and sac usually grow large too. The functions of the endolymphatic duct and sac are not completely understood. Scientists believe that the endolymphatic duct and sac help to ensure that the fluid in the inner ear contains the correct amounts of certain chemicals called "ions." Ions are needed to help start the nerve signals that send sound and balance information to the brain.

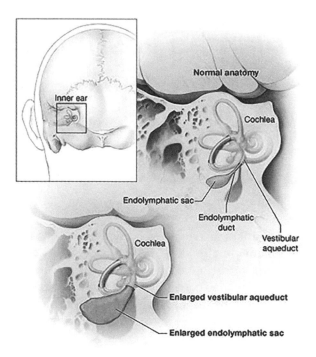

Figure 25.1. *Illustration of Vestibular Aqueducts*

How Are Enlarged Vestibular Aqueducts Related to Childhood Hearing Loss?

Research suggests that most children with EVA will develop some amount of hearing loss. Scientists also are finding that 5 to 15 percent of children with sensorineural hearing loss (hearing loss caused by damage to sensory cells inside the cochlea) have EVA. However, scientists do not think that EVA causes the hearing loss, but that both are caused by the same underlying defect. EVA can be an important clue pointing to what is actually causing the hearing loss.

How Are Enlarged Vestibular Aqueducts Related to Pendred Syndrome?

EVA can be a sign of a genetic disorder called "Pendred syndrome," a cause of childhood hearing loss. According to a study by the National Institute on Deafness and Other Communication Disorders (NIDCD), approximately one-fourth of the people with EVA and hearing loss have Pendred syndrome. Hearing loss associated with Pendred syndrome is usually progressive, which means that a child will lose hearing over time. Some children may become totally deaf.

In addition to its association with hearing loss, EVA also may be linked to balance problems in a small percentage of people. However, the brain is very good at making up for a weak vestibular system, and most children and adults with EVA do not have balance disorders or difficulty doing routine tasks.

What Causes Enlarged Vestibular Aqueducts

EVA has many causes, not all of which are fully understood. The most well-known cause of EVA and hearing loss is mutations in a gene called "*SLC26A4*" (previously known as the "PDS gene"). Two mutations in the *SLC26A4* gene can result in Pendred syndrome. Scientists believe that other, currently unknown, genetic or environmental factors also may lead to EVA.

How Are Enlarged Vestibular Aqueducts Diagnosed?

Medical professionals use different clues to help them determine the cause of hearing loss. Two tests that are often used to identify the cause of hearing loss are magnetic resonance imaging (MRI) and computed tomography (CT) imaging of the inner ear. One or both tests are often recommended to evaluate a child with sensorineural hearing loss. This is particularly true when a child's hearing loss occurs suddenly, is greater in one ear than the other, or varies or gets worse over time. Although most CT scans of children with hearing loss are normal, EVA is the most commonly observed abnormality.

Can Enlarged Vestibular Aqueducts Be Treated to Reduce Hearing Loss?

No treatment has been proven effective in reducing the hearing loss associated with EVA or in slowing its progression. Although some otolaryngologists (a doctor or surgeon who specializes in diseases of the ears, nose, throat, and head and neck) recommend steroids to treat sudden sensorineural hearing loss, there are no scientific studies to show that this is an effective treatment for EVA. In addition, surgery to drain liquid out of the endolymphatic duct and sac or to remove the endolymphatic duct and sac is not only ineffective in treating EVA, it can be harmful. Research has shown conclusively that these surgeries can destroy hearing.

To reduce the likelihood of progression of hearing loss, people with EVA should avoid contact sports that might lead to head injury; wear head protection when engaged in activities, such as bicycle riding or skiing that might lead to head injury; and avoid situations that can lead to barotrauma (extreme, rapid changes in air pressure), such as scuba diving or hyperbaric oxygen treatment. The pressure changes associated with flying in airplanes have also been reported to cause hearing loss in people with EVA. However, this is a rare event in commercial aircraft with pressurized cabins. If you have EVA, you can minimize your risk of hearing loss associated with air travel by taking nasal decongestants if you have sinus or nasal congestion, such as during a cold or flu.

Identifying hearing loss as early as possible is the best way to reduce EVA's impact. The earlier hearing loss is identified in children, the sooner they can develop skills that will help them learn and communicate with others. Children with permanent and progressive hearing loss, which is often linked with EVA, will benefit from learning other forms of communication, such as sign language or cued speech, or using assistive devices, such as a hearing aid or cochlear implant.

Chapter 26

Vertigo

Our body balance is directly related to gravity; the signals regarding gravity are sent by our inner ear to the brain. Any disruption of this inner ear function affects the signals sent by the inner ear and through sensory nerve pathways to the brain, which gives rise to a symptom called "vertigo." Vertigo is a sensation of feeling off-balance. This feeling is barely noticeable, and the attacks of vertigo can develop suddenly and last for a few seconds or minutes, based on its severity. It is considered a symptom of a range of conditions rather than a condition itself. Other symptoms that can occur in association with vertigo are:

- Loss of balance, causing difficulty with standing or walking
- Feeling sick (nausea or vomiting)
- Fullness or ringing in the ear (tinnitus)
- Lightheadedness or dizziness—Episodes in which a room feels as if it is rotating or our surrounding environment feels as if it is spinning are called "dizzy spells."

Types of Vertigo

There are two types of vertigo

- Peripheral vertigo
- Central vertigo

Peripheral Vertigo

Benign paroxysmal positional vertigo (BPPV) involves short, recurrent, episodic attacks of vertigo that are triggered by certain movements of the head. It is caused by the buildup of canaliths (tiny calcium particles) inside the inner canal that blocks the signal sent by the ears to the brain, which leads to imbalance, uncontrolled eye movements (nystagmus). It usually affects older people and may occur due to:

- Head injury
- An ear infection
- After an ear surgery

Labyrinthitis—inflammations of the fluid-filled channels that send gravitation signals from the ear to the brain are called "labyrinths." The inflammation may be due to the common cold or flu (viral-related). Vertigo caused by labyrinthitis may occasionally be accompanied by nausea, tinnitus with ear pain, and high temperature.

Vestibular neuritis—inflammation of the vestibular nerve that connects the labyrinth and the brain. This is also caused by a viral infection and can cause unsteadiness, nausea, and vomiting. It may last for a few hours to a few days.

Ménière disease—also causes vertigo, along with tinnitus, fullness in the ears, and hearing loss.

Taking certain types of medication can cause vertigo as a side effect. Speak with your healthcare provider if you notice any vertigo symptoms due to your medication usage so that they can arrange for an alternative medication. Never discontinue your medication use without your doctor's advice.

Central Vertigo

Central vertigo is caused by problems in the part of the brain, such as the cerebellum (located at the bottom of the brain) or the brainstem (lower part of the brain connecting to the spinal cord). Causes include:

- **Migraines**—severe headaches felt as a throbbing pain in the center or on one side of the head. Migraines are common in younger people due to lack of sleep, stress, etc.

- **Multiple sclerosis**—a condition that affects the brain and spinal cord (the central nervous system (CNS))

- **Acoustic neuroma**—noncancerous brain tumor growing in the acoustic nerve, which controls hearing and balance

- **Transient ischemic attack (TIA) or stroke**—blood supply to the brain will be partly cut off.

Diagnosing Vertigo

- A physical examination of the eyes for uncontrolled eye movement. If it is severe, a videonystagmography (VNG) will be conducted, in which special goggles record your eye movement.

- Checking your balance while changing positions to identify triggers of vertigo

- Hearing tests, such as an audiometry test or a tuning fork test, to check for hearing loss or tinnitus

- Caloric testing, which involves running cool or warm air into the ear for about 30 seconds to check for dizziness

- Posturography, which checks your balance with a machine that collects sensations from your feet, joints, and the ear signals that help maintain your stability

- A magnetic resonance imaging (MRI) scan and a computed tomography (CT) scan of the head to rule out the possibility of a brain tumor (acoustic neuroma), which can be the cause of vertigo.

Treating Vertigo

Some types of vertigo resolve without treatment, but other underlying medical problems may need attention.

- A bacterial infection would likely need antibiotic therapy.

- Early stages of vertigo, such as in motion sickness, can be treated with prochlorperazine and antihistamines, and nausea can be treated with antiemetics.

- Vestibular neuritis is a disorder that may need antiviral drugs, antibiotics, or steroids. Additionally, vestibular rehabilitation training (VRT)—a series of exercises—is also used to treat dizziness and balance problems. It is also called "brain retraining," as it attempts to adapt the brain to the abnormal messages sent by your ears.

- Nystagmus and BPPV can be cured using inner surgery, in which a bone plug will be inserted into the inner ear to block the area where vertigo is triggered. The plug prevents the ear from responding to the movements inside of the ear that triggers vertigo, as well as the head movements that lead to vertigo. Also for BPPV, a series of simple head movements called "Epley manoeuver" is used for treatment.

- Brandt-Daroff exercises are used if the Epley maneuver does not work. These are a set of exercises that involve the movement of the neck and back.

- Sound therapy for treating ringing in the ears

- Use of hearing aids to manage hearing loss

- Physiotherapy to help with balance problems

Tips for Managing Vertigo

- Do simple exercises that are recommended to correct the symptoms.

- Avoid bending down suddenly or picking something up.

- Avoid extending your neck, especially when you are reaching for something high up, such as shelves.

- Move the head slowly and carefully while doing daily activities.

- Sleep with your head slightly raised with two to three pillows.

- Get up slowly from your bed while changing from the sleeping position to the sitting position.

- Sit on the edge of your bed before standing up to avoid dizziness.

References

1. "Benign Paroxysmal Positional Vertigo (BPPV)," Mayoclinic, June 30, 2018.

2. Tucci, Debara L. MD, MS, MBA. "Dizziness and Vertigo," Merck Manual, June 2017.

3. Ambardekar, Nayana. MD. "Vertigo," WebMD, December 22, 2018.

Chapter 27

Dizziness and Motion Sickness

Motion sickness is a common condition characterized by a feeling of unwellness brought on by certain kinds of movement. The usual symptoms include dizziness, pale skin (pallor), and sweating, followed by nausea and vomiting. Affected individuals may also experience rapid breathing (hyperventilation), headache, restlessness, and drowsiness. These symptoms can be triggered by many kinds of motion, particularly traveling in a car, bus, train, airplane, or boat. Amusement park rides, skiing, and virtual reality environments can also induce motion sickness.

Frequency

Motion sickness is very common. About one in three people are considered highly susceptible to motion sickness. However, almost everyone will become motion sick if exposed to motion that is intense enough.

Motion sickness is more common in some groups of people than in others for reasons that are not fully understood. The condition is more common in women (particularly during menstruation or pregnancy) than in men and more common in children than in adults. People who have migraines, including a balance disorder called "vestibular

This chapter includes text excerpted from "Motion Sickness," Genetics Home Reference (GHR), National Institutes of Health (NIH), March 19, 2019.

migraine," have a higher risk of motion sickness than those who do not have these conditions. People in some ethnic and geographic groups are more likely to report being susceptible to motion sickness; for example, studies suggest that there is a higher prevalence of motion sickness among Asians than among Europeans.

Causes

The factors that contribute to motion sickness are not well understood, but susceptibility to the condition does seem to be partly genetic. When motion sickness occurs, it likely results from a mismatch in signals about movement coming from different parts of the body. The brain senses movement by combining signals from the inner ears, eyes, muscles, and joints. When the eyes signal to the brain that the body is still (for example, a moving car appears stationary to the person riding in it), but the inner ears and other parts of the body signal that the body is in motion, a conflict occurs. Researchers believe it is this sensory conflict that triggers the symptoms of motion sickness. The mechanism by which a sensory mismatch could lead to dizziness, nausea, and related symptoms is unclear, and other explanations for motion sickness are also being explored.

Common, complex conditions, such as motion sickness, are often polygenic, which means they involve variations in many genes. However, little is known about the specific genes involved in motion sickness because few studies have been done to identify them.

One study compared genetic variations in a large number of people with and without a susceptibility to motion sickness. The researchers found common genetic variations in or near 35 genes that may be associated with the condition. These genes play a wide variety of roles in the body: some are involved in eye and ear development, and others in the formation of otoliths, which are tiny structures in the inner ear that are involved in sensing gravity and movement. Still, other identified genes play roles in the development and function of junctions between nerve cells (synapses) where cell-to-cell communication takes place, and in the way that the body processes the simple sugar glucose and the hormone insulin, which helps regulate blood sugar levels. Additional research will be necessary to confirm the association between variations in specific genes and motion sickness susceptibility.

Inheritance Pattern

Motion sickness does not have a clear pattern of inheritance, although it does tend to cluster in families. People who have a first-degree relative (for example, a parent or sibling) who is highly susceptible to motion sickness are more likely than the general public to get motion sick themselves.

Other Names for This Condition

- Airsickness
- Carsickness
- Ciders' vertigo
- Seasickness

Chapter 28

Ménière Disease

What Is Ménière Disease?

Ménière disease is a disorder of the inner ear that causes severe dizziness (vertigo), ringing in the ears (tinnitus), hearing loss, and a feeling of fullness or congestion in the ear. Ménière disease usually affects only one ear.

Attacks of dizziness may come on suddenly or after a short period of tinnitus or muffled hearing. Some people will have single attacks of dizziness separated by long periods of time. Others may experience many attacks closer together over a number of days. Some people with Ménière disease have vertigo so extreme that they lose their balance and fall. These episodes are called "drop attacks."

Ménière disease can develop at any age, but it is more likely to happen to adults between 40 and 60 years of age. The National Institute on Deafness and Other Communication Disorders (NIDCD) estimates that approximately 615,000 individuals in the United States are currently diagnosed with Ménière disease and that 45,500 cases are newly diagnosed each year.

This chapter includes text excerpted from "Ménière's Disease," National Institute on Deafness and Other Communication Disorders (NIDCD), February 13, 2017.

What Causes the Symptoms of Ménière Disease

The symptoms of Ménière disease are caused by the buildup of fluid in the compartments of the inner ear, called the "labyrinth." The labyrinth contains the organs of balance (the semicircular canals and otolithic organs) and of hearing (the cochlea). It has two sections: the bony labyrinth and the membranous labyrinth. The membranous labyrinth is filled with a fluid called "endolymph" that, in the balance organs, stimulates receptors as the body moves. The receptors then send signals to the brain about the body's position and movement. In the cochlea, fluid is compressed in response to sound vibrations, which stimulate sensory cells that send signals to the brain.

In Ménière disease, the endolymph buildup in the labyrinth interferes with the normal balance and hearing signals between the inner ear and the brain. This abnormality causes vertigo and other symptoms of Ménière disease.

Why Do People Get Ménière Disease?

Many theories exist about what happens to cause Ménière disease, but no definite answers are available. Some researchers think that Ménière disease is the result of constrictions in blood vessels similar to those that cause migraine headaches. Others think Ménière disease could be a consequence of viral infections, allergies, or autoimmune reactions. Because Ménière disease appears to run in families, it could also be the result of genetic variations that cause abnormalities in the volume or regulation of endolymph fluid.

How Does a Doctor Diagnose Ménière Disease?

Ménière disease is most often diagnosed and treated by an otolaryngologist (commonly called an "ear, nose, and throat doctor," or "ENT"). However, there is no definitive test or single symptom that a doctor can use to make the diagnosis. Diagnosis is based upon your medical history and the presence of:

- 2 or more episodes of vertigo, lasting at least 20 minutes each
- Tinnitus
- Temporary hearing loss
- A feeling of fullness in the ear

Some doctors will perform a hearing test to establish the extent of hearing loss caused by Ménière disease. To rule out other diseases, a doctor also might request magnetic resonance imaging (MRI) or computed tomography (CT) scans of the brain.

How Is Ménière Disease Treated?

Ménière disease does not have a cure yet, but your doctor might recommend some of the treatments below to help you cope with the condition.

- **Medications.** The most disabling symptom of an attack of Ménière disease is dizziness. Prescription drugs, such as meclizine, diazepam, glycopyrrolate, and lorazepam, can help relieve dizziness and shorten the attack.

- **Salt restriction and diuretics.** Limiting dietary salt and taking diuretics (water pills) help some people control dizziness by reducing the amount of fluid the body retains, which may help lower fluid volume and pressure in the inner ear.

- **Other dietary and behavioral changes.** Some people claim that caffeine, chocolate, and alcohol make their symptoms worse and either avoid or limit them in their diet. Not smoking also may help lessen the symptoms.

- **Cognitive therapy.** Cognitive therapy is a type of talk therapy that helps people focus on how they interpret and react to life experiences. Some people find that cognitive therapy helps them cope better with the unexpected nature of attacks and reduces their anxiety about future attacks.

- **Injections.** Injecting the antibiotic gentamicin into the middle ear helps control vertigo but significantly raises the risk of hearing loss because gentamicin can damage the microscopic hair cells in the inner ear that help us hear. Some doctors inject a corticosteroid instead, which often helps reduce dizziness and has no risk of hearing loss.

- **Pressure pulse treatment.** The U.S. Food and Drug Administration (FDA) approved a device for Ménière disease that fits into the outer ear and delivers intermittent air pressure pulses to the middle ear. The air pressure pulses appear to act on endolymph fluid to prevent dizziness.

- **Surgery.** Surgery may be recommended when all other treatments have failed to relieve dizziness. Some surgical procedures are performed on the endolymphatic sac to decompress it. Another possible surgery is to cut the vestibular nerve, although this occurs less frequently.

- **Alternative medicine.** Although scientists have studied the use of some alternative medical therapies in Ménière disease treatment, there is still no evidence to show the effectiveness of such therapies as acupuncture or acupressure; tai chi; or herbal supplements, such as ginkgo biloba, niacin, or ginger root. Be sure to tell your doctor if you are using alternative therapies since they sometimes can impact the effectiveness or safety of conventional medicines.

What Is the Outlook for Someone with Ménière Disease?

Scientists estimate that 9 out of 10 people either get better on their own or can control their vertigo with diet, drugs, or devices. However, a small group of people with Ménière disease will get relief only by undergoing surgery.

What Research about Ménière Disease Is Being Done?

Insights into the biological mechanisms in the inner ear that cause Ménière disease will guide scientists as they develop preventive strategies and more effective treatment. The NIDCD is supporting scientific research across the country that is:

- Determining the most effective dose of gentamicin with the least amount of risk for hearing loss

- Developing an in-ear device that uses a programmable microfluid pump (the size of a computer chip) to precisely deliver vertigo-relieving drugs to the inner ear

- Studying the relationship between endolymph volume and inner ear function to determine how much endolymph is "too much." Researchers are hoping to develop methods for manipulating inner ear fluids and treatments that could lower endolymph volume and reduce or eliminate dizziness.

Chapter 29

Perilymph Fistula

Perilymph fistula (PLF) occurs when there is an abnormal opening in the thin membrane (either in the oval or round window) that separates the fluid-filled inner ear and the air-filled middle ear. The opening leads to the leakage of perilymph fluid from the inner ear and to the middle ear, causing a disturbance to the air pressure in the middle ear.

Causes

The most common causes of PLF are listed below.

- Head trauma
- Ear trauma
- Perforated ear drum
- Barotrauma that occurs on airplane or while scuba diving
- Rapid increase in the intracranial pressure that may occur during weightlifting or childbirth

Symptoms

The symptoms of PLF include:

- Ear fullness or pressure buildup within the ear

- Sensitive hearing

- Vertigo

- Tullio phenomenon (experiencing vertigo when exposed to loud sounds)

- Tinnitus

- Hearing loss

- Dizziness

- Nausea and vomiting

The symptoms of perilymph fistula may worsen with coughing, sneezing, straining, or a change in altitude.

Diagnosis

As of now, there is not any positive test that can confirm the presence of PLF. There is considerable difficulty in diagnosing PLF as the symptoms overlap with other ear disorders, such as Ménière disease. Some tests that can possibly increase the chance of an accurate diagnosis are:

- Audiometry

- Computed tomography (CT) scan

- Electrocochleography (ECOG)

- Electronystagmography (ENG)

- Fistula test

- Fraser test

- Magnetic resonance imaging (MRI) scan

- Valsalva test

- Vestibular evoked myogenic potential (VEMP)

- Videonystagmography (VNG)

Since none of the above-mentioned methods can give an exact result, a physician has to analyze the medical history of the patient thoroughly and perform a combination of diagnostic tests to arrive at a conclusive diagnosis of PLF.

Treatment

There are certain medications to treat the symptoms of PLS, but these medications will have no effect on the fistula itself. In some cases, PLF can heal on its own when certain activities, such as bending, straining, weightlifting, airplane travel, scuba diving, etc., are restricted. Therefore, strict bed rest is often recommended to cure PLF. But if the bed rest does not help, the only possible treatment is a surgical repair. The surgery involves using soft tissue grafts to repair the opening in the round window. The surgery is usually performed under general anesthesia and may last around 45 to 60 minutes. Even after the surgery, patients are advised to have restricted activities in order to avoid recurring PLF.

References

1. "Perilymph Fistula," Vestibular Disorders Association (VeDA), May 13, 2014.

2. Hayes, Kristin. "What Causes a Perilymph Fistula?" Verywell Health, November 14, 2018.

3. Hain, Timothy C. "Perilymph Fistula," Chicago Dizziness and Hearing (CDH), December 11, 2017.

Part Five

Disorders of the Nose and Sinuses

Chapter 30

Your Stuffy Nose

Chapter Contents

Section 30.1

The Common Cold

This section contains text excerpted from the following sources:
Text in this section begins with excerpts from "Common Cold and
Runny Nose," Centers for Disease Control and Prevention (CDC),
September 26, 2017; Text under the heading "Summertime
Sniffles" is excerpted from "Catching a Cold When It's Warm," *NIH
News in Health*, National Institutes of Health (NIH), June 2012.
Reviewed April 2019; Text under the heading "Common
Colds: Protect Yourself and Others " is excerpted from "Common
Colds: Protect Yourself and Others," Centers for Disease
Control and Prevention (CDC), February 11, 2019.

Antibiotics cannot cure the common cold, one of the most frequent reasons children miss school and adults miss work. Every
year, adults have an average of two to three colds, and children
have even more.

Causes

More than 200 viruses can cause the common cold, and infections
can spread from person to person through the air and close personal
contact. Antibiotics do not work against these viruses and do not help
you feel better if you have a cold. Rhinovirus is the most common type
of virus that causes colds.

Risk Factors

There are many things that can increase your risk for the common
cold, including:

- Exposure to someone with the common cold

- Age (infants and young children are at higher risk for colds)

- A weakened immune system or taking drugs that weaken the
  immune system

- Season (colds are more common during the fall and winter)

Signs and Symptoms

When germs that cause colds first infect the nose and sinuses
(air-filled pockets in the face), the nose makes clear mucus. This helps

wash the germs from the nose and sinuses. After two or three days, mucus may change to a white, yellow, or green color. This is normal and does not mean you or your child needs antibiotics. Other signs and symptoms of the common cold can include:

- Sneezing

- Stuffy nose

- Sore throat

- Coughing

- Postnasal drip (mucus dripping down your throat)

- Watery eyes

- Mild headache

- Mild body aches

These symptoms usually peak within 2 to 3 days, but they can last for up to 10 to 14 days.

When to Seek Medical Care

See a healthcare professional if you or your child has any of the following symptoms:

- Symptoms that last more than 10 days without improvement

- Symptoms that are severe or unusual

If your child is younger than three months of age and has a fever, it is important to call your healthcare professional right away.

Diagnosis and Treatment

Antibiotics are not needed to treat a cold or runny nose, which almost always gets better on its own. Your healthcare professional will determine what type of illness you or your child has by asking about symptoms and doing a physical examination. Sometimes they will also swab the inside of your nose or mouth.

Since the common cold is caused by viruses, antibiotics will not help it get better and may even cause harm in both children and adults. Your healthcare professional can give you tips to help with symptoms, such as fever and coughing.

Symptom Relief

Rest, over-the-counter (OTC) medicines, and other self-care methods may help you or your child feel better. For more information about symptomatic relief, talk to your healthcare professional, including your pharmacist. Remember, always use over-the-counter products as directed. Many over-the-counter products are not recommended for children of certain ages.

Prevention

There are steps you can take to help prevent getting a cold, including:

- Practice good hand hygiene

- Avoid close contact with people who have colds or other upper respiratory infections

Summertime Sniffles

Most everyone looks forward to summer; it is a time to get away, get outside, and have some fun. So, what could be more unfair than catching a cold when it is warm? How can cold symptoms arise when it is not cold and flu season? Is there any way to dodge the summertime sniffles?

Cold symptoms can be caused by more than 200 different viruses. Each can bring the sneezing, scratchy throat, and runny nose that can be the first signs of a cold. The colds we catch in winter are usually triggered by the most common viral infections in humans, a group of germs called "rhinoviruses." Rhinoviruses and a few other cold-causing viruses seem to survive best in cooler weather. Their numbers surge in September and begin to dwindle in May.

During summer months, the viral landscape begins to shift. "Generally speaking, summer and winter colds are caused by different viruses," says Dr. Michael Pichichero, a pediatrician and infectious disease researcher at the Rochester General Hospital Research Institute (RGHRI) in New York. "When you talk about summer colds, you are probably talking about a nonpolio enterovirus infection."

Enteroviruses can infect the tissues in your nose and throat, eyes, digestive system and elsewhere. A few enteroviruses can cause polio, but vaccines have mostly eliminated these viruses from Western countries. Far more widespread are more than 60 types of nonpolio enteroviruses. They are the second most common type of virus—after rhinovirus—that infects humans. About half of people with enterovirus infections do not get sick at all. But nationwide, enteroviruses cause an estimated 10 to 15 million illnesses each year, usually between June and October.

Enteroviruses can cause a fever that comes on suddenly. Body temperatures may range from 101°F to 104°F. Enteroviruses can also cause mild respiratory symptoms, sore throat, headache, muscle aches, and gastrointestinal issues, such as nausea or vomiting.

"All age groups can be affected, but like most viral infections, enterovirus infections predominate in childhood," says Pichichero. Adults may be protected from enterovirus infections if they have developed antibodies from previous exposures. But, adults can still get sick if they encounter a new type of enterovirus.

Less common enteroviruses can cause other symptoms. Some can lead to conjunctivitis, or pinkeye—a swelling of the outer layer of the eye and eyelid. Others can cause an illness with rash. In rare cases, enteroviruses can affect the heart or brain.

To prevent enterovirus infections, says Pichichero, "it is all about blocking viral transmission." The viruses travel in respiratory secretions, similar to saliva or mucus, or in the stool of an infected person. You can become infected by direct contact. Or you might pick up the virus by touching contaminated surfaces or objects, such as a telephone, doorknob, or a baby's diaper. "Frequent hand washing and avoiding exposure to people who are sick with fever can help prevent the spread of infection," says Pichichero.

The summer colds caused by enteroviruses generally clear up without treatment within a few days or even a week. But see a healthcare provider if you have concerning symptoms, such as a high fever or a rash.

Common Colds: Protect Yourself and Others

Sore throat and runny nose are usually the first signs of a cold, followed by coughing and sneezing. Most people recover in about 7 to 10 days. You can help reduce your risk of getting a cold by washing your hands often, avoiding close contact with sick people, and not touching your face with unwashed hands.

Common colds are the main reason that children miss school and adults miss work. Each year in the United States, there are millions of cases of the common cold. Adults have an average of two to three colds per year, and children have even more.

Most people get colds in the winter and spring, but it is possible to get a cold any time of the year. Symptoms usually include:

- Sore throat

- Runny nose

- Coughing

- Sneezing

- Headaches

- Body aches

Most people recover within about 7 to 10 days. However, people with weakened immune systems, asthma, or respiratory conditions may develop serious illness, such as bronchitis or pneumonia.

How to Protect Yourself

Viruses that cause colds can spread from infected people to others through the air and close personal contact. You can also get infected through contact with stool or respiratory secretions from an infected person. This can happen when you shake hands with someone who has a cold or when you touch a surface, such as a doorknob, that has respiratory viruses on it, then touch your eyes, mouth, or nose.

You can help reduce your risk of getting a cold:

- Wash your hands often with soap and water. Wash them for 20 seconds, and help young children do the same. If soap and water are not available, use an alcohol-based hand sanitizer. Viruses that cause colds can live on your hands, and regular hand washing can help protect you from getting sick.

- Avoid touching your eyes, nose, and mouth with unwashed hands. Viruses that cause colds can enter your body this way and make you sick

- Stay away from people who are sick. Sick people can spread viruses that cause the common cold through close contact with others.

How to Protect Others

If you have a cold, you should follow these tips to help prevent spreading it to other people:

- Stay at home while you are sick, and keep children out of school or day care while they are sick.

- Avoid close contact with others, such as hugging, kissing, or shaking hands.

- Move away from people before coughing or sneezing.

- Cough and sneeze into a tissue then throw it away, or cough and sneeze into your upper shirt sleeve, completely covering your mouth and nose.

- Wash your hands after coughing, sneezing, or blowing your nose.

- Disinfect frequently touched surfaces and objects, such as toys and doorknobs.

There is no vaccine to protect you against the common cold.

How to Feel Better

There is no cure for a cold. To feel better, you should get lots of rest and drink plenty of fluids. Over-the-counter medicines may help ease symptoms, but they will not make your cold go away any faster. Always read the label and use medications as directed. Talk to your doctor before giving your child nonprescription cold medicines, since some medicines contain ingredients that are not recommended for children.

Antibiotics will not help you recover from a cold caused by a respiratory virus. They do not work against viruses, and they may make it harder for your body to fight future bacterial infections if you take them unnecessarily.

Section 30.2

Cold, Flu, or Allergy

This section contains text excerpted from the following sources: Text
in this section begins with excerpts from "Cold, Flu, or Allergy?"
NIH News in Health, National Institutes of Health (NIH), October 7,
2014. Reviewed April 2019; Text under the heading "Cold versus Flu"
is excerpted from "Cold versus Flu," Centers for Disease Control and
Prevention (CDC), February 8, 2019.

You are feeling pretty lousy. You have got sniffles, sneezing, and
a sore throat. Is it a cold, flu, or allergies? It can be hard to tell them
apart because they share so many symptoms. But understanding the
differences will help you choose the best treatment.

"If you know what you have, you won't take medications that you
don't need, that aren't effective, or that might even make your symptoms worse," says Nationa Institutes of Health's (NIH) Dr. Teresa
Hauguel, an expert on infectious diseases that affect breathing.

Cold, flu, and allergies all affect your respiratory system, which
can make it hard to breathe. Each condition has key symptoms that
set them apart.

Colds and flu are caused by different viruses. "As a rule of thumb,
the symptoms associated with the flu are more severe," says Hauguel.
Both illnesses can lead to a runny, stuffy nose; congestion; cough; and
sore throat. But the flu can also cause high fever that lasts for three to
four days, along with a headache, fatigue, and general aches and pain.
These symptoms are less common when you have a cold.

"Allergies are a little different, because they aren't caused by a
virus," Hauguel explains. "Instead, it's your body's immune system
reacting to a trigger, or allergen, which is something you're allergic
to." If you have allergies and breathe in things such as pollen or pet
dander, the immune cells in your nose and airways may overreact to
these harmless substances. Your delicate respiratory tissues may then
swell, and your nose may become stuffed up or runny.

"Allergies can also cause itchy, watery eyes, which you don't normally have with a cold or flu," Hauguel adds.

Allergy symptoms usually last as long as you are exposed to the
allergen, which may be about six weeks during pollen seasons in the
spring, summer, or fall. Colds and flu rarely last beyond two weeks.

Most people with a cold or flu recover on their own without medical
care. But check with a healthcare provider if symptoms last longer than
10 days or if symptoms are not relieved by over-the-counter medicines.

To treat colds or flu, get plenty of rest and drink lots of fluids. If you have the flu, pain relievers such as aspirin, acetaminophen, or ibuprofen can reduce fever or aches. Allergies can be treated with antihistamines or decongestants.

Be careful to avoid "drug overlap" when taking medicines that list two or more active ingredients on the label. For example, if you take two different drugs that contain acetaminophen—one for a stuffy nose and the other for headache—you may be getting too much acetaminophen.

"Read medicine labels carefully—the warnings, side effects, dosages. If you have questions, talk to your doctor or pharmacist, especially if you have children who are sick," Hauguel says. "You don't want to overmedicate, and you don't want to risk taking a medication that may interact with another."

Table 30.1. Difference among Cold, Flu, and Airborne Allergy

Symptoms	Cold	Flu	Airborne Allergy
Fever	Rare	Usual, high (100-102 °F), sometimes higher, especially in young children); lasts 3-4 days	Never
Headache	Uncommon	Common	Uncommon
General Aches, Pains	Slight	Usual; often severe	Never
Fatigue, Weakness	Sometimes	Usual, can last up to 3 weeks	Sometimes
Extreme Exhaustion	Never	Usual, at the beginning of the illness	Never
Stuffy, Runny Nose	Common	Sometimes	Common
Sneezing	Usual	Sometimes	Usual
Sore Throat	Common	Sometimes	Sometimes
Cough	Common	Common, can become severe	Sometimes
Chest Discomfort	Mild to moderate	Common	Rare, except for those with allergic asthma

Table 30.1. Continued

Symptoms	Cold	Flu	Airborne Allergy
Treatment	Get plenty of rest. Stay hydrated. (Drink plenty of fluids.) Decongestants. Aspirin (ages 18 and up), acetaminophen, or ibuprofen for aches and pains	Get plenty of rest. Stay hydrated. Aspirin (ages 18 and up), acetaminophen, or ibuprofen for aches, pains, and fever Antiviral medicines (see your doctor)	Avoid allergens (things that you're allergic to) Antihistamines Nasal steroids Decongestants
Prevention	Wash your hands often. Avoid close contact with anyone who has a cold.	Get the flu vaccine each year. Wash your hands often. Avoid close contact with anyone who has the flu.	Avoid allergens, such as pollen, house dust mites, mold, pet dander, cockroaches.
Complications	Sinus infection middle ear infection, asthma	Bronchitis, pneumonia; can be life-threatening	Sinus infection, middle ear infection, asthma

Cold versus Flu

Flu and the common cold are both respiratory illnesses, but they are caused by different viruses. Because these two types of illnesses have similar symptoms, it can be difficult to tell the difference between them based on symptoms alone. In general, flu is worse than the common cold, and symptoms are more intense. Colds are usually milder than flu. People with colds are more likely to have a runny or stuffy nose. Colds generally do not result in serious health problems, such as pneumonia, bacterial infections, or hospitalizations. Flu can have very serious associated complications.

How Can You Tell the Difference between a Cold and the Flu?

Because colds and flu share many symptoms, it can be difficult (or even impossible) to tell the difference between them based on symptoms alone. Special tests that usually must be done within the first few days of illness can tell if a person has the flu.

What Are the Symptoms of the Flu versus the Symptoms of a Cold?

The symptoms of flu can include fever or feeling feverish/chills, cough, sore throat, runny or stuffy nose, muscle or body aches, headaches and fatigue (tiredness). Cold symptoms are usually milder than the symptoms of flu. People with colds are more likely to have a runny or stuffy nose. Colds generally do not result in serious health problems.

Section 30.3

Complementary Health Approaches for Colds

This section includes text excerpted from "Flu and Colds:
In Depth," National Center for Complementary and
Integrative Health (NCCIH), March 8, 2019.

Each year, Americans get more than 1 billion colds, and between 5 and 20 percent of Americans get the flu. The 2 diseases have some symptoms in common, and both are caused by viruses. However, they are different conditions, and the flu is more severe. Unlike the flu, colds generally do not cause serious complications, such as pneumonia, or lead to hospitalization. No vaccine can protect you against the common cold, but vaccines can protect you against the flu. Everyone over the age of 6 months should be vaccinated against the flu each year. Vaccination is the best protection against getting the flu.

What the Science Says about Complementary Health Approaches for Colds

The following complementary health approaches have been studied for colds:

American Ginseng

- Several studies have evaluated the use of American ginseng (Panax quinquefolius) to prevent colds. A 2011 evaluation of these studies concluded that the herb has not been shown to reduce the number of colds that people catch, although it may shorten the length of colds. The researchers who conducted the evaluation concluded that there was insufficient evidence to support the use of American ginseng for preventing colds.

• Taking American ginseng in an effort to prevent colds means taking it for prolonged periods of time. However, little is known about the herb's long-term safety. American ginseng may interact with the anticoagulant (blood-thinning) drug warfarin.

Echinacea

• At least 24 studies have tested echinacea to see whether it can prevent colds or relieve cold symptoms. A comprehensive 2014 assessment of this research concluded that echinacea has not been convincingly shown to be beneficial. However, at least some echinacea products might have a weak effect.

• One reason why it is hard to reach definite conclusions about this herb is that echinacea products vary greatly. They may contain different species (types) of the plant and be made from different plant parts (the above-ground parts, the root, or both). They also may be manufactured in different ways, and some products contain other ingredients in addition to echinacea. Research findings on one echinacea product may not apply to other products.

• Few side effects have been reported in studies of echinacea. However, some people are allergic to this herb, and in one study in children, taking echinacea was linked to an increase in rashes.

Garlic

• A 2014 evaluation of the research on garlic concluded that there is not enough evidence to show whether this herb can help prevent colds or relieve their symptoms.

• Garlic can cause bad breath, body odor, and other side effects. Because garlic may interact with anticoagulant drugs (blood-thinners), people who take these drugs should consult their healthcare providers before taking garlic.

Honey

Honey's traditional reputation as a cough remedy has some science to back it up. A small amount of research suggests that honey may help to decrease nighttime coughing in children.

Honey should never be given to infants under the age of one year because it may contain spores of the bacterium that causes infant botulism. Honey is considered safe for older children.

Meditation

- Reducing stress and improving general health may protect against colds and other respiratory infections. In a 2012 study funded by the National Center for Complementary and Integrative Health (NCCIH), adults 50 years of age and older were randomly assigned to training in mindfulness meditation, which can reduce stress; an exercise training program, which may improve physical health; or a control group that did not receive any intervention. The study participants kept track of their illnesses during the cold and flu season. People in the meditation group had shorter and less severe acute respiratory infections (most of which were colds) and lost fewer days of work because of these illnesses than those in the control group. Exercise also had some benefit, but not as much as meditation.

- This study is the first to suggest that meditation may reduce the impact of colds. Because it is the only study of its kind, its results should not be regarded as conclusive.

- Meditation is generally considered to be safe for healthy people. However, there have been reports that it might worsen symptoms in people with certain chronic physical or mental-health problems. If you have an ongoing health issue, talk with your healthcare provider before starting meditation.

Probiotics

- A 2015 evaluation of 13 studies found some evidence suggesting that probiotics might reduce the number of colds or other upper respiratory tract infections that people catch and the length of the illnesses, but the quality of the evidence was low or very low.

- In people who are generally healthy, probiotics have a good safety record. Side effects, if they occur at all, usually consist only of mild digestive symptoms, such as gas. However, information on the long-term safety of probiotics is limited, and safety may differ from one type of probiotic to another. Probiotics have been linked to severe side effects, such as dangerous infections, in people with serious underlying medical problems.

Saline Nasal Irrigation

• Saline nasal irrigation means rinsing your nose and sinuses with salt water. People may do this with a neti pot (a device that comes from the Ayurvedic tradition) or with other devices, such as bottles, sprays, pumps, or nebulizers. Saline nasal irrigation may be used for sinus congestion, allergies, or colds.

• There is limited evidence that saline nasal irrigation can help relieve cold symptoms. Studies of this technique have been too small to allow researchers to reach definite conclusions.

• Saline nasal irrigation used to be considered safe, with only minor side effects, such as nasal discomfort or irritation. However, in 2011, a severe disease caused by an amoeba (a type of microorganism) was linked to nasal irrigation with tap water. The U.S. Food and Drug Administration (FDA) has warned that tap water that is not filtered, treated, or processed in specific ways is not safe for use in nasal rinsing devices, and the FDA has explained how to use and clean these devices safely.

Vitamin C

• An evaluation of the large amount of research done on vitamin C and colds (29 studies involving more than 11,000 people) concluded that taking vitamin C does not prevent colds in the general population and shortens colds only slightly. Taking vitamin C only after you start to feel cold symptoms does not affect the length or severity of the cold.

• Unlike the situation in the general population, vitamin C does seem to reduce the number of colds in people exposed to short periods of extreme physical stress (such as marathon runners and skiers). In studies of these groups, taking vitamin C cut the number of colds in half.

• Taking too much vitamin C can cause diarrhea, nausea, and stomach cramps. People with the iron-storage disease hemochromatosis should avoid high doses of vitamin C. People who are being treated for cancer or taking cholesterol-lowering medications should talk with their healthcare providers before taking vitamin C supplements.

Zinc

- Zinc has been used for colds in forms that are taken orally (by mouth), such as lozenges, tablets, or syrup, or used intranasally (in the nose), such as swabs or gels.

- **Oral Zinc**

  - A 2012 evaluation of 17 studies of various types of zinc lozenges, tablets, or syrup found that zinc can reduce the duration of colds in adults. 2 evaluations of 3 studies of high-dose zinc acetate lozenges in adults, conducted in 2015 and 2016, found that they shortened colds.

  - Some participants in studies that tested zinc for colds reported that the zinc caused a bad taste or nausea.

  - Long-term use of high doses of zinc can cause low copper levels, reduced immunity, and low levels of HDL cholesterol (the "good" cholesterol). Zinc may interact with drugs, including antibiotics and penicillamine (a drug used to treat rheumatoid arthritis).

- **Intranasal Zinc**

  - The use of zinc products inside the nose, such as gels or swabs, may cause loss of the sense of smell, which may be long-lasting or permanent. In 2009, the FDA warned consumers to stop using several intranasal zinc products marketed as cold remedies because of this risk.

  - Prior to the warnings about effects on the sense of smell, a few studies of intranasal zinc had suggested a possible benefit against cold symptoms. However, the risk of a serious and lasting side effect outweighs any possible benefit in the treatment of a minor illness.

Other Complementary Approaches

In addition to the complementary approaches described above, several other approaches have been studied for colds. In all instances, there is insufficient evidence to show whether these approaches help to prevent colds or relieve cold symptoms.

- Andrographis (*Andrographis paniculata*)
- Chinese herbal medicines
- Green tea
- Guided imagery
- Hydrotherapy
- Vitamin D
- Vitamin E

Section 30.4

Coughing and Sneezing: Hygiene Etiquette

This section includes text excerpted from "Coughing and Sneezing," Centers for Disease Control and Prevention (CDC), July 26, 2016.

Hygiene etiquette involves practices that prevent the spread of illness and disease. A critical time to practice good hygiene etiquette is when you are sick, especially when you are coughing or sneezing. Serious respiratory illnesses, such as influenza, respiratory syncytial virus (RSV), whooping cough, and severe acute respiratory syndrome (SARS) are spread by:

- Coughing or sneezing
- Unclean hands
  - Touching your face after touching contaminated objects
  - Touching objects after contaminating your hands

To help stop the spread of germs:

- Cover your mouth and nose with a tissue when you cough or sneeze.
- Put your used tissue in a wastebasket.

- If you do not have a tissue, cough or sneeze into your upper sleeve, not your hands.

Remember to wash your hands after coughing or sneezing:

- Wash with soap and water

- Keeping hands clean through improved hand hygiene is one of the most important steps we can take to avoid getting sick and spreading germs to others. Many diseases and conditions are spread by not washing hands with soap and clean, running water. If clean, running water is not accessible, as is common in many parts of the world, use soap and available water. If soap and water are unavailable, use an alcohol-based hand sanitizer that contains at least 60 percent alcohol to clean your hands.

Cough etiquette is especially important for infection control measures in healthcare settings, such as emergency departments, doctor's offices, and clinics.

One final practice that helps prevent the spread of respiratory disease is avoiding close contact with people who are sick. If you are ill, you should try to distance yourself from others so you do not spread your germs. Distancing includes staying home from work or school when possible.

Section 30.5

Allergic Rhinitis

This section contains text excerpted from the following sources: Text
in this section begins with excerpts from "Seasonal Allergies (Allergic
Rhinitis)," National Center for Complementary and Integrative
Health (NCCIH), September 24, 2017; Text under the heading
"Symptoms" is excerpted from "Hay Fever," MedlinePlus, National
Institutes of Health (NIH), January 30, 2019; Text under the
heading "Complementary Health Approaches for Seasonal Allergy
Relief" is excerpted from "6 Things To Know About Complementary
Health Approaches for Seasonal Allergy Relief," National Center for
Complementary and Integrative Health (NCCIH), March 21, 2017.

Allergic rhinitis (hay fever) is a common health problem; about
eight percent of adults and children in the United States have it. If
you have an allergy, your immune system reacts to something that
does not cause problems for most people. Many complementary health
approaches, including both mind and body practices and natural products, have been studied for allergic rhinitis.

Symptoms

Each spring, summer, and fall, trees, weeds, and grasses release
tiny pollen grains into the air. Some of the pollen ends up in your
nose and throat. This can trigger a type of allergy called "hay
fever."

Symptoms can include:

- Sneezing, often with a runny or clogged nose

- Coughing and postnasal drip

- Itchy eyes, nose, and throat

- Red and watery eyes

- Dark circles under the eyes

Your healthcare provider may diagnose hay fever based on a physical exam and your symptoms. Sometimes, skin or blood tests are used.
Taking medicines and using nasal sprays can relieve symptoms. You
can also rinse out your nose, but be sure to use distilled or sterilized
water with saline. Allergy shots can help make you less sensitive to
pollen and provide long-term relief.

Complementary Health Approaches for Seasonal Allergy Relief

Seasonal allergies are triggered each spring, summer, and fall when trees, weeds, and grasses release pollen into the air. When the pollen ends up in your nose and throat, it can bring on sneezing, runny nose, coughing, and itchy eyes and throat. People manage seasonal allergies by taking medication, avoiding exposure to the substances that trigger their allergic reactions, or having a series of "allergy shots" (a form of immunotherapy).

People also try various complementary approaches to manage their allergies. If you are considering any complementary health approach for the relief of seasonal allergy symptoms, here are some things you need to know.

- **Nasal saline irrigation.** There is some good evidence that saline nasal irrigation (putting salt water into one nostril and draining it out the other) can be useful for modest improvement of allergy symptoms. Nasal irrigation is generally safe; however, neti pots and other rinsing devices must be used and cleaned properly. According to the U.S. Food and Drug Administration (FDA), tap water that is not filtered, treated, or processed in specific ways is not safe for use as a nasal rinse.

- **Butterbur extract.** There are hints that the herb butterbur may decrease the symptoms associated with nasal allergies. However, there are concerns about its safety.

- **Honey.** Only a few studies have looked at the effects of honey on seasonal allergy symptoms, and there is no convincing scientific evidence that honey provides symptom relief. Eating honey is generally safe; however, children under one year of age should not eat honey. People who are allergic to pollen or bee stings may also be allergic to honey.

- **Acupuncture.** A 2015 evaluation of 13 studies of acupuncture for allergic rhinitis, involving a total of 2,365 participants, found evidence that this approach may be helpful.

- **Probiotics.** There is some evidence that suggests that probiotics may improve some symptoms, as well as the quality of life (QOL), in people with allergic rhinitis, but because probiotic formulations vary from study to study, it is difficult to make firm conclusions about its effectiveness.

Talk to your healthcare provider. If you suffer from seasonal allergies and are considering a complementary health approach, talk to your healthcare provider about the best ways to manage your symptoms. You may find that when the pollen count is high, staying indoors, wearing a mask, or rinsing off when you come inside can help.

Chapter 31

Common Nasal Concerns and Treatments

Chapter Contents

Section 31.1

Nasal Polyps

What Is a Nasal Polyp?

Nasal polyps are small, polypoidal, noncancerous growths that can occur anywhere in the mucous membranes lining the nose or the paranasal sinuses. They are overgrowths of the mucosa that frequently accompany allergic rhinitis. They are not tender and are freely movable. They may occur singly or in clusters, and they usually form where the sinuses open into the nasal cavity. While small polyps may not cause problems, larger ones can block the sinuses or the nasal airway.

Nasal polyps can develop at any age, but they are most common in adults over the age of 40, and men are more affected than women. They are uncommon in children under 10 years of age. When young children are diagnosed with nasal polyps, in fact, doctors should conduct further tests to rule out cystic fibrosis, a genetic disorder characterized by a buildup of mucus in the lungs. Nasal polyps occur in nearly two-thirds of cystic fibrosis patients.

Causes

It is not entirely clear why some people develop nasal polyps and others do not. Although there is no definite cause of nasal polyposis, some factors may contribute to an increased risk of developing nasal polyps. One of the most common triggers is nasal congestion arising from chronic inflammation of the sinuses, which may be caused by allergies or recurring sinus infections. A certain degree of genetic predisposition has been observed in patients with nasal polyps, and it may explain why the mucosa in some people reacts differently to inflammation. Polyps are also commonly seen in patients with late onset of asthma and aspirin sensitivity, allergic rhinitis, sinusitis, a foreign body in the nose.

Types of Nasal Polyp

It is classified as antrochoanal or ethmoidal. Antrochoanal nasal polyp is single, unilateral. It will originate from maxillary sinus and is usually found in children. Ethmoidal polyps are bilateral and usually found in adults.

Symptoms and Diagnosis

Polyposis may be asymptomatic in some people, particularly if the polyps are small. Larger polyps are usually associated with catarrh (excessive secretion of mucus), breathing difficulties, inflammation of the paranasal cavities, and loss of smell and taste. Other symptoms of nasal polyps may include postnasal drip (drainage of mucous down the back of the throat) and a dull, achy feeling in the face because of fluid buildup.

Diagnosis of nasal polyps is generally made using a procedure called "nasal endoscopy." Although a routine examination with a rhinoscope (a lighted device fitted with a lens that can be inserted into the nose) can find polyps located in the nasal cavity, an endoscope (a long, flexible tool fitted with a miniature camera on its end) is required to find polyps that are deep-seated in the sinuses. The doctor may also request a computerized tomography (CT) scan to diagnose polyps and additional tests, such as a biopsy, to rule out nasal and sinus cancer and nonmalignant conditions, such as nasal papilloma.

Pathogenesis of Nasal Polyp

The exact pathogenesis of nasal polyps is unknown. Nasal mucosa first becomes oedematous due to collection of extracellular fluid, causing polypoidal change. Polyps which are sessile in the beginning become pedunculated due to gravity and excessive sneezing. In early stages, surfaces of nasal polyps are covered by ciliated columnar epithelium, but later on, it undergoes metaplastic change to squamous type on atmospheric irritation. Submucosa shows large intercellular spaces filled with serous fluid.

The following are some diseases associated with polyp formation:

1. Chronic rhinosinusitis

2. Cystic fibrosis

3. Asthma

4. Aspirin-induced asthma

5. Nasal mastocytosis

6. Kartagener syndrome, etc.

341

Exposure to some forms of chromium can cause nasal polyps and associated diseases.

Treatment Options

Although various forms of medicine can alleviate symptoms associated with nasal polyps, they may provide only temporary relief. The first line of treatment is usually nasal drops or sprays containing steroids. Steroid treatment is often beneficial if the polyps are small, and the patient is likely to experience marked improvement in breathing as the polyps shrink and free up the airways. Tapered oral steroid medications can prevent sinus inflammation associated with allergies and effectively reduce the size of inflammatory polyps, but these drugs are used sparingly because they may increase the risk of health concerns, such as diabetes, high blood pressure, and osteoporosis. Steroids, both topical and oral, are also frequently used after surgery to prevent the recurrence of polyps. Doctors may also prescribe antibiotics to treat chronic sinusitis that may be associated with nasal polyps.

Endoscopic nasal surgery is the most commonly used treatment option for polyposis when the polyps are too large to respond to corticosteroids. This minimally invasive surgical procedure, known as a "polypectomy," is performed with a nasal endoscope and can be done on an outpatient basis. The procedure is carried out under general anesthesia and with a suction device or a microdebrider (a minuscule, motorized shaver) to remove the polyps. The removal of nasal polyps by nasal endoscopy surgery lasts approximately 45 minutes to 1 hour. Recovery from the disease is anywhere from 1 to 3 weeks. If there is no bleeding, the patient is discharged after a few hours of observation. Antibiotics are usually prescribed to prevent infection at the site of surgery. Although surgery can provide symptomatic relief for a few years, the nasal polyps grow back in at least 15 percent of patients. In such cases, postoperative use of steroidal sprays and saline washes is usually prescribed to extend the period before the polyps recur.

References

1. Case-Lo, Christine. "Nasal Polyps," Healthline, October 5, 2015.

2. "Nasal Polyps—Treatment," NHS Choices, February 12, 2015.

Section 31.2

Nosebleeds

"Nosebleeds," © 2017 Omnigraphics. Reviewed April 2019.

A nosebleed, also known as "epistaxis," is a common condition that occurs when one of the small, delicate blood vessels inside the nose bursts open. Many children under the age of 10 are prone to nosebleeds. Although blood streaming from the nose can seem alarming, nosebleeds are usually harmless and easy to manage at home with simple first-aid techniques.

Blood vessels on the nasal septum—the tissue that separates the nostrils—are responsible for most nosebleeds. Those that occur in the front part of the nose are known as "anterior nosebleeds," and they are the most common among children and the easiest to stop. Posterior nosebleeds, on the other hand, occur deep inside the nasal cavity. They usually affect older adults, people with high blood pressure, and people who have experienced facial injuries.

Causes of Nosebleeds

Irritation of the membranes lining the inside of the nose is the cause of most nosebleeds. Breathing cold, dry, or overheated air can cause irritation of nasal membranes, as can the accumulation of mucus from allergies, colds, sinus infections, or the flu. Medications used to dry out the sinuses, such as decongestants or antihistamines, can also cause irritation of the nasal membranes. Irritation causes crusts to form inside the nose, which can bleed when they are removed by blowing or picking the nose.

Injuries or bumps to the nose can also cause surface capillaries to burst and create nosebleeds. Children may also get nosebleeds by inserting foreign objects into their nose. In rare cases, repeated nosebleeds may be symptomatic of an underlying disorder, such as high blood pressure, hemophilia, or a tumor in the nose or sinuses.

First Aid at Home

The first step in treating a nosebleed is to remain calm and reassuring. Children often become upset at the sight or taste of blood, and it is important to let them know that everything will be fine. The next step is to stop the bleeding by applying pressure to the soft part of the nose. With the child sitting down and leaning forward slightly, use the fingers, a tissue, or a soft cloth to hold the nostrils closed for 10 minutes. Do not release the pressure to check whether the bleeding has stopped until the full time has passed. Encourage the child to spit out any blood in the mouth, as swallowing blood can cause vomiting and make the nosebleed worse. It may also be helpful to apply an ice pack or cold compress to the bridge of the nose. If the bleeding has not stopped after 10 minutes, repeat the above procedures for 10 more minutes.

Once the bleeding stops, it is important to have the child pursue quiet activities for a few hours instead of running around. The child should also avoid taking hot baths or showers and drinking hot liquids for the next 24 hours to prevent dilation of blood vessels in the nose. Finally, the child should not be allowed to sniff, blow, or pick their nose for at least 24 hours following a nosebleed.

Medical Treatment

In most cases, nosebleeds can be treated successfully at home. It may be necessary to seek medical treatment, however, under the following conditions:

- The bleeding continues for more than 20 minutes

- The nosebleed accompanies a head injury

- The nose may have been fractured by a fall or blow to the face

- A foreign object may have been inserted into the nose

- The child tends to bruise easily or bleed profusely from minor wounds

- The child has recently begun taking a new medication

For a persistent nosebleed, the doctor is likely to apply a medicated cream or ointment to the inside of the nose to help stop the bleeding. The doctor may also use heat, electric current, or silver nitrate sticks to cauterize the blood vessel and stop the bleeding. Finally, the doctor may pack the child's nose with gauze, which should remain in place for 24 to 48 hours. Once the bleeding has stopped, the doctor can take steps to address any underlying causes of the nosebleed. The doctor may remove a foreign object from the nose, for instance, or reset a broken nose. If nosebleeds are related to medication, a change in prescription may be recommended.

Although it is rare, frequent, severe nosebleeds can create enough blood loss to cause anemia in children. Doctors may perform blood tests to determine whether hemoglobin levels are low. They may also check for signs of low blood pressure due to blood loss. Children who have frequent nosebleeds may also be referred to an ear, nose, and throat (ENT) specialist for further testing, such as nasal endoscopy or computerized tomography (CT) scan of the nose and sinuses.

Preventing Nosebleeds

To prevent nosebleeds caused by dry air, it may be helpful to use a vaporizer at home to add moisture. In addition, using a saline nasal spray, water-based lubricating gel, or antibiotic ointment can help prevent nasal membranes from drying out. Cutting children's fingernails can help discourage nose-picking. Finally, wearing appropriate protective headgear during sports and activities can help prevent head and facial injuries that cause nosebleeds.

References

1. Jothi, Sumana. "Nosebleed," MedlinePlus, August 5, 2015.

2. "Nosebleeds," The Nemours Foundation/KidsHealth®, 2016.

3. "Nosebleeds," Royal Children's Hospital Melbourne, August 2015.

Section 31.3

Deviated Septum, Septoplasty, and Rhinoplasty

"Deviated Septum, Septoplasty, and Rhinoplasty," © 2019
Omnigraphics. Reviewed April 2019.

Deviated Septum

Inside the nose is a hollow cavity called the "nasal cavity," which is separated into two parts by a wall-like structure called the "septum."

The septum extends from the nostril to the back of the nose and is made of bone and cartilage. It is positioned in the middle of the nose and is intended to be straight to give good support to the nose and also to maintain the facial features of an individual cosmetically. The condition in which the nasal septum deviates from the center or looks bent or crooked, which can lead to disfigurement of the nose, is referred to as a "deviated septum."

Displacement of the septum ranges from minor to major—when one nostril becomes tighter than the other. When the degree of deviation is severe, it can even block one side of the breathing passage and cause difficulty breathing due to reduced air flow; this is called a "nasal obstruction."

Causes of Deviated Septum

Septal deviation can be the result of:

- **Trauma**—injury to the nose or a broken nose caused by:
  - Injury during childbirth that resulted in septal displacement
  - Accidental injury to the nose from contact sports, roughhousing, active play, or automobile accidents
  - An intentional injury that may result from getting hit in the nose with force

- **Birth defect (congenital)**—in which the fetus develops a nasal septal deviation (defect) that becomes apparent at birth

Symptoms of Deviated Septum

In most people, the deviated septum may not cause problems but in some, it can cause any of the following symptoms:

- Nosebleeds
- Postnasal drip accompanied by headache
- Recurrent sinus infections
- Nasal congestion, or a stuffy nose, more severe on one side than the other
- Difficulty breathing through the nose
- Sleep problems that contribute to loud breathing (snoring) or sleep apnca

346

The symptoms, as well as the degree of septal deviation, worsens:

- With age—the aging process worsens septal deviation over time

- With infection of the nose (rhinitis/rhinosinusitis)—infection leads to swelling of nasal tissues, which accentuates the narrowing of the nasal passage from a deviated septum

Diagnosis of Deviated Septum

This condition can be easily diagnosed during a physical examination. Your doctor will open the nostril with a nasal speculum (a medical tool for investigating body orifices) and use a bright light to examine your nasal septum. Your doctor may need to view deeper deviations with the aid of an endoscope or small telescope. Your doctor or a medical professional will use computed tomography (CT) of the nose in some cases to view the extent of the deviation or to rule out other associated findings.

Treatment of a Deviated Septum

Septal deviation is an extremely common condition that does not need treatment in most cases. Septal repair may be suggested if the deviation is severe enough to cause breathing problems and contribute to sleep apnea and snoring. For children with a deviated septum, it is best to opt for surgery after the nose has completely grown (i.e., around or after the age of 15).

Symptoms such as postnasal drip or stuffy nose/nasal congestion (blocked nose) can be treated using decongestants, antihistamines, or nasal sprays.

The surgical method of repairing a malpositioned septum is called "septoplasty." The surgeon makes a small cut in the nasal septum and then trims the cartilage or bone to even out the breathing space of the nostrils. Septoplasty can also be performed in combination with sinus surgery when there is damage to the sinuses.

Rhinoplasty, or a "nose job," is performed on occasion along with the septoplasty in order to achieve a better cosmetic outcome of the nasal appearance. This procedure is called "septorhinoplasty."

Other surgical septal corrections such as "septal reconstruction" and "submucous resection of the septum" can also be done in some cases.

Septoplasty and Turbinate Reduction

Septoplasty is a procedure that is performed as a treatment option for conditions that blocks the breathing passage such as:

- Deviated septum or septal deviation

- Chronic sinusitis

- Nasal polyp removal

- Recurrent nosebleeds (sometimes)

Risks and complications of the surgery include:

- Bleeding

- Infection

- Hole (perforation) of the septum

- Loss of ability to smell (rare) or decreased sense of smell (rare)

This procedure is done under local or general anesthesia in an outpatient setting. The procedure takes around one to two hours, depending on the severity of the deviation and the need to combine other procedures for a better outcome.

During the surgery, the surgeon will first lift the mucosa that covers the cartilage and bone, then attempt to straighten the septum by trimming or shaving the cartilage or bone.

Balloon septoplasty may also be performed for mild cases; this procedure is also performed in an office setting and is not a surgical procedure.

In some cases, enlarged bone structures (turbinates) can cause blockage of the breathing passage. In such cases, the surgeon may perform a septoplasty as well as a turbinate correction to remove a portion of the turbinate, or reduce the enlargement, using radiofrequency. This is called "turbinate reduction."

Once the reshaping has been performed, the surgeon will put the mucosal lining back in place. A dressing of soft packing material will be applied to avoid excess postsurgical bleeding. Patients may need to breathe through their mouths immediately after the surgery as both nostrils will be packed with dressing to support the healing process.

The dressing will be removed by the nurse three to four hours after postoperative recovery. Then the doctor will inspect the site. If the surgical site is stable, then the patient will be sent home.

Rarely, internal splints will be put in place in the appropriate position to help the septum heal; in such cases, a follow-up appointment will be scheduled after seven days for removal of the splints.

If a septoplasty is only performed, there will be little to no swelling or bruising after surgery. If septoplasty in combination with sinus surgery or rhinoplasty is performed, mild swelling along with bruising will remain for a week or two after surgery, which is normal.

For a safe and speedy recovery, it is best to avoid:

- Blowing the nose for three to four days

- Using alcohol

- Smoking (or coming into contact with secondhand smoke)

- Returning to work too soon

- Crowds or individuals who have a cough or cold, which will increase the chances of the patient getting sick

Rhinoplasty, or a "Nose Job"

This surgery is performed to change the shape and size of the nose and can be done for:

- **Medical reasons**—to correct breathing problems or disfigurement due to trauma or a birth defect.

- **Cosmetic reasons**—to change the shape of the nose and enhance facial appearance.

Once the patient is placed under general or local anesthesia, the surgeon makes a small cut (incision) inside the nostrils or externally at the base of the nose and then reshapes the cartilage and bones in order to obtain a pleasing anatomical structure of the nose.

For small changes, the surgeon may use cartilage inside the nose for reshaping. For large changes, the surgeon may remove cartilage from the ribs or bones from other parts of the body, or sometimes use implants placed inside the nose for reshaping. The amount of work performed depends on the availability of materials and the amount of reshaping needed.

Once the reshaping is complete, the surgeon will stitch the incision closed and pack the nostrils with a dressing that reduces excess bleeding. A protective splint may also be used to support and maintain the shape of the nose as it heals. The patient may feel swelling inside the nose due to the presence of the splint. The dressing and splint will be removed in seven days during a postsurgical follow-up appointment. A "drip pad"—a small piece of gauze held with tape—will then be placed in the nose to absorb further drainage.

Postsurgery Do's and Don'ts

- Do not blow the nose.

- Avoid extreme facial expressions, such as laughing or wide smiling.

- Avoid strenuous activities, such as jogging or aerobics.

- Do not use ice/cold packs after surgery to reduce swelling of the nose, which could take a longer time to heal. Also, do not panic if you notice black-and-blue discoloration of the eyelids due to nasal swelling; this is is normal.

- Take baths instead of showers to accommodate the bandaged nose.

- Brush teeth gently to avoid vigorous movement of the upper lip.

- Do not wear clothing that needs to be removed over the head; instead, wear clothes that fasten in the front.

- Do not rest eyeglasses or sunglasses on the nose for at least a month after surgery. If you have to wear glasses, use cheek rests or tape the glasses on the forehead.

- Use SPF30 sunscreen, especially on the nose, while in sun to avoid permanent discoloration of the nose.

- Limit dietary intake of sodium to help the swelling heal faster.

- Eat a high-fiber diet to avoid constipation, as this will put pressure on the surgical site.

How Is Rhinoplasty Different from Septoplasty?

Rhinoplasty is performed to change the way that the nose looks (the cosmetic shape of the nose) or to improve breathing through the nose. Septoplasty is done to straighten the wall (septum) that divides nasal passages inside the nose when it is crooked and makes it harder to breathe through the nose. Often, a septoplasty is combined with rhinoplasty.

References

1. Cunha, John P DO, FACOEP; Balentine, Jerry R DO, FACEP. "Deviated Septum Facts," MedicineNet, May 7, 2011.

2. Robinson, Jennifer MD. "Deviated Septum," WebMD, December 12, 2018.

3. "Septoplasty," Mayoclinic, January 3, 2018.

Chapter 32

Sinus Problems

Chapter Contents

Section 32.1

Sinusitis

This section includes text excerpted from "Sinus
Infection (Sinusitis)," Centers for Disease Control
and Prevention (CDC), September 25, 2017.

A sinus infection (sinusitis) does not typically need to be treated
with antibiotics in order to get better. If you or your child is diagnosed
with a sinus infection, your healthcare professional can decide if antibiotics are needed.

Causes

Sinus infections occur when fluid is trapped or blocked in the
sinuses, allowing germs to grow. Sinus infections are usually (9 out
of 10 cases in adults; 5 to 7 out of 10 cases in children) caused by a
virus. They are less commonly (1 out of 10 cases in adults; 3 to 5 out
of 10 cases in children) caused by bacteria.

Other conditions can cause symptoms similar to a sinus infection,
including:

- Allergies
- Pollutants (airborne chemicals or irritants)
- Fungal infections

Risk Factors

Several conditions can increase your risk of getting a sinus infection:

- A previous respiratory tract infection, such as the common cold
- Structural problems within the sinuses
- A weak immune system or taking drugs that weaken the
  immune system
- Nasal polyps
- Allergies

In children, the following are also risk factors for a sinus infection:

- Going to day care
- Using a pacifier

- Drinking a bottle while laying down
- Being exposed to secondhand smoke

Signs and Symptoms

Common signs and symptoms of a sinus infection include:

- Headache
- Stuffy or runny nose
- Loss of sense of smell
- Facial pain or pressure
- Postnasal drip (mucus drips down the throat from the nose)
- Sore throat
- Fever
- Coughing
- Fatigue (being tired)
- Bad breath

When to Seek Medical Care

See a healthcare professional if you or your child has any of the following:

- Temperature higher than 100.4°F
- Symptoms that are getting worse or lasting longer than 10 days
- Multiple sinus infections in the past year
- Symptoms that are not relieved with over-the-counter (OTC) medicines

If your child is younger than three months of age and has a fever, it is important to call your healthcare professional right away.

You may have chronic sinusitis if your sinus infection lasts more than eight weeks or if you have more than four sinus infections each year. If you are diagnosed with chronic sinusitis, or believe you may have chronic sinusitis, you should visit your healthcare professional for evaluation. Chronic sinusitis can be caused by nasal growths, allergies, or respiratory tract infections (viral, bacterial, or fungal).

Diagnosis and Treatment

Your healthcare professional will determine if you or your child has a sinus infection by asking about symptoms and doing a physical examination. Sometimes, they will also swab the inside of your nose.

Antibiotics may be needed if the sinus infection is likely to be caused by bacteria. Antibiotics will not help a sinus infection caused by a virus or an irritation in the air (such as secondhand smoke). These infections will almost always get better on their own. Antibiotic treatment in these cases may even cause harm in both children and adults.

If symptoms continue for more than 10 days, schedule a follow-up appointment with your healthcare professional for re-evaluation.

Symptom Relief

Rest, over-the-counter medicines, and other self-care methods may help you or your child feel better. For more information about symptomatic relief, talk to your healthcare professional, including your pharmacist. Always use over-the-counter products as directed, since many over-the-counter products are not recommended for children of certain ages.

Prevention

There are several steps you can take to help prevent a sinus infection, including:

- Practice good hand hygiene
- Keep you and your child up to date with recommended immunizations
- Avoid close contact with people who have colds or other upper respiratory infections
- Avoid smoking and exposure to secondhand smoke
- Use a clean humidifier to moisten the air at home

Section 32.2

Sinus Surgery

This section includes text excerpted from "Endoscopic
Sinus Surgery," U.S. Department of Veterans Affairs (VA),
July 2013. Reviewed April 2019.

Your sinuses are air-filled spaces in the bones of the face and head.
The sinuses drain mucous through small openings that are linked to
the inside of the nose. They play a big role in how we breathe and
make mucous. Mucous does not drain well when you have swelling of
the lining of the nose and sinuses; an acute or chronic infection can
result. When medical therapies and sinus rinses do not clear up the
swelling, surgery may be needed to open up the sinuses and allow
them to drain. Some people grow polyps (a small growth sticking out
from the mucous lining). Surgery may be needed to remove the polyps.

Endoscopic Sinus Surgery

You will be given medicine to keep you asleep and free from pain
during surgery. There will be no incisions (cuts) made on the outside
of your nose. All surgery is done through your nostrils, using scopes.
Your doctor can see the images on a monitor. The opening to each
sinus that is blocked will be opened. Any polyps are removed. This is
a detailed surgery and must be done carefully. The surgery may take
three to four hours. If the divider between the two sides of your nose
(the nasal septum) is too crooked, it may have to be straightened. This
will allow drainage of all the sinuses. This is called "septoplasty" and
will add an extra hour to the procedure.

At the end of the surgery, your sinuses will still be oozing a little
blood. Nasal packings or foam are placed in your nostrils to stop the
bleeding. If you have nasal packing (such as a nasal tampon), you will
revisit your healthcare provider within a few days so that it can be
taken out. You need to stop taking aspirin, ibuprofen (Advil or Motrin),
naproxen (Aleve) and similar meds at least one week before surgery.
These meds can cause bleeding.

Sinus surgery is usually safe. There is a one percent risk of a major
complication. Problems that may happen due to sinus surgery may
include blindness, double vision, injury to brain tissue, and leakage of
fluid from around the brain. More common minor problems are scarring, need for more surgery, decreased sense of smell, and nosebleeds.

You can go home the same day of surgery. You will need someone to drive you home.

After Your Surgery Instructions
Nosebleed Safety Measures

You may have a slow trickle of blood down your throat or out of the front of your nose for a few days. You need to see your surgeon right away if you are having a lot of bleeding or it seems too much to you. If you are having bothersome oozing, it can help to spray oxymetazoline (Afrin), two sprays in each nostril. You can use the spray up to four times a day during the first week. Only use the spray for one week. Oxymetazoline constricts blood vessels and can decrease bleeding. However, if used longer than a week, it can hurt the lining of your nose and cause nasal congestion that is only relieved by more oxymetazoline. To decrease the risk of nosebleeds after surgery:

• Sneeze with your mouth open.

• Do not blow your nose for at least one week after surgery. You may gently wipe the front of your nose or use a sinus rinse bottle to cleanse the inside of your nose.

• Keep your head elevated to lessen swelling. This is especially important at night. You could raise the head of your bed, sleep with two to three pillows, or sleep in a recliner. Avoid bending over.

• If you take meds to control your blood pressure, make sure to take them as ordered. High blood pressure will make nosebleeds more likely.

• Do not lift anything more than 10 pounds. Do not strain yourself in any way with vigorous activity, sex, or exercise for 2 weeks after surgery.

• You need to stop taking aspirin, ibuprofen (Advil or Motrin), naproxen (Aleve) and similar meds at least one week after surgery. These meds can increase risk of nosebleeds.

Nasal / Sinus Rinses

After surgery, you need to keep your nasal cavities moist, to help blood clots dissolve and loosen crusting. Your surgeon may ask you to use nasal saline (salt water). You should use it as often during the day as you remember, or at least four to five times per day.

Your surgeon may ask you to do saline sinus rinses after surgery. You can use an over-the-counter system, such as Neil Med Sinus Rinse (you can buy it for about $11 at Walgreens, CVS, Walmart, Target, and other pharmacies). Start gentle rinses the evening after surgery. If the nose seems to be blocked, stop rinsing and gently try again the next day. This will really help dissolve clots and help nasal breathing and healing.

Activity

You need to avoid activity that raises your blood pressure for two weeks. Things that can raise your blood pressure are heavy lifting, hard exercise, and sex. This could cause a nosebleed.

Diet

You may eat your regular diet after surgery, as long as your stomach is not upset from the anesthesia. If it is, wait until you feel better before you start eating solid foods.

Pain

Pain is usually mild to moderate the first 24–48 hours. Then it will decrease. You may not need a strong narcotic pain med. The sooner you reduce your narcotic pain med use, the faster you will heal. As your pain lessens, try using extra-strength acetaminophen (Tylenol) instead of your narcotic med. It is best to reduce your pain to a level you can manage, rather than to get rid of the pain completely. Start at a lower of narcotic pain med, and increase the dose only if the pain remains uncontrolled. Decrease the dose if the side effects are too severe.

Do not drive, operate dangerous machinery, or do anything dangerous if you are taking narcotic pain medication (such as oxycodone, hydrocodone, morphine, etc.) This medication affects your reflexes and responses, similar to alcohol.

When to Call Your Surgeon

Call a surgeon if you have:

- Any concerns
- Fever over 101.5°F
- Any changes in your vision

- Headaches

- Leakage of clear fluid from your nose

- Excessive bleeding

- Pain that continues to increase instead of decrease

- Problem urinating

- If you have chest pain or difficulty breathing, do not call—go to the nearest emergency room right away

Section 32.3

Is Rinsing Your Sinuses with Neti Pots Safe?

This section includes text excerpted from "Is Rinsing Your Sinuses with Neti Pots Safe?" U.S. Food and Drug Administration (FDA), November 6, 2017.

Little teapots with long spouts have become a fixture in many homes to flush out clogged nasal passages and help people breathe easier.

Along with other nasal irrigation systems, these devices—commonly called "neti pots"—use a saline, or saltwater, solution to treat congested sinuses, colds, and allergies. They are also used to moisten nasal passages exposed to dry indoor air. But be careful. According to the U.S. Food and Drug Administration (FDA), improper use of these neti pots and other nasal rinsing devices can increase your risk of infection.

These nasal rinse devices—which include bulb syringes, squeeze bottles, and battery-operated pulsed water devices—are usually safe and effective products when used and cleaned properly, says Eric A. Mann, MD, Ph.D., a doctor at the FDA.

What does safe use mean? First, rinse only with distilled, sterile, or previously boiled water.

Tap water is not safe for use as a nasal rinse because it is not adequately filtered or treated. Some tap water contains low levels of organisms—such as bacteria and protozoa, including amoebas—that may

360

be safe to swallow because stomach acid kills them. But in your nose, these organisms can stay alive in nasal passages and cause potentially serious infections. They can even be fatal in some rare cases, according to the Centers for Disease Control and Prevention (CDC).

What Types of Water Are Safe to Use?

- Distilled or sterile water, which you can buy in stores. The label will state "distilled" or "sterile."

- Boiled and cooled tap water—boiled for 3 to 5 minutes, then cooled until it is lukewarm. Previously boiled water can be stored in a clean, closed container for use within 24 hours.

- Water passed through a filter designed to trap potentially infectious organisms. The CDC has information on selecting these filters.

Safely Use Nasal Irrigation Systems

Second, make sure you follow instructions.

"There are various ways to deliver saline to the nose. Nasal spray bottles deliver a fine mist and might be useful for moisturizing dry nasal passages. But, irrigation devices are better at flushing the nose and clearing out mucus, allergens, and bacteria," Mann says.

Information included with the irrigation device might give more specific instructions about its use and care. These devices all work in basically the same way:

- Leaning over a sink, tilt your head sideways with your forehead and chin roughly level to avoid liquid flowing into your mouth.

- Breathing through your open mouth, insert the spout of the saline-filled container into your upper nostril so that the liquid drains through the lower nostril.

- Clear your nostrils. Then repeat the procedure, tilting your head sideways, on the other side.

Sinus rinsing can remove dust, pollen, and other debris, as well as help to loosen thick mucus. It can also help relieve nasal symptoms of sinus infections, allergies, colds, and flu. Plain water can irritate your nose. The saline allows the water to pass through delicate nasal membranes with little or no burning or irritation.

361

And if your immune system is not working properly, consult your healthcare provider before using any nasal irrigation systems.

To use and care for your device:

- Wash and dry your hands.

- Check that the device is clean and completely dry.

- Prepare the saline rinse, either with the prepared mixture supplied with the device or one you make yourself.

- Follow the manufacturer's directions for use.

- Wash the device, and dry the inside with a paper towel or let it air dry between uses.

Talk with a healthcare provider or pharmacist if the instructions on your device do not clearly state how to use it or if you have any questions.

Nasal Rinsing Devices and Children

Finally, make sure the device fits the age of the person using it. Some children are diagnosed with nasal allergies as early as two years of age and could use nasal rinsing devices at that time, if a pediatrician recommends it. But, very young children might not tolerate the procedure.

Whether for a child or adult, talk to your healthcare provider to determine whether nasal rinsing will be safe or effective for your condition. If symptoms are not relieved or worsen after nasal rinsing, then return to your healthcare provider, especially if you have fever, nosebleeds or headaches while using the nasal rinse.

Healthcare professionals and patients can report problems about nasal rinsing devices to the FDA's MedWatch Safety Information and Adverse Event Reporting Program.

Chapter 33

Snoring and Sleep Apnea

Snoring

Snoring is the sound you make when your breathing is blocked while you are asleep. The sound is caused by tissues at the top of your airway that strike each other and vibrate. Snoring is common, especially among older people and people who are overweight.

When severe, snoring can cause frequent awakenings at night and daytime sleepiness. It can disrupt your bed partner's sleep. Snoring can also be a sign of a serious sleep disorder called "sleep apnea." You should see your healthcare provider if you are often tired during the day, do not feel that you sleep well, or wake up gasping.

To reduce snoring

- Lose weight if you are overweight. It may help, but thin people snore too.

- Cut down or avoid alcohol and other sedatives at bedtime.

- Do not sleep flat on your back.

This chapter contains text excerpted from the following sources: Text under the heading "Snoring" is excerpted from "Snoring," MedlinePlus, National Institutes of Health (NIH), August 4, 2016; Text beginning with the heading "What Is Sleep Apnea?" is excerpted from "Sleep Apnea," National Heart, Lung, and Blood Institute (NHLBI), December 10, 2018.

What Is Sleep Apnea?

Sleep apnea is a common condition in the United States. It can occur when the upper airway becomes blocked repeatedly during sleep, reducing or completely stopping airflow. This is known as "obstructive sleep apnea." If the brain does not send the signals needed to breathe, the condition may be called "central sleep apnea."

Healthcare providers use sleep studies to diagnose sleep apnea. They record the number of episodes of slow or stopped breathing and the number of central sleep apnea events detected in an hour. They also determine whether oxygen levels in the blood are lower during these events.

Breathing devices, such as continuous positive air pressure (CPAP) machines, and lifestyle changes are common sleep apnea treatments. Undiagnosed or untreated sleep apnea can lead to serious complications, such as heart attack, glaucoma, diabetes, cancer, and cognitive and behavioral disorders.

Causes of Sleep Apnea

Sleep apnea can be caused by a person's physical structure or medical conditions. These include obesity, large tonsils, endocrine disorders, neuromuscular disorders, heart or kidney failure, certain genetic syndromes, and premature birth.

Obesity

Obesity is a common cause of sleep apnea in adults. People with this condition have increased fat deposits in their necks that can block the upper airway.

Large Tonsils

Large tonsils may contribute to sleep apnea because they narrow the upper airway.

Endocrine Disorders

The endocrine system produces hormone that can affect sleep-related breathing. The following are examples of endocrine disorders associated with sleep apnea.

- **Hypothyroidism:** People with this condition have low levels of thyroid hormones. This affects the part of the brain that controls breathing, as well as the nerves and muscles used to breathe. People with hypothyroidism can also be diagnosed with obesity, which can cause sleep apnea.

- **Acromegaly:** People with this condition have high levels of growth hormone. This condition is associated with changes in the facial bones, swelling of the throat, and increased size of the tongue. These changes can obstruct the upper airway and lead to sleep apnea.

- **Polycystic ovary syndrome (PCOS):** Sleep apnea is also seen in women with PCOS, an endocrine condition that causes large ovaries and prevents proper ovulation. PCOS is also associated with being overweight or obese, which can cause sleep apnea.

Neuromuscular Conditions

Conditions interfering with brain signals to airway and chest muscles can cause sleep apnea. Some of these conditions are stroke, amyotrophic lateral sclerosis (ALS), Chiari malformations, myotonic dystrophy, postpolio syndrome, dermatomyositis, myasthenia gravis (MG), and Lambert-Eaton myasthenic syndrome (LEMS).

Heart or Kidney Failure

Sleep apnea is commonly found in people who have advanced heart or kidney failure. These patients may have fluid buildup in their neck, which can obstruct the upper airway and cause sleep apnea.

Genetic Syndromes

Genetic syndromes that affect the structure of the face or skull, particularly syndromes that cause smaller facial bones or cause the tongue to sit further back in the mouth, may cause sleep apnea. These genetic syndromes include cleft lip and cleft palate, Down syndrome, and congenital central hypoventilation syndrome (CCHS).

Premature Birth

Babies born before 37 weeks of pregnancy have a higher risk of breathing problems during sleep. In most cases, the risk decreases as the brain matures.

Risk Factors of Sleep Apnea

There are many risk factors for sleep apnea. Some risk factors, such as unhealthy lifestyle habits and environments, can be changed. Other risk factors, such as age, family history and genetics, race and ethnicity, and sex, cannot be changed. Healthy lifestyle changes can decrease your risk for developing sleep apnea.

Age

Sleep apnea can occur at any age. The risk for sleep apnea increases as you get older. In younger adults, sleep apnea is more common in men than in women, but the difference decreases later in life. Normal age-related changes in how the brain controls breathing during sleep partially explain the increased risk as you get older. Another possible reason is that as we age, more fatty tissue builds up in the neck and the tongue.

Unhealthy Lifestyle Habits

Drinking alcohol, smoking, and being overweight or obese can increase your risk for sleep apnea.

- Alcohol can increase relaxation of the muscles in the mouth and throat, closing the upper airway. It can also affect how the brain controls sleep or the muscles involved in breathing.

- Smoking can cause inflammation in the upper airway, affecting breathing, or it can affect how the brain controls sleep or the muscles involved in breathing.

- Unhealthy eating patterns and lack of physical activity can lead to one being overweight or obese, which can result in sleep apnea.

Family History and Genetics

Researchers have identified family history as a risk factor for sleep apnea, but maintaining a healthy lifestyle can decrease this risk. Studies in twins have shown that sleep apnea can be inherited. Some of the genes related to sleep apnea are associated with the structural development of the face and skull and with how the brain controls sleep and breathing during sleep. Some genes are also associated with obesity and inflammation.

Race or Ethnicity

In the United States, sleep apnea is more common among Blacks, Hispanics, and Native Americans than among Whites.

Signs, Symptoms, and Complications of Sleep Apnea

Common sleep apnea signs and symptoms are snoring or gasping during sleep; reduced or absent breathing, which is called "apnea events"; and sleepiness. Undiagnosed or untreated sleep apnea prevents restful sleep and can cause complications that may affect many parts of your body.

Signs and Symptoms

Common signs of sleep apnea:

- Reduced or absent breathing, known as "apnea events"
- Frequent loud snoring
- Gasping for air during sleep

Common symptoms of sleep apnea:

- Excessive daytime sleepiness and fatigue
- Decreases in attention, vigilance, concentration, motor skills, and verbal and visuospatial memory
- Dry mouth or headaches when waking
- Sexual dysfunction or decreased libido
- Waking up often during the night to urinate

Did you know that sleep apnea symptoms may be different for women and children when compared with men?

Women who have sleep apnea more often report headache, fatigue, depression, anxiety, insomnia, and sleep disruption. Children may experience bedwetting, asthma exacerbations, hyperactivity, and learning and academic performance issues.

Screening and Prevention of Sleep Apnea

To screen for sleep apnea, your doctor will review your medical history and symptoms. To prevent sleep apnea, your doctor may recommend healthy lifestyle changes.

Screening for Sleep Apnea

To screen for sleep apnea or other sleep disorders, your doctor may ask you about common signs and symptoms of this condition, such as how sleepy you feel during the day or when driving and whether you or your partner has noticed that you snore, stop breathing, or gasp during your sleep. Your doctor may ask questions to assess your risk for developing this condition and take your physical measurements. Your doctor will also want to see whether you have any complications of undiagnosed sleep apnea, such as high blood pressure, that is difficult to control. If the screening suggests a sleep breathing disorder, you may get a referral to a sleep specialist to help confirm a diagnosis.

Healthy Lifestyle Changes to Prevent Sleep Apnea

If you are concerned about having risk factors for developing sleep apnea, ask your doctor to recommend healthy lifestyle changes, including eating a heart-healthy diet, aiming for a healthy weight, quitting smoking, and limiting alcohol intake. Your doctor may recommend that you sleep on your side and adopt healthy sleep habits, such as getting the recommended amount of sleep.

Complications

Sleep apnea may increase your risk of the following disorders:

- Asthma

- Atrial fibrillation

- Cancers, such as pancreatic, renal, and skin cancers

- Chronic kidney disease (CKD)

- Cognitive and behavioral disorders, such as decreases in attention, vigilance, concentration, motor skills, and verbal and visuospatial memory, as well as dementia in older adults. In children, sleep apnea has been associated with learning disabilities.

- Diseases of the heart and blood vessels, such as atherosclerosis, heart attacks, heart failure, difficult-to-control high blood pressure, and stroke

- Eye disorders, such as glaucoma, dry eye, or keratoconus

- Metabolic disorders, including glucose intolerance and type 2 diabetes

- Pregnancy complications, including gestational diabetes and gestational high blood pressure, as well as having a baby with low birth weight

Did you know that sleep apnea can cause inflammation and lead to complications?

When blood oxygen levels drop due to obstructive sleep apnea, your body and brain trigger the "fight or flight" response. This increases your blood pressure and heart rate and wakes you from sleep so that your upper airway can open. These cycles of decreased and increased blood oxygen levels can cause inflammation that may contribute to atherosclerosis, the buildup of plaque in blood vessels, which can increase the risk of heart attack or stroke. Chronic inflammation can also damage the pancreas and lead to type 2 diabetes.

Diagnosis of Sleep Apnea

Your doctor may diagnose sleep apnea based on your medical history, a physical exam, and results from a sleep study. Before diagnosing you with sleep apnea, your doctor will rule out other medical reasons or conditions that may be causing your signs and symptoms.

Medical History

To help diagnose sleep apnea, your doctor may consider the following:

- Information that you provide, such as signs and symptoms that you are experiencing

- Whether you have a family history of sleep apnea or another sleep disorder

- Whether you have risk factors for sleep apnea

- Whether you have complications of undiagnosed or untreated sleep apnea, such as atrial fibrillation, type 2 diabetes, or hard-to-control high blood pressure

Physical Exam

During the physical exam, your doctor will look for signs of other conditions that can increase your risk for sleep apnea, such as obesity, large tonsils, narrowing of the upper airway, or a large neck circumference. A neck circumference greater than 17 inches for men or 16 inches for women is considered large. Your doctor may also look at your jaw size and structure, the size of your tongue, and your tongue's position in your mouth. Your doctor will check your lungs, heart, and neurological systems to see whether you have any common complications of sleep apnea.

Sleep Studies

To diagnose sleep apnea or another sleep disorder, your doctor may refer you to a sleep specialist or a center for a sleep study. Sleep studies can be done in a special center or at home. Studies at a sleep center can:

- Detect apnea events

- Detect low or high levels of activity in muscles that control breathing

- Monitor blood oxygen levels during sleep

- Monitor brain and heart activity during sleep

Your doctor may be able to diagnose mild, moderate, or severe sleep apnea based on the number of sleep apnea events you have in an hour during the sleep study.

- **Mild:** 5 to 14 apnea events in an hour

- **Moderate:** 15 to 29 apnea events in an hour

- **Severe:** 30 or more apnea events in an hour

Did you know that sleep studies can help determine which type of sleep apnea you have?

Sleep studies can monitor the movement of your muscles and help determine breathing patterns and whether you have obstructive or central sleep apnea. Sleep studies of patients with obstructive sleep apnea often show an increase in breathing muscle activity when muscles try to open an obstructed upper airway. In contrast, sleep studies of patients with central sleep apnea tend to show decreased activity in chest muscles, which can lead to periods of slowed or no breathing.

Ruling Out Other Medical Reasons or Conditions

Your doctor may order the following tests to help rule out other medical conditions that can cause sleep apnea:

- **Blood tests** to check the levels of certain hormones and to rule out endocrine disorders that could be contributing to sleep apnea. Thyroid hormone can rule out hypothyroidism. Growth hormone tests can rule out acromegaly. Total testosterone and dehydroepiandrosterone sulfate (DHEAS) tests can help rule out polycystic ovary syndrome (PCOS).

- **Pelvic ultrasound** to examine the ovaries and detect cysts. This can rule out PCOS.

Your doctor will also want to know whether you are using medicines, such as opioids, that could be affecting your sleep or causing breathing symptoms of sleep apnea. Your doctor may want to know whether you have traveled recently to altitudes greater than 6,000 feet, because these low-oxygen environments can cause symptoms of sleep apnea for a few weeks after traveling.

Treatment of Sleep Apnea

If you are diagnosed with sleep apnea, your doctor may make recommendations to help you maintain an open airway during sleep. These could include healthy lifestyle changes or a breathing device, such as a positive airway pressure (PAP) machine, mouthpiece, or implant. Talk to your doctor. Depending on the type and severity of your sleep apnea and your needs and preferences, other treatments may be possible.

Healthy Lifestyle Changes

To help control or treat your sleep apnea, your doctor may recommend that you adopt lifelong healthy lifestyle changes.

- **Make heart-healthy eating choices.** This also includes limiting your alcohol intake, especially before bedtime.

- **Get regular physical activity.**

- **Aim for a healthy weight.** Research has shown that losing weight can reduce sleep apnea in people who were also diagnosed with obesity.

- **Develop healthy sleeping habits.** Your doctor may recommend general healthy sleep habits, which include getting the recommended amount of sleep based on your age.

- **Quit smoking.** For free help and support to quit smoking, call the National Cancer Institute's (NCI) smoking quitline at 877-44U-QUIT (877-448-7848).

Breathing Devices

A breathing device, such as a CPAP machine, is the most commonly recommended treatment for patients with sleep apnea. If your doctor prescribes a CPAP or other breathing device, be sure to continue your doctor-recommended healthy lifestyle changes.

Mouthpieces

Mouthpieces, or oral appliances, are typically custom-fit devices that you wear while you sleep. There are two types of mouthpieces that work differently to open the upper airway. Some hybrid mouthpieces have features of both types.

- **Mandibular repositioning mouthpieces** are devices that cover the upper and lower teeth and hold the jaw in a position that prevents it from blocking the upper airway.

- **Tongue retaining devices** are mouthpieces that hold the tongue in a forward position to prevent it from blocking the upper airway.

Your doctor may prescribe a mouthpiece if you have mild sleep apnea or if your apnea occurs only when you are lying on your back. To get your mouthpiece, your doctor may recommend that you visit a dentist or an orthodontist, a type of dentist who specializes in correcting teeth or jaw problems. These specialists will ensure that the oral appliance is custom fit to your mouth and jaw.

Implants

Implants can benefit some people with sleep apnea. Some devices treat both obstructive and central sleep apnea. You must have surgery to place an implant in your body. The U.S. Food and Drug Administration (FDA) has approved one implant as a treatment for sleep apnea. The device senses breathing patterns and delivers mild stimulation to certain muscles that open the airways during sleep. More research is needed to determine how effective the implant is in treating central sleep apnea.

A nerve stimulator can also treat sleep apnea. This treatment also involves surgery. A surgeon will insert a stimulator for the hypoglossal nerve, which controls tongue movement. Increasing stimulation of this nerve helps position the tongue to keep the upper airway open.

Therapy for Mouth and Facial Muscles

Children and adults with sleep apnea may benefit from therapy for mouth and facial muscles, known as "orofacial therapy." This therapy helps improve tongue positioning and strengthen muscles that control the lips, tongue, soft palate, lateral pharyngeal wall, and face.

Surgical Procedures

You may need surgery if you have severe obstructive sleep apnea (OSA) that does not respond to breathing devices, such as a CPAP machine, or that is caused by visible obstruction to the upper airway, perhaps due to large tonsils. Possible surgical procedures include:

- **Tonsillectomy:** a surgery to remove the tonsils, which are organs at the back of your throat

- **Maxillary or jaw advancement:** a surgery to move the upper jaw (maxilla) and lower jaw (mandible) forward, to enlarge the upper airway

- **Tracheostomy:** a surgery to make a hole through the front of your neck into your trachea, or windpipe. A breathing tube, called a "trach tube," is placed through the hole and directly into your windpipe to help you breathe.

If surgery is considered as a possible treatment, talk to your doctor about the different types of surgical procedures, the risks and benefits of the procedures, potential discomfort, and the recovery time you will need after surgery.

Living with Sleep Apnea

If you have been diagnosed with sleep apnea, it is important that you adopt and maintain healthy lifestyle habits and use your prescribed treatment. Learn about how to use and care for your breathing device or mouthpiece, how your doctor may monitor whether your treatment is working, when you may need a repeat sleep study, and other tips to keep you safe if you have sleep apnea.

Using and Caring for Your Breathing Device or Mouthpiece

It is important that you properly use and care for your prescribed breathing device or mouthpiece. If your doctor prescribed a breathing device or CPAP machine:

- **Be patient with your breathing device or CPAP machine.** It may take time to adjust to breathing with the help of a CPAP machine.

- **Use your breathing device or CPAP machine for all sleep, including naps.** To benefit fully from your treatment, you should wear your device whenever and wherever you sleep. If you are traveling, be sure to bring your breathing device with you. Call your doctor or sleep specialist right away if your device stops working correctly.

- **Talk to your doctor or supplier if you experience discomfort or have difficulty using your prescribed breathing device.** Let the team or supplier know if you are having irritation from the mask, if your mask is not staying on or fitting well, if it leaks air, if you are having difficulty falling or staying asleep, if you wake with dry mouth, or if you have a stuffy or runny nose. Your doctor can explore options to improve the treatment, such as trying different masks or nasal pillows, adjusting the machine's pressure timing and settings, or trying a different breathing device that has a humidifier chamber or provides bi-level or auto-adjusting pressure settings. Cleaning the mask and washing your face before putting your mask on can help make a better seal between the mask and your skin.

- **Properly care for your breathing device or CPAP machine.** Know how to set up and properly clean all parts of your machine. Be sure to refill prescriptions on time for all of the device's replaceable parts, including the tubes, masks, and air filters.

- **Properly care for your mouthpiece.** If you were prescribed a mouthpiece, ask your dentist how to properly care for it. If it does not fit right or your signs and symptoms do not improve, let your dentist know so that she or he can adjust the device. It is common to feel some discomfort after a device is adjusted until your mouth and facial muscles get used to the new fit.

Monitor Your Condition

You should visit your doctor to monitor your response to treatment and see whether you have any complications that, if left untreated, can be life-threatening. Your doctor may do any of the following to monitor your condition.

- **If your doctor prescribed a breathing device, your doctor and possibly your insurance company will want to check the data card from the machine.** The data card shows how often you use the breathing device and whether the device and its pressure settings are helping to reduce or eliminate apnea events while you sleep. Your doctor may also check to see whether you still experience excessive sleepiness during the day, how you feel about your quality of life, whether you are still snoring, or whether have experienced weight loss or changes in your lifestyle.

- **If you were prescribed a mouthpiece, you should follow up with your dental specialist after six months and then at least every year.** This is to see whether the mouthpiece is working correctly, whether it needs adjustment, and whether a replacement device is needed.

Repeat Sleep Studies

Sometimes, repeat sleep studies are necessary. Your doctor may have you repeat a sleep study to monitor your response to the treatment, especially if your sleep symptoms continue, if you are using a mouthpiece, if your weight changes significantly, or if your employer requires these tests.

Learn the Warning Signs of Some Continuous Positive Air Pressure Side Effects

Side effects of CPAP treatment may include congestion, runny nose, dry mouth, dry eyes, or nosebleeds. If you experience stomach discomfort or bloating, you should stop using your CPAP machine and contact your doctor.

Learn about Other Precautions to Help You Stay Safe

Sleep apnea can increase your risks of complications if you are having surgery, and it can affect your ability to drive.

375

- **Before surgery.** If you are having any type of surgery that requires medicine to put you to sleep or for pain management, let your surgeon and doctors know that you have sleep apnea. They might have to take extra steps to make sure that your upper airway stays open during the surgery and when selecting your pain medicines.

- **Driving precautions.** Undiagnosed and untreated sleep apnea can decrease learning capabilities, slow down decision-making, and decrease attention span, which can result in drowsy driving.

Chapter 34

Smell and Taste Disorders

Chapter Contents

Section 34.1

Smell Disorders

This section includes text excerpted from "Smell Disorders,"
National Institute on Deafness and Other Communication
Disorders (NIDCD), May 12, 2017.

Your sense of smell helps you enjoy life. You may delight in the
aromas of your favorite foods or the fragrance of flowers. Your sense
of smell is also a warning system, alerting you to danger signals such
as a gas leak, spoiled food, or a fire. Any loss in your sense of smell
can have a negative effect on your quality of life (QOL). It can also be
a sign of more serious health problems.

1 to 2 percent of North Americans report problems with their sense
of smell. Problems with the sense of smell increase as people get older,
and they are more common in men than women. In one study, nearly
one-quarter of men between the ages of 60 and 69 had a smell disorder,
while about 11 percent of women in that age range reported a problem.

Many people who have smell disorders also notice problems with
their sense of taste.

What Are the Smell Disorders?

People who have smell disorders either have a decrease in their
ability to smell or changes in the way they perceive odors.

- Hyposmia is a reduced ability to detect odors.

- Anosmia is the complete inability to detect odors. In rare cases,
  someone may be born without a sense of smell, a condition called
  "congenital anosmia."

- Parosmia is a change in the normal perception of odors, such
  as when the smell of something familiar is distorted or when
  something that normally smells pleasant now smells foul.

- Phantosmia is the sensation of an odor that is not there.

What Causes Smell Disorders

Smell disorders have many causes, with some more obvious than
others. Most people who develop a smell disorder have experienced a
recent illness or injury. Common causes of smell disorders are:

- Aging

- Sinus and other upper respiratory infections

- Smoking

- Growths in the nasal cavities

- Head injury

- Hormonal disturbances

- Dental problems

- Exposure to certain chemicals, such as insecticides and solvents

- Numerous medications, including some common antibiotics and antihistamines

- Radiation for treatment of head and neck cancers

- Conditions that affect the nervous system, such as Parkinson disease (PD) or Alzheimer disease (AD)

How Are Smell Disorders Diagnosed and Treated?

Both smell and taste disorders are treated by an otolaryngologist, a doctor who specializes in diseases of the ear, nose, throat, head, and neck (sometimes called an "ENT"). An accurate assessment of a smell disorder will include, among other things, a physical examination of the ears, nose, and throat; a review of your health history, such as exposure to toxic chemicals or injury; and a smell test supervised by a healthcare professional.

There are two common ways to test smell. Some tests are designed to measure the smallest amount of odor that someone can detect. Another common test consists of a paper booklet of pages that contain tiny beads filled with specific odors. People are asked to scratch each page and identify the odor. If they cannot smell the odor, or they identify it incorrectly, it could indicate a smell disorder or an impaired ability to smell.

Diagnosis by a doctor is important to identify and treat the underlying cause of a potential smell disorder. If your problem is caused by medications, talk to your doctor to see if lowering the dosage or changing the medicine could reduce its effect on your sense of smell. If nasal obstructions, such as polyps, are restricting the airflow in your nose, you might need surgery to remove them and restore your sense of smell.

Some people recover their ability to smell when they recover from the illness causing their loss of smell. Some people recover their sense of smell spontaneously, for no obvious reason. If your smell disorder cannot be successfully treated, you might want to seek counseling to help you adjust.

Are Smell Disorders Serious?

Like all of your senses, your sense of smell plays an important part in your life. Your sense of smell often serves as a first warning signal, alerting you to the smoke of a fire, spoiled food, or the odor of a natural gas leak or dangerous fumes.

When their smell is impaired, some people change their eating habits. Some may eat too little and lose weight, while others may eat too much and gain weight. As food becomes less enjoyable, you might use too much salt to improve the taste. This can be a problem if you have or are at risk for certain medical conditions, such as high blood pressure or kidney disease. In severe cases, loss of smell can lead to depression.

Problems with your chemical senses may be a sign of other serious health conditions. A smell disorder can be an early sign of Parkinson disease, Alzheimer disease, or multiple sclerosis (MS). It can also be related to other medical conditions, such as obesity, diabetes, hypertension, and malnutrition. If you are experiencing a smell disorder, talk with your doctor.

What Research Is Being Done on Smell Disorders?

The National Institute on Deafness and Other Communication Disorders (NIDCD) supports basic and clinical research of smell and taste disorders at its laboratories in Bethesda, Maryland and at universities and chemosensory research centers across the country. These chemosensory scientists are exploring how to:

- Promote the regeneration of sensory nerve cells

- Understand the effects of the environment (such as gasoline fumes, chemicals, and extremes of humidity and temperature) on smell and taste

- Prevent the effects of aging on smell and taste

- Develop new diagnostic tests for taste and smell disorders

- Understand associations between smell disorders and changes in diet and food preferences in the elderly or among people with chronic illnesses

Section 34.2

Taste Disorders

This section includes text excerpted from "Taste Disorders,"
National Institute on Deafness and Other Communication
Disorders (NIDCD), May 12, 2017.

Many of us take our sense of taste for granted, but a taste disorder can have a negative effect on your health and quality of life (QOL). If you are having a problem with your sense of taste, you are not alone. More than 200,000 people visit a doctor each year for problems with their ability to taste or smell. Scientists believe that up to 15 percent of adults might have a taste or smell problem, but many do not seek a doctor's help.

The senses of taste and smell are very closely related. Most people who go to the doctor because they think they have lost their sense of taste are surprised to learn that they have a smell disorder instead.

How Does Your Sense of Taste Work?

Your ability to taste comes from tiny molecules released when you chew, drink, or digest food; these molecules stimulate special sensory cells in the mouth and throat. These taste cells, or gustatory cells, are clustered within the taste buds of the tongue and roof of the mouth and are along the lining of the throat. Many of the small bumps on the tip of your tongue contain taste buds. At birth, you have about 10,000 taste buds, but after the age of 50, you may start to lose them.

When the taste cells are stimulated, they send messages through three specialized taste nerves to the brain, where specific tastes are identified. Taste cells have receptors that respond to one of at least five basic taste qualities: sweet, sour, bitter, salty, and umami. Umami, or savory, is the taste you get from glutamate, which is found in chicken broth, meat extracts, and some cheeses. A common misconception is that taste cells that respond to different tastes are found in separate regions of the tongue. In humans, the different types of taste cells are scattered throughout the tongue.

Taste quality is just one way that you experience a certain food. Another chemosensory mechanism, called the "common chemical sense," involves thousands of nerve endings, especially on the moist surfaces of the eyes, nose, mouth, and throat. These nerve endings give rise to sensations such as the coolness of mint and the burning or irritation of chili peppers. Other specialized nerves create the sensations

381

of heat, cold, and texture. When you eat, the sensations from the five taste qualities, together with the sensations from the common chemical sense and the sensations of heat, cold, and texture, combine with a food's aroma to produce a perception of flavor. It is the flavor that lets you know whether you are eating a pear or an apple.

Most people who think they have a taste disorder actually have a problem with smell. When you chew food, aromas are released that activate your sense of smell by way of a special channel that connects the roof of the throat to the nose. If this channel is blocked, such as when your nose is stuffed up by a cold or flu, odors cannot reach sensory cells in the nose that are stimulated by smells. As a result, you lose much of your enjoyment of flavor. Without smell, foods tend to taste bland and have little or no flavor.

What Are the Taste Disorders

The most common taste disorder is phantom taste perception: a lingering, often unpleasant taste even though there is nothing in your mouth. People can also experience a reduced ability to taste sweet, sour, bitter, salty, and umami—a condition called "hypogeusia." Some people cannot detect any tastes, which is called "ageusia." True taste loss, however, is rare. Most often, people are experiencing a loss of smell instead of a loss of taste.

In other disorders of the chemical senses, an odor, a taste, or a flavor may be distorted. Dysgeusia is a condition in which a foul, salty, rancid, or metallic taste sensation persists in the mouth. Dysgeusia is sometimes accompanied by burning mouth syndrome, a condition in which a person experiences a painful burning sensation in the mouth. Although it can affect anyone, burning mouth syndrome is most common in middle-aged and older women.

What Causes Taste Disorders

Some people are born with taste disorders, but most develop them after an injury or illness. Among the causes of taste problems are:

- Upper respiratory and middle ear infections
- Radiation therapy for cancers of the head and neck
- Exposure to certain chemicals, such as insecticides and some medications, including some common antibiotics and antihistamines
- Head injury

- Some surgeries to the ear, nose, and throat (such as middle ear surgery) or extraction of the third molar (wisdom tooth)

- Poor oral hygiene and dental problems

How Are Taste Disorders Diagnosed?

Both taste and smell disorders are diagnosed by an otolaryngologist (sometimes called an "ENT doctor"), a doctor of the ear, nose, throat, head, and neck. An otolaryngologist can determine the extent of your taste disorder by measuring the lowest concentration of a taste quality that you can detect or recognize. You may be asked to compare the tastes of different substances or to note how the intensity of a taste grows when a substance's concentration is increased.

Scientists have developed taste tests in which the patient responds to different chemical concentrations. This may involve a simple "sip, spit, and rinse" test, or chemicals may be applied directly to specific areas of the tongue.

An accurate assessment of your taste loss will include, among other things, a physical examination of your ears, nose, and throat; a dental examination and assessment of oral hygiene; a review of your health history; and a taste test supervised by a healthcare professional.

Can Taste Disorders Be Treated?

Diagnosis by an otolaryngologist is important to identify and treat the underlying cause of your disorder. If a certain medication is the cause, stopping or changing your medicine may help eliminate the problem. (Do not stop taking your medications unless directed by your doctor, however.) Often, the correction of a general medical problem can correct the loss of taste. For example, people who lose their sense of taste because of respiratory infections or allergies may regain it when these conditions resolve. Occasionally, a person may recover her or his sense of taste spontaneously. Proper oral hygiene is important to regaining and maintaining a well-functioning sense of taste. If your taste disorder cannot be successfully treated, counseling may help you adjust to your problem.

If you lose some or all of your sense of taste, here are things you can try to make your food taste better:

- Prepare foods with a variety of colors and textures.

- Use aromatic herbs and hot spices to add more flavor; however, avoid adding more sugar or salt to foods.

- If your diet permits, add small amounts of cheese, bacon bits, butter, olive oil, or toasted nuts on vegetables.

- Avoid combination dishes, such as casseroles, that can hide individual flavors and dilute taste.

Are Taste Disorders Serious?

Taste disorders can weaken or remove an early warning system that most of us take for granted. Taste helps you detect spoiled food or liquids and, for some people, the presence of ingredients to which they are allergic.

Loss of taste can create serious health issues. A distorted sense of taste can be a risk factor for heart disease, diabetes, stroke, and other illnesses that require sticking to a specific diet. When taste is impaired, a person may change his or her eating habits. Some people may eat too little and lose weight, while others may eat too much and gain weight.

Loss of taste can cause you to add too much sugar or salt to make food taste better. This can be a problem for people with certain medical conditions, such as diabetes or high blood pressure. In severe cases, loss of taste can lead to depression.

If you are experiencing a taste disorder, talk with your doctor.

What Research Is Being Done about Taste Disorders?

The National Institute on Deafness and Other Communication Disorders (NIDCD) supports basic and clinical investigations of smell and taste disorders at its laboratories in Bethesda, Maryland and at universities and chemosensory research centers across the country. These chemosensory scientists are exploring how to:

- Prevent the effects of aging on taste and smell

- Develop new diagnostic tests

- Understand associations between taste disorders and changes in diet and food preferences in the elderly or among people with chronic illnesses

- Improve treatment methods and rehabilitation strategies

Some recent chemosensory research focuses on identifying the key receptors expressed by taste cells and understanding how those receptors send signals to the brain. Researchers are also working to develop a better understanding of how sweet and bitter substances attach to their targeted receptors. This research holds promise for the development of sugar or salt substitutes that could help combat obesity or hypertension, as well as the development of bitter blockers that could make life-saving medicines more acceptable to children. Taste cells—as well as sensory cells that help you smell—are the only sensory cells in the human body that are regularly replaced throughout life. Researchers are exploring how and why this happens so that they might find ways to replace other damaged sensory cells.

NIDCD-funded researchers have shown that small variations in our genetic code can raise or lower our sensitivity to sweet tastes, which might influence our desire for sweets. Scientists are also working to find out why some medications and medical procedures can have a harmful effect on our senses of taste and smell. They hope to develop treatments to help restore the sense of taste to people who have lost it.

Scientists are gaining a better understanding of why the same receptor that helps your tongue detect sweet taste can also be found in the human stomach. NIDCD-funded scientists have shown that the sweet receptor helps the intestine to sense and absorb sugar and turn up the production of blood sugar-regulation hormones, including the hormone that regulates insulin release. Further research may help scientists develop drugs targeting the gut taste receptors to treat obesity and diabetes.

Section 34.3

Taste and Smell-Related Statistics

This section includes text excerpted from "Quick Statistics about Taste and Smell," National Institute on Deafness and Other Communication Disorders (NIDCD), February 27, 2019.

Taste

The following are the statistics related to taste disorders:

- Almost 1 in 5 Americans (or 19 percent) over the age of 40 reports some alteration in their sense of taste.

- The prevalence of reported alterations in the sense of taste increases with age, and is at 27 percent for people 80 years of age and older.

- Risk factors include dry mouth, nose/facial injury, lower educational attainment, and fair/poor health.

- 1 in 20 Americans (or 5 percent) reports experiencing dysgeusia, a disorder characterized by distorted taste. This disorder is often persistent.

  - Dysgeusia is more commonly reported in women (64 percent of reported cases).

- Based on their genetics, certain people can taste the bitterness of phenylthiocarbamide (PTC) or a related substance called "6-n-propylthiouracil" (PROP). In the U.S., about 25 percent are super-tasters who describe PTC as extremely bitter, 50 percent are medium tasters of PTC, and 25 percent cannot taste PTC. Medium tasters and especially super-tasters tend to dislike more types of food, particularly if they are strongly flavored.

  - The ability to taste PTC/PROP varies around the world and among different ethnic and racial groups.

Smell

The following are the statistics related to smell disorders:

- Nearly 1 in 4 Americans (or 23 percent) over the age of 40 reports some alteration in their sense of smell.

  - Rates increase in older populations and are highest for those over 80 years of age, at 32 percent.

  - Risk factors include sinonasal symptoms (of the nose and sinuses), heavy drinking, previous loss of consciousness from head injury, poverty, and dry mouth.

- Approximately 1 in 15 Americans (or 6.5 percent) over the age of 40 reports sometimes experiencing phantom odor perception.

  - Women are more likely to report phantom odors, particularly if they are between the ages of 40 and 60, compared to individuals older than 60 years of age.

  - Those with a history of head injury or poor overall health are more likely to report phantom odors.

- Approximately 1 in 8 Americans over the age of 40 (up to 13.3 million people, or 12.4 percent of the population) have measurable smell dysfunction.

  - Approximately 3 percent of Americans have anosmia (no sense of smell) or severe hyposmia (minimal sense of smell).

  - The prevalence of any type of smell impairment increases with age: 4 percent in Americans between the ages of 40 and 49, 11 percent in Americans between the ages of 50 and 59, 13 percent in Americans between the ages of 60 and 69, 25 percent in Americans between 70 and 79 years of age, and 39 percent in Americans 80 years of age and older.

  - The prevalence of smell impairment is higher in men, ethnic minorities (non-Hispanic Black and Mexican American), and in those with lower educational attainment and/or family income.

Part Six

Disorders of the Throat and Vocal Cords

Chapter 35

Sore Throat

Chapter Contents

Section 35.1

Understanding Sore Throat

This section includes text excerpted from "Sore Throat,"
Centers for Disease Control and Prevention (CDC),
April 17, 2015. Reviewed April 2019.

Most sore throats will go away on their own without antibiotics. In some cases (such as for strep throat), a lab test will need to be done to see if you or your child need antibiotics.

Causes

Most sore throats are caused by viruses, such as the ones that cause a cold or the flu, and do not need antibiotic treatment.

Some sore throats are caused by bacteria, such as group A Streptococcus (group A strep). Sore throats caused by these bacteria are known as "strep throat." In children, 20 to 30 out of every 100 sore throats are strep throat. In adults, only 5 to 15 out of every 100 sore throats is strep throat.

Other common causes of sore throats include:

- Allergies

- Dry air

- Pollution (airborne chemicals or irritants)

- Smoking or exposure to secondhand smoke

Risk Factors

There are many things that can increase your risk for a sore throat, including:

- Age (children and teens between 5 and 15 years of age are most likely to get a sore throat)

- Exposure to someone with a sore throat or strep throat

- Time of year (winter and early spring are common times for strep throat)

- Weather (cold air can irritate your throat)

- Irregularly shaped or large tonsils

- Pollution or smoke exposure

- A weak immune system or taking drugs that weaken the immune system

- Postnasal drip or allergies

- Acid reflux disease

Signs and Symptoms

A sore throat can make it painful to swallow. A sore throat can also feel dry and scratchy and may be a symptom of the common cold or other upper respiratory tract infections.

The following symptoms are often associated with sore throats caused by a viral infection or due to allergies:

- Sneezing

- Coughing

- Watery eyes

- Mild headache or body aches

- Runny nose

- Low fever (less than 101°F)

Symptoms more commonly associated with strep throat include:

- Red and swollen tonsils, sometimes with white patches or streaks of pus

- Tiny red spots (petechiae) on the soft or hard palate (the roof of the mouth)

- High fever (101°F or above)

- Nausea

- Vomiting

- Swollen lymph nodes in the neck

- Severe headache or body aches

- Rash

When to Seek Medical Care

See a healthcare professional if you or your child has any of the following:

- Sore throat that lasts longer than one week

- Difficulty swallowing or breathing

- Excessive drooling (young children)

- Temperature higher than 100.4°F

- Pus on the back of the throat

- Rash

- Joint pain

- Hoarseness lasting longer than two weeks

- Blood in saliva or phlegm

- Dehydration (symptoms include a dry, sticky mouth; sleepiness or tiredness; thirst; decreased urination or fewer wet diapers; few or no tears when crying; muscle weakness; headache; and dizziness or lightheadedness)

- Recurring sore throats

Diagnosis and Treatment

Antibiotics are not needed to treat most sore throats, which usually improve on their own within one to two weeks. Antibiotics will not help if a sore throat is caused by a virus or irritation from the air. Antibiotic treatment in these cases may cause harm in both children and adults. Your healthcare professional may prescribe other medicine or give you tips to help with other symptoms, such as fever and coughing.

Antibiotics are needed if a healthcare professional diagnoses you or your child with strep throat, which is caused by bacteria. This diagnosis can be done using a quick swab of the throat. Strep throat cannot be diagnosed by looking in the throat—a lab test must be done.

Antibiotics are prescribed for strep throat to prevent rheumatic fever. If diagnosed with strep throat, an infected patient should stay home from work, school, or day care until 24 hours after starting an antibiotic.

Symptom Relief

Rest, over-the-counter (OTC) medicines, and other self-care methods may help you or your child feel better. Remember, always use over-the-counter products as directed. Many over-the-counter products are not recommended for children of certain ages.

Prevention

There are steps you can take to help prevent getting a sore throat, including:

- Practice good hand hygiene

- Avoid close contact with people who have sore throats, colds, or other upper respiratory infections

- Avoid smoking and exposure to secondhand smoke

Section 35.2

Strep Throat

This section includes text excerpted from "Strep Throat: All You Need to Know," Centers for Disease Control and Prevention (CDC), November 2018.

Strep throat is a common type of sore throat in children, but it is not very common in adults. Doctors can do a quick test to see if a sore throat is strep throat. If so, antibiotics can help you feel better faster and prevent spreading it to others.

Bacteria Cause Strep Throat

Viruses are the most common cause of a sore throat. However, strep throat is an infection in the throat and tonsils caused by bacteria called "group A *Streptococcus*" (group A strep).

How You Get Strep Throat

Group A strep live in the nose and throat and can easily spread to other people. It is important to know that all infected people do not have symptoms or seem sick. People who are infected spread the bacteria by coughing or sneezing, which creates small respiratory droplets that contain the bacteria.

People can get sick if they:

- Breathe in those droplets

- Touch something with droplets on it and then touch their mouth or nose

- Drink from the same glass or eat from the same plate as a sick person

- Touch sores on the skin caused by group A strep (impetigo)

Rarely, people can spread group A strep through food that is not handled properly. Experts do not believe pets or household items, such as toys, spread these bacteria.

Pain and Fever without a Cough Are Common Signs and Symptoms

In general, strep throat is a mild infection, but it can be very painful. The most common symptoms of strep throat include:

- Sore throat that can start very quickly

- Pain when swallowing

- Fever

- Red and swollen tonsils, sometimes with white patches or streaks of pus

- Tiny, red spots on the roof of the mouth (the soft or hard palate)

- Swollen lymph nodes in the front of the neck

Other symptoms may include a headache, stomach pain, nausea, or vomiting—especially in children. Someone with strep throat may also have a rash known as "scarlet fever" (also called "scarlatina").

The following symptoms suggest a virus is the cause of the illness instead of strep throat:

- Cough

- Runny nose

- Hoarseness (changes in your voice that makes it sound breathy, raspy, or strained)

- Conjunctivitis (also called "pink eye")

It usually takes two to five days for someone exposed to group A strep to become ill.

Children and Certain Adults Are at Increased Risk

Anyone can get strep throat, but there are some factors that can increase the risk of getting this common infection.

Strep throat is more common in children than adults. It is most common in children between the ages of 5 and 15. It is rare in children younger than 3 years of age. Adults who are at increased risk for strep throat include:

- Parents of school-aged children

- Adults who are often in contact with children

Close contact with another person with strep throat is the most common risk factor for illness. For example, if someone has strep throat, it often spreads to other people in their household.

Infectious illnesses tend to spread wherever large groups of people gather together. Crowded conditions can increase the risk of getting a group A strep infection. These settings include:

- Schools

- Day care centers

- Military training facilities

A Simple Test Gives Fast Results

Only a rapid strep test or throat culture can determine if group A strep is the cause. A doctor cannot tell if someone has strep throat just by looking at his or her throat.

A rapid strep test involves swabbing the throat and running a test on the swab. The test quickly shows if group A strep is causing the illness. If the test is positive, doctors can prescribe antibiotics. If the test is negative, but a doctor still suspects strep throat, then the doctor can take a throat culture swab. A throat culture takes time to see if group A strep bacteria grow from the swab. While it takes more time, a throat culture sometimes finds infections that the rapid strep test misses. Culture is important to use in children and teens since they can get rheumatic fever from an untreated strep throat infection. For adults, it is usually not necessary to do a throat culture following a negative rapid strep test. Adults are generally not at risk of getting rheumatic fever following a strep throat infection.

Someone with strep throat should start feeling better in just a day or two after starting antibiotics. Call the doctor if you or your child are not feeling better after taking antibiotics for 48 hours.

Antibiotics Get You Well Fast

Doctors treat strep throat with antibiotics. Either penicillin or amoxicillin are recommended as a first choice for people who are not allergic to penicillin. Doctors can use other antibiotics to treat strep throat in people who are allergic to penicillin.

Benefits of antibiotics include:

- Decreasing how long someone is sick

- Decreasing symptoms (feeling better)

- Preventing the bacteria from spreading to others

- Preventing serious complications, such as rheumatic fever

Someone who tests positive for strep throat but has no symptoms (called a "carrier") usually does not need antibiotics. They are less likely to spread the bacteria to others and very unlikely to get complications. If a carrier gets a sore throat illness caused by a virus, the rapid strep test can be positive. In these cases, it can be hard to know what is causing the sore throat. If someone keeps getting a sore throat after taking the right antibiotics, they may be a strep carrier and have a viral throat infection. Talk to a doctor if you think you or your child may be a strep carrier.

Serious Complications Are Not Common but Can Happen

Complications can occur after a strep throat infection. This can happen if the bacteria spread to other parts of the body. Complications can include:

- Abscesses (pockets of pus) around the tonsils
- Swollen lymph nodes in the neck
- Sinus infections
- Ear infections
- Rheumatic fever (a heart disease)
- Poststreptococcal glomerulonephritis (a kidney disease)

Protect Yourself and Others

People can get strep throat more than once. Having strep throat does not protect someone from getting it again in the future. While there is no vaccine to prevent strep throat, there are things people can do to protect themselves and others.

Good Hygiene Helps Prevent Group A Strep Infections

The best way to keep from getting or spreading group A strep is to wash your hands often. This is especially important after coughing or sneezing and before preparing foods or eating. To practice good hygiene you should:

- Cover your mouth and nose with a tissue when you cough or sneeze.
- Put your used tissue in the wastebasket.
- Cough or sneeze into your upper sleeve or elbow, not your hands, if you do not have a tissue.
- Wash your hands often with soap and water for at least 20 seconds.
- Use an alcohol-based hand rub if soap and water are not available.

You should also wash glasses, utensils, and plates after someone who is sick uses them. These items are safe for others to use once washed.

Antibiotics Help Prevent Spreading the Infection to Others

People with strep throat should stay home from work, school, or day care until they:

- No longer have a fever

399

- Have taken antibiotics for at least 24 hours

Take the prescription exactly as the doctor says to. Do not stop taking the medicine, even if you or your child feel better, unless the doctor says to stop.

Wash your hands often to help prevent germs from spreading.

Section 35.3

Candida Infections of the Mouth, Throat, and Esophagus

This section includes text excerpted from "Candida Infections of the Mouth, Throat, and Esophagus," Centers for Disease Control and Prevention (CDC), August 4, 2017.

Candidiasis is an infection caused by a yeast (a type of fungus) called "*Candida.*" *Candida* normally lives in the digestive tract and on skin without causing any problems. Sometimes, *Candida* can multiply and cause an infection if the environment inside the mouth, throat, or esophagus changes in a way that encourages fungal growth.

Candidiasis in the mouth and throat is also called "thrush" or "oropharyngeal candidiasis." Candidiasis in the esophagus (the tube that connects the throat to the stomach) is called "esophageal candidiasis" or "Candida esophagitis." Esophageal candidiasis is one of the most common infections in people living with human immunodeficiency virus (HIV) or acquired immunodeficiency syndrome (AIDS).

Symptoms

Candidiasis in the mouth and throat can have many different symptoms, including:

- White patches on the inner cheeks, tongue, roof of the mouth, and throat

- Redness or soreness

- Cottony feeling in the mouth
- Loss of taste
- Pain while eating or swallowing
- Cracking and redness at the corners of the mouth

Symptoms of candidiasis in the esophagus usually include pain when swallowing and difficulty swallowing. Contact your healthcare provider if you have symptoms that you think are related to candidiasis in the mouth, throat, or esophagus.

Risk

Candidiasis in the mouth, throat, or esophagus is uncommon in healthy adults. People who are at higher risk for getting candidiasis in the mouth and throat include babies, especially those younger than one month of age, and people who:

- Wear dentures
- Have diabetes
- Have cancer
- Have HIV/AIDS
- Take antibiotics or corticosteroids, including inhaled corticosteroids for conditions such as asthma
- Take medications that cause dry mouth or have medical conditions that cause dry mouth
- Smoke

Most people who get candidiasis in the esophagus have weakened immune systems, meaning that their bodies do not fight infections well. This includes people living with HIV/AIDS and people who have blood cancers, such as leukemia and lymphoma. People who get candidiasis in the esophagus often also have candidiasis in the mouth and throat.

Prevention

Ways to help prevent candidiasis in the mouth and throat include:

- Maintain good oral health
- Rinse your mouth or brush your teeth after using inhaled corticosteroids

- Some studies have shown that chlorhexidine mouthwash may help to prevent oral candidiasis in people undergoing cancer treatment

Sources

Candida normally lives in the mouth, throat, and the rest of the digestive tract without causing any problems. Sometimes, *Candida* can multiply and cause an infection if the environment inside the mouth, throat, or esophagus changes in a way that encourages its growth. This can happen when a person's immune system becomes weakened, if antibiotics affect the natural balance of microbes in the body, or for a variety of other reasons in other groups of people.

Diagnosis and Testing

Healthcare providers can usually diagnose candidiasis in the mouth or throat simply by looking inside. Sometimes a healthcare provider will take a small sample from the mouth or throat. The sample is sent to a laboratory for testing, usually to be examined under a microscope.

Healthcare providers usually diagnose candidiasis in the esophagus by doing an endoscopy. An endoscopy is a procedure to examine the digestive tract using a tube with a light and a camera. A healthcare provider might prescribe antifungal medication without doing an endoscopy to see if the patient's symptoms get better.

Treatment

Candidiasis in the mouth, throat, or esophagus is usually treated with antifungal medicine. The treatment for mild to moderate infections in the mouth or throat is usually an antifungal medicine applied to the inside of the mouth for 7 to 14 days. These medications include clotrimazole, miconazole, or nystatin. For severe infections, the treatment is usually fluconazole or another type of antifungal medicine given by mouth or through a vein for people who do not get better after taking fluconazole. The treatment for candidiasis in the esophagus is usually fluconazole. Other types of prescription antifungal medicines can also be used for people who cannot take fluconazole or who do not get better after taking fluconazole.

Statistics

The exact number of cases of candidiasis in the mouth, throat, and esophagus in the United States is difficult to determine because there is no national surveillance for these infections. The risk of these infections varies based on the presence of certain underlying medical conditions. For example, candidiasis in the mouth, throat, or esophagus is uncommon in healthy adults. However, they are some of the most common infections in people living with HIV/AIDS. In one study, approximately one-third of patients with advanced HIV infection had candidiasis in the mouth and throat.

Chapter 36

Tonsils and Adenoids

Chapter Contents

Section 36.1

Tonsils and Tonsillectomies

This section includes text excerpted from "Tonsillitis," MedlinePlus, National Institutes of Health (NIH), April 1, 2019.

What Are Tonsils?

Tonsils are lumps of tissue at the back of the throat. There are two of them, one on each side. Along with the adenoids, tonsils are part of the lymphatic system. The lymphatic system clears away infection and keeps body fluids in balance. Tonsils and adenoids work by trapping the germs coming in through the mouth and nose.

What Is Tonsillitis?

Tonsillitis is an inflammation (swelling) of the tonsils. Sometimes along with tonsillitis, the adenoids are also swollen.

What Causes Tonsillitis

The cause of tonsillitis is usually a viral infection. Bacterial infections, such as strep throat, can also cause tonsillitis.

Who Is at Risk for Tonsillitis?

Tonsillitis is most common in children over the age of two. Almost every child in the United States gets it at least once. Tonsillitis caused by bacteria is more common in kids between the ages of 5 and 15. Tonsillitis caused by a virus is more common in younger children.

Adults can get tonsillitis, but it is not very common.

Is Tonsillitis Contagious?

Although tonsillitis is not contagious, the viruses and bacteria that cause it are contagious. Frequent handwashing can help prevent spreading or catching the infections.

What Are the Symptoms of Tonsillitis?

The symptoms of tonsillitis include:

- A sore throat, which may be severe

- Red, swollen tonsils
- Trouble swallowing
- A white or yellow coating on the tonsils
- Swollen glands in the neck
- Fever
- Bad breath

When Should I Get Medical Help for My Child?

You should call your healthcare provider if your child:

- Has a sore throat for more than two days
- Has trouble or pain when swallowing
- Feels very sick or very weak

You should get emergency care right away if your child:

- Has trouble breathing
- Starts drooling
- Has a lot of trouble swallowing

How Is Tonsillitis Diagnosed?

To diagnose tonsillitis, your child's healthcare provider will first ask you about your child's symptoms and medical history. The provider will look at your child's throat and neck, checking for things such as redness or white spots on the tonsils and swollen lymph nodes.

Your child will probably also have one or more tests to check for strep throat, since it can cause tonsillitis and it requires treatment. It could be a rapid strep test, a throat culture, or both. For both tests, the provider uses a cotton swab to collect a sample of fluids from your child's tonsils and the back of the throat. With the rapid strep test, testing is done in the office, and you get the results within minutes. The throat culture is done in a lab, and it usually takes a few days to get the results. The throat culture is a more reliable test. So, sometimes if the rapid strep test is negative (meaning that it does not show any strep bacteria), the provider will also do a throat culture just to make sure that your child does not have strep.

What Are the Treatments for Tonsillitis?

Treatment for tonsillitis depends on the cause. If the cause is a virus, there is no medicine to treat it. If the cause is a bacterial infection, such as strep throat, your child will need to take antibiotics. It is important for your child to finish the antibiotics even if she or he feels better. If treatment stops too soon, some bacteria may survive and re-infect your child.

No matter what is causing the tonsillitis, there are some things you can do to help your child feel better. Make sure that your child

- Gets a lot of rest

- Drinks plenty of fluids

- Tries eating soft foods if it hurts to swallow

- Tries consuming warm liquids or cold foods, such as popsicles, to soothe the throat

- Is not around cigarette smoke or anything else that could irritate the throat

- Sleeps in a room with a humidifier

- Gargles with salt water

- Sucks on a lozenge (but do not give them to children under four years of age; they can choke on them)

- Takes an over-the-counter pain reliever such as acetaminophen. Children and teenagers should not take aspirin.

In some cases, your child may need a tonsillectomy.

What Is a Tonsillectomy and Why Might My Child Need One?

A tonsillectomy is surgery to remove the tonsils. Your child might need it if he or she:

- Keeps getting tonsillitis

- Has bacterial tonsillitis that does not get better with antibiotics

- Has tonsils that are too big and are causing trouble breathing or swallowing

Your child usually gets the surgery and goes home later that day. Very young children and people who have complications may need to stay in the hospital overnight. It can take a week or two before your child completely recovers from the surgery.

Section 36.2

Adenoids and Adenoidectomies

This section includes text excerpted from "Adenoids," MedlinePlus, National Institutes of Health (NIH), February 7, 2019.

What Are Adenoids?

Adenoids are a patch of tissue that is high up in the throat, just behind the nose. They, along with the tonsils, are part of the lymphatic system. The lymphatic system clears away infection and keeps body fluids in balance. The adenoids and tonsils work by trapping germs coming in through the mouth and nose.

Adenoids usually start to shrink after about five years of age. By the teenage years, they are almost completely gone. By then, the body has other ways to fight germs.

What Are Enlarged Adenoids?

Enlarged adenoids are adenoids that are swollen. It is a common problem in children.

What Causes Enlarged Adenoids

Your child's adenoids can be enlarged, or swollen, for different reasons. It may just be that your child had enlarged adenoids at birth. Adenoids can also become enlarged when they are trying to fight off an infection. They might stay enlarged even after the infection is gone.

What Problems Can Enlarged Adenoids Cause?

Enlarged adenoids can make it hard to breathe through the nose. Your child might end up breathing only through the mouth. This may cause:

- A dry mouth, which can also lead to bad breath

- Cracked lips

- A runny nose

Other problems that enlarged adenoids can cause include:

- Loud breathing

- Snoring

- Restless sleep

- Sleep apnea, where you repeatedly stop breathing for a few seconds while sleeping

- Ear infections

How Can Enlarged Adenoids Be Diagnosed?

Your child's healthcare provider will take a medical history; check your child's ears, throat, and mouth; and feel your child's neck.

Since the adenoids are higher up than the throat, the healthcare provider cannot see them just by looking through your child's mouth. To check the size of your child's adenoids, your provider may use:

- A special mirror in the mouth

- A long, flexible tube with a light (an endoscope)

- An X-ray

What Are the Treatments for Enlarged Adenoids?

The treatment depends on what is causing the problem. If your child's symptoms are not too bad, she or he may not need treatment. Your child might get nasal spray to reduce the swelling, or antibiotics if the healthcare provider thinks that your child has a bacterial infection.

In some cases your child may need an adenoidectomy.

What Is an Adenoidectomy and Why Might My Child Need One?

An adenoidectomy is surgery to remove the adenoids. Your child might need it if:

- She or he has repeated infections of the adenoids. Sometimes, the infections can also cause ear infections and fluid buildup in the middle ear.

- Antibiotics cannot get rid of a bacterial infection

- The enlarged adenoids block the airways

If your child also has problems with his or her tonsils, she or he will probably have a tonsillectomy (removal of the tonsils) at the same time that the adenoids are removed.

After having the surgery, your child usually goes home the same day. She or he will probably have some throat pain, bad breath, and a runny nose. It can take several days to feel better.

Chapter 37

Laryngeal Problems

Chapter Contents

Section 37.1

Gastroesophageal Reflux Disease

This section includes text excerpted from "GERD," MedlinePlus,
National Institutes of Health (NIH), February 7, 2019.

Your esophagus is the tube that carries food from your mouth to your stomach. Gastroesophageal reflux disease (GERD) happens when a muscle at the end of your esophagus does not close properly. This allows stomach contents to leak back, or reflux, into the esophagus and irritate it.

You may feel a burning in the chest or throat called "heartburn." Sometimes, you can taste stomach fluid in the back of the mouth. If you have these symptoms more than twice a week, you may have GERD. You can also have GERD without having heartburn. Your symptoms could include a dry cough, asthma symptoms, or trouble swallowing.

Anyone, including infants and children, can have GERD. If not treated, it can lead to more serious health problems. In some cases, you might need medicines or surgery. However, many people can improve their symptoms by:

- Avoiding alcohol and spicy, fatty, or acidic foods that trigger heartburn

- Eating smaller meals

- Not eating close to bedtime

- Losing weight if needed

- Wearing loose-fitting clothes

Section 37.2

Recurrent Respiratory Papillomatosis/ Laryngeal Papillomatosis

This section includes text excerpted from "Recurrent Respiratory Papillomatosis or Laryngeal Papillomatosis," National Institute on Deafness and Other Communication Disorders (NIDCD), November 28, 2017.

What Is Recurrent Respiratory Papillomatosis?

Recurrent respiratory papillomatosis (RRP) is a disease in which benign (noncancerous) tumors called "papillomas" grow in the air passages, leading from the nose and mouth and into the lungs (respiratory tract). Although the tumors can grow anywhere in the respiratory tract, they most commonly grow in the larynx (voice box)—a condition called "laryngeal papillomatosis." The papillomas may vary in size and grow very quickly. They often grow back after they have been removed.

What Causes Recurrent Respiratory Papillomatosis

Recurrent respiratory papillomatosis (RRP) is caused by two types of human papillomavirus (HPV): HPV 6 and HPV 11. There are more than 150 types of HPV, and they do not all have the same symptoms.

Most people who encounter HPV never develop a related illness. However, in a small number of people exposed to the HPV 6 or 11 virus, respiratory tract papillomas and genital warts can form. Although scientists do not fully understand why some people develop the disease and others do not, the virus is thought to be spread through sexual contact or when a mother with genital warts passes the HPV 6 or 11 virus to her baby during childbirth.

Who Is Affected by Recurrent Respiratory Papillomatosis?

Recurrent respiratory papillomatosis (RRP) may occur in adults (adult-onset RRP), as well as in infants and small children (juvenile-onset RRP) who may have contracted the virus during childbirth. The RRP Foundation estimates that there are roughly 20,000 active cases in the United States. According to the Centers for Disease Control and Prevention (CDC), estimates of the incidence for juvenile-onset RRP are imprecise but range from 2 or fewer cases per 100,000 children under the age of 18. Even less is known about the incidence of the adult form of RRP. Estimates of the incidence for adult-onset RPP range between 2 to 3 cases per 100,000 adults in the United States.

What Are the Symptoms of Recurrent Respiratory Papillomatosis?

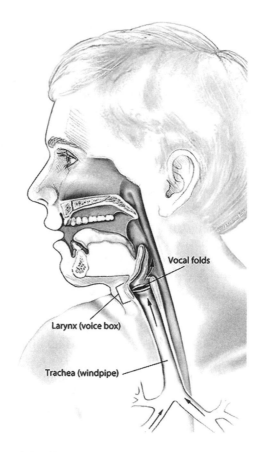

Figure 37.1. *Parts of the Respiratory Tract Affected by Recurrent Respiratory Papillomatosis (National Institutes of Health (NIH)/The National Institute on Deafness and Other Communication Disorders (NIDCD).)*

Normally, the human voice is produced when air from the lungs is pushed through two side-by-side specialized muscles—called "vocal folds"—with enough pressure to cause them to vibrate (see figure 37.1).

Hoarseness, the most common RRP symptom, is caused when RRP papillomas interfere with the normal vibrations of the vocal folds. Eventually, RRP tumors may block the airway passage and cause difficulty breathing.

Recurrent respiratory papillomatosis (RRP) symptoms tend to be more severe in children than in adults. Because the tumors grow quickly, young children with the disease may find it difficult to breathe when sleeping, or they may have difficulty swallowing. Some children experience some relief or remission of the disease when they begin puberty. Both children and adults may experience hoarseness, chronic coughing, or breathing problems. Because of the similarity of the symptoms, RRP is sometimes misdiagnosed as asthma or chronic bronchitis.

How Is Recurrent Respiratory Papillomatosis Diagnosed?

Health professionals use two routine tests for RRP: indirect and direct laryngoscopy. In an indirect laryngoscopy, an otolaryngologist—a doctor who specializes in diseases of the ear, nose, throat, head, and neck—or speech-language pathologist will typically insert a fiberoptic telescope, called an "endoscope," into a patient's nose or mouth and then view the larynx on a monitor. Some medical professionals use a video camera attached to this endoscope to view and record the exam. An older, less common method is for the otolaryngologist to place a small mirror in the back of the throat and angle the mirror down toward the larynx to inspect it for papillomas.

A direct laryngoscopy is conducted in the operating room with the use of general anesthesia. This method allows the otolaryngologist to view the vocal folds and other parts of the larynx under high magnification. This procedure is usually used to minimize discomfort, especially with children, or to enable the doctor to biopsy tissue samples from the larynx or other parts of the throat to obtain a diagnosis of RRP.

How Is Recurrent Respiratory Papillomatosis Prevented or Treated?

Vaccination with the HPV vaccine could prevent the development of RRP. The CDC currently recommends that all children (both boys and girls) receive the HPV vaccine at 11 or 12 years of age. Ask your child's doctor whether the type of HPV vaccine your child will receive will protect against HPV 6 and 11. As more young people receive the vaccine, future research will reveal its effectiveness in preventing HPV-associated diseases, such as RRP.

Once RRP develops, there is currently no cure. Surgery is the primary method for removing tumors from the larynx or airway. Because traditional surgery can cause problems, due to scarring of the larynx tissue, many surgeons now use laser surgery. Carbon dioxide (CO_2) or potassium titanyl phosphate (KTP) lasers are frequently used for this purpose. Surgeons also commonly use a device called a "microdebrider," which uses suction to hold the tumor in place while a small internal rotary blade removes the growth.

Once the tumors have been removed, they can still return. It is common for patients to require multiple surgeries. With some patients, surgery may be required every few weeks in order to keep the breathing passage open, while others may require surgery only once a year or even less frequently.

In the most extreme cases of aggressive tumor growth, a tracheotomy may be performed. A tracheotomy is a surgical procedure in which an incision is made in the front of the patient's neck and a breathing tube (trach tube) is inserted through an opening, called a "stoma," into the trachea (windpipe). Rather than breathing through the nose and mouth, the patient will now breathe through the trach tube. Although the trach tube keeps the breathing passage open, doctors try to remove it as soon as possible.

Some patients may be required to keep a trach tube indefinitely in order to keep the breathing passage open. Because the trach tube re-routes all or some of the exhaled air away from the vocal folds, the patient may find it difficult to use his or her voice. With the help of a voice specialist or speech-language pathologist who specializes in voice, the patient can learn to use her or his voice with the use of a speaking valve.

In severe cases of RRP, therapies in addition to surgery may be used. Drug treatments may include antivirals, such as interferon and cidofovir, which block the virus from making copies of itself; indole-3-carbinol, a cancer-fighting compound found in cruciferous vegetables, such as broccoli and brussels sprouts; or bevacizumab, which targets the blood vessel growth of papilloma. To date, the results of these and other nonsurgical therapies have been mixed or not yet fully proven.

What Research Is Being Conducted on Recurrent Respiratory Papillomatosis?

Scientists and clinicians are working to discover more about RRP. While HPV 6 and HPV 11 are known causes, millions of people are exposed to these two viruses without developing the disease. It is not known why some people are more at risk than others or why some cases are much more serious than others.

Researchers funded by the National Institute on Deafness and Other Communication Disorders (NIDCD) are conducting research studies to explore how HVP 6 and HVP 11 evade the immune system and cause RRP. In another NIDCD-supported study, scientists aim to decipher the precise ways in which cells infected with HVP 6 and HVP 11 multiply and grow into tumors. Eventually, research may help to develop new vaccine strategies to treat or prevent RRP.

New clinical trials, one of which is being conducted at the National Institutes of Health (NIH) Clinical Center, are investigating whether immunotherapies originally developed to treat patients with cancer (immune checkpoint inhibitors) can be used to activate the immune system against HPV-infected papilloma cells.

Section 37.3

Laryngoscopy and Esophagoscopy

This section includes text excerpted from "Laryngoscopy, Esophagoscopy, and Bronchoscopy," U.S. Department of Veterans Affairs (VA), April 2013. Reviewed April 2019.

The respiratory (breathing) system is made up of the nose, larynx (voice box), trachea (windpipe), bronchial tubes, and lungs. When air is breathed in, it goes through the nose and mouth. The air then goes to the larynx and then through the trachea. From the trachea, air passes through the bronchial tubes and into the lungs.

The esophagus is the soft swallowing tube that carries food and liquids from your throat to your stomach.

Laryngoscopy

This means looking at your larynx, or voice box. The doctor places tools inside your mouth to keep it open and to keep your tongue out of the way. Your doctor can look at other parts of the throat using the same tools. Your doctor may see a mass or lesion. If so, a small amount of tissue (biopsy) is taken and sent to a lab for tests. The doctor uses tools to stop the bleeding in the areas where tissue was taken out. Rarely, a tooth can be chipped or dislodged, even though tooth protectors are used during surgery. You may have tongue numbness after surgery, which sometimes can takes weeks to improve. If a lesion is removed from the vocal cords, you may have hoarseness after surgery.

Esophagoscopy

A test that helps the doctor look at the inside your esophagus (swallowing tube). The test is done using a special tube (scope) that has a camera and light. The doctor can remove growths (polyps) if they are found. Small pieces of tissue can also be removed (biopsy) if needed. The lab can then check the tissue for disease. The test is safe. There is a one percent risk of a puncture of the esophagus, which could cause a severe chest infection.

After Surgery Care
Activity

You can resume your usual activity the day after surgery. If you have had surgery on your vocal cords, please rest your voice for one week. You must only talk five minutes every hour of one-on-one conversation. You must not talk on the phone, sing, whisper, or yell.

Diet

You may eat your regular diet after surgery, as long as your stomach is not upset from the anesthesia. If it is, wait until you feel better before you start eating solid foods. If you had biopsies of your throat, you should follow a soft diet for a week.

Pain

Pain is usually mild. You may not need strong narcotic medicine, unless deep biopsies were taken. The sooner you reduce your narcotic pain medication use, the faster you will heal. As your pain lessens, try using extra-strength acetaminophen (Tylenol) instead of your narcotic medication. Never take more than three grams (or 3000 milligrams) of acetaminophen within 24 hours. You can hurt your liver if you take too much. Please check the medication bottle to see how many milligrams of acetaminophen are in each tablet.

It is best to reduce your pain to a level you can manage, rather than to get rid of the pain completely. Please start at a lower of narcotic pain medicine, and increase the dose only if the pain remains uncontrolled. Decrease the dose if the side effects are too severe.

Do not drive, operate dangerous machinery, or do anything dangerous if you are taking narcotic pain medication (such as oxycodone, hydrocodone, morphine, etc.) This medication affects your reflexes and responses, similar to alcohol.

When to Call Your Surgeon: If you have...

1. Any concerns

2. Persistent fever over 101.5°F

3. Excessive bleeding

4. Cannot eat or drink

5. Problem urinating

If you have chest pain or problems breathing, do not call—go to the closest emergency room right away.

If it is urgent, call 911 or go directly to the emergency room without calling.

Postoperative Appointment

Your follow-up appointment date will depend on your surgery and biopsy results. You may have been given the results of your biopsy, but still do not when to go back.

Chapter 38

Swallowing Problems

Chapter Contents

Section 38.1

Dysphagia

This section includes text excerpted from "Dysphagia,"
National Institute on Deafness and Other Communication
Disorders (NIDCD), March 6, 2017.

What Is Dysphagia?

People with dysphagia have difficulty swallowing and may even experience pain while swallowing (odynophagia). Some people may be completely unable to swallow or may have trouble safely swallowing liquids, foods, or saliva. When that happens, eating becomes a challenge. Often, dysphagia makes it difficult to take in enough calories and fluids to nourish the body and can lead to additional serious medical problems.

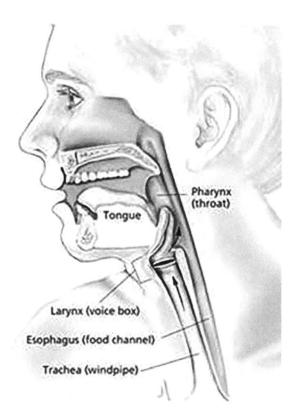

Figure 38.1. Parts of the Mouth and Neck Involved in Swallowing

How Does Dysphagia Occur?

Dysphagia occurs when there is a problem with the neural control or the structures involved in any part of the swallowing process. Weak tongue or cheek muscles may make it hard to move food around in the mouth for chewing. A stroke or other nervous system disorder may make it difficult to start the swallowing response, a stimulus that allows food and liquids to move safely through the throat. Another difficulty can occur when weak throat muscles, such as after cancer surgery, cannot move all of the food toward the stomach. Dysphagia may also result from disorders of the esophagus.

What Are Some Problems Caused by Dysphagia?

Dysphagia can be serious. Someone who cannot swallow safely may not be able to eat enough of the right foods to stay healthy or maintain an ideal weight.

Food pieces that are too large for swallowing may enter the throat and block the passage of air. In addition, when foods or liquids enter the airway of someone who has dysphagia, coughing or throat clearing sometimes cannot remove it. Food or liquid that stays in the airway may enter the lungs and allow harmful bacteria to grow, resulting in a lung infection called "aspiration pneumonia."

Swallowing disorders may also include the development of a pocket outside the esophagus, which is caused by weakness in the esophageal wall. This abnormal pocket traps some food being swallowed. While lying down or sleeping, someone with this problem may draw undigested food into the throat. The esophagus may also be too narrow, causing food to stick. This food may prevent other food or even liquids from entering the stomach.

What Causes Dysphagia

Dysphagia has many possible causes and happens most frequently in older adults. Any condition that weakens or damages the muscles and nerves used for swallowing may cause dysphagia. For example, people with diseases of the nervous system, such as cerebral palsy or Parkinson's disease (PD), often have problems swallowing. Additionally, stroke or head injury may weaken or affect the coordination of the swallowing muscles or limit sensation in the mouth and throat.

People born with abnormalities of the swallowing mechanism may not be able to swallow normally. Infants who are born with an opening in the roof of the mouth (cleft palate) are unable to suck properly, which complicates nursing and drinking from a regular baby bottle.

In addition, cancer of the head, neck, or esophagus may cause swallowing problems. Sometimes the treatment for these types of cancers can cause dysphagia. Injuries of the head, neck, and chest may also create swallowing problems. An infection or irritation can cause narrowing of the esophagus. Finally, dementia, memory loss, and cognitive decline may make it difficult for individuals to chew and swallow.

How Is Dysphagia Treated?

There are different treatments for various types of dysphagia. Medical doctors and speech-language pathologists who evaluate and treat swallowing disorders use a variety of tests that allow them to look at the stages of the swallowing process. One test, the Flexible Endoscopic Evaluation of Swallowing with Sensory Testing (FEESST), uses a lighted fiberoptic tube, or endoscope, to view the mouth and throat while examining how the swallowing mechanism responds to such stimuli as a puff of air, food, or liquids.

A videofluoroscopic swallow study (VFSS) is a test in which a clinician takes a videotaped X-ray of the entire swallowing process by having you consume several foods or liquids along with the mineral barium to improve visibility of the digestive tract. Such images help identify where in the swallowing process you are experiencing problems. Speech-language pathologists use this method to explore what changes can be made to offer a safe strategy when swallowing. The changes may be in food texture, size, head and neck posture, or behavioral maneuvers, such as "chin tuck," a strategy in which you tuck your chin so that food and other substances do not enter the trachea when swallowing. If you are unable to swallow safely, despite rehabilitation strategies, then medical or surgical intervention may be necessary for the short term as you recover. In progressive conditions such as amyotrophic lateral sclerosis (ALS), (or Lou Gehrig's disease), a feeding tube in the stomach may be necessary for the long-term.

For some people, treatment may involve muscle exercises to strengthen weak facial muscles or to improve coordination. For others, treatment may involve learning to eat in a special way. For example, some people may have to eat with their head turned to one side or looking straight ahead. Preparing food in a certain way or avoiding certain foods may help in some situations. For instance, people who cannot swallow thin liquids may need to add special thickeners to their drinks. Other people may have to avoid hot or cold foods or drinks.

For some, however, consuming enough foods and liquids by mouth may no longer be possible. These individuals must use other methods to nourish their bodies. Usually, this involves a feeding system, such as a feeding tube, that bypasses or supplements the part of the swallowing mechanism that is not working normally.

What Research Is Being Done on Dysphagia?

Scientists are conducting research that will improve the ability of physicians and speech-language pathologists to evaluate and treat swallowing disorders. Every aspect of the swallowing process is being studied in people of all ages, including those who do not have dysphagia, to give researchers a better understanding of how normal and disordered processes compare.

Research has also led to new, safe ways to study tongue and throat movements during the swallowing process. These methods will help physicians and speech-language pathologists safely evaluate a patient's progress during treatment.

Studies of treatment methods are helping scientists discover why some forms of treatment work with some people and not with others. This knowledge will help some people avoid serious lung infections and help others avoid tube feedings.

Where Can I Get Help?

If you have a sudden or gradual change in your ability to swallow, you should consult with your physician. She or he may refer you to an otolaryngologist—a doctor who specializes in diseases of the ear, nose, throat, head, and neck—and a speech-language pathologist. You may be referred to a neurologist if a stroke or other neurologic disorder is the cause of the swallowing problem.

Section 38.2

Achalasia

This section includes text excerpted from "Idiopathic
Achalasia," Genetic and Rare Diseases Information
Center (GARD), National Center for Advancing
Translational Sciences (NCATS), March 15, 2016.

Achalasia is a disorder of the esophagus, the tube that carries food
from the mouth to the stomach. It is characterized by enlargement of
the esophagus, impaired ability of the esophagus to push food down
toward the stomach (peristalsis), and failure of the ring-shaped muscle at the bottom of the esophagus (the lower esophageal sphincter)
to relax. Achalasia is typically diagnosed in individuals between 25
and 60 years of age. The exact etiology is unknown however, symptoms are caused by damage to the nerves of the esophagus. Familial
studies have shown evidence of a potential genetic influence. When
a genetic influence is suspected, achalasia is called "familial esophageal achalasia." Treatment is aimed at reducing the pressure at the
lower esophageal sphincter and may include Botox, medications, or
surgery.

Symptoms

Most people with achalasia experience difficulty with swallowing,
also known as "dysphagia," and heartburn. Other symptoms might
include regurgitation or vomiting, noncardiac chest pain, odynophagia (painful swallowing), and pain in the upper central region
of the abdomen. Nonesophageal symptoms might include coughing
or asthma, chronic aspiration (breathing a foreign object, such as
food, into the airway), hoarseness or sore throat, and unintentional
weight loss.

Cause

The lower esophageal sphincter normally relaxes during swallowing. In people with achalasia, this muscle ring does not relax as well.
The reason for this problem is damage to the nerves of the esophagus.
In some people, this problem appears to be inherited. There is additionally a suspected autoimmune component involved in the development
of achalasia, as individuals with achalasia are more likely to have a
concomitant autoimmune disease than the general population.

Diagnosis

Achalasia is suspected in individuals with dysphagia and in instances where regurgitation symptoms are not responsive to protein pump inhibitor medication.

The diagnosis of achalasia is confirmed by manometry (test that measures how well the esophagus is working); however, other tests, such as upper endoscopy and upper GI X-ray, can additionally be useful.

Treatment

The aim of treatment is to reduce the pressure at the lower esophageal sphincter. Therapy may involve:

- Injection with botulinum toxin (Botox) to help relax the sphincter muscles (used as a temporary fix)

- Medications, such as long-acting nitrates (i.e., isosorbide dinitrate) or calcium channel blockers (i.e., nifedipine), to relax the lower esophagus sphincter

- Surgery (Heller myotomy) to decrease the pressure in the lower sphincter

- Pneumatic balloon dilation of the esophagus at the location of the narrowing (done during esophagogastroduodenoscopy)

A doctor should help to determine the best treatment for each individual situation.

Prognosis

Although there is no cure for achalasia, treatment options are estimated to be effective in 90 percent of cases. Without treatment, individuals with achalasia develop progressive dilation of the esophagus. This then leads to late- or end-stage achalasia, characterized by esophageal tortuosity (twisting and turning), angulation, and severe dilation.

Approximately 10 to 15 percent of individuals who have undergone treatment will progress to late- or end-stage achalasia. Treatment for late- or end-stage achalasia is typically esophagectomy (surgery to remove all or part of the esophagus).

Chapter 39

Voice and Vocal Cord Disorders

Chapter Contents

Section 39.1

Hoarseness

This section includes text excerpted from "Hoarseness,"
National Institute on Deafness and Other Communication
Disorders (NIDCD), March 6, 2017.

What Is Hoarseness?

If you are hoarse, your voice will sound breathy, raspy, or strained, or will be softer in volume or lower in pitch. Your throat might feel scratchy. Hoarseness is often a symptom of problems in the vocal folds of the larynx.

How Does Our Voice Work?

The sound of our voice is produced by vibration of the vocal folds, which are two bands of smooth muscle tissue that are positioned opposite each other in the larynx. The larynx is located between the base of the tongue and the top of the trachea, which is the passageway to the lungs.

When we are not speaking, the vocal folds are open so that we can breathe. When it is time to speak, however, the brain orchestrates a series of events. The vocal folds snap together while air from the lungs blows past, making them vibrate. The vibrations produce sound waves that travel through the throat, nose, and mouth, which act as resonating cavities to modulate the sound. The quality of our voice—its pitch, volume, and tone—is determined by the size and shape of the vocal folds and the resonating cavities. This is why people's voices sound so different.

Individual variations in our voices are the result of how much tension we put on our vocal folds. For example, relaxing the vocal folds makes a voice deeper; tensing them makes a voice higher.

If My Voice Is Hoarse, When Should I See My Doctor?

You should see your doctor if your voice has been hoarse for more than three weeks, especially if you have not had a cold or the flu. You should also see a doctor if you are coughing up blood or if you have difficulty swallowing, feel a lump in your neck, experience pain when speaking or swallowing, have difficulty breathing, or lose your voice completely for more than a few days.

How Will My Doctor Diagnose What Is Wrong?

Your doctor will ask you about your health history and how long you have been hoarse. Depending on your symptoms and general health, your doctor may send you to an otolaryngologist (a doctor who specializes in diseases of the ears, nose, and throat). An otolaryngologist will usually use an endoscope (a flexible, lighted tube designed for looking at the larynx) to get a better view of the vocal folds. In some cases, your doctor might recommend special tests to evaluate voice irregularities or vocal airflow.

What Are Some of the Disorders That Cause Hoarseness and How Are They Treated?

Hoarseness can have several possible causes and treatments, as described below:

- **Laryngitis.** Laryngitis is one of the most common causes of hoarseness. It can be due to temporary swelling of the vocal folds from a cold, an upper respiratory infection, or allergies. Your doctor will treat laryngitis according to its cause. If it is due to a cold or upper respiratory infection, your doctor might recommend rest, fluids, and nonprescription pain relievers. Allergies might be treated similarly, with the addition of over-the-counter (OTC) allergy medicines.

- **Misusing or overusing your voice.** Cheering at sporting events, speaking loudly in noisy situations, talking for too long without resting your voice, singing loudly, or speaking with a voice that is too high or too low can cause temporary hoarseness. Resting, reducing voice use, and drinking lots of water should help relieve hoarseness from misuse or overuse. Sometimes, people whose jobs depend on their voices—such as teachers, singers, or public speakers—develop hoarseness that will not go away. If you use your voice for a living and you regularly experience hoarseness, your doctor might suggest seeing a speech-language pathologist for voice therapy. In voice therapy, you will be given vocal exercises and tips for avoiding hoarseness by changing the ways in which you use your voice.

- **Gastroesophageal reflux (GERD).** GERD—commonly called "heartburn"—can cause hoarseness when stomach acid rises up the throat and irritates the tissues. Usually, hoarseness caused by GERD is worse in the morning and improves throughout the day. In some people, the stomach acid rises all the way up to the throat and larynx and irritates the vocal folds. This is called "laryngopharyngeal reflux" (LPR). LPR can happen during the day or night. Some people will have no heartburn with LPR, but they may feel as if they constantly have to cough to clear their throat, and they may become hoarse. GERD and LPR are treated with dietary modifications and medications that reduce stomach acid.

- **Vocal nodules, polyps, and cysts.** Vocal nodules, polyps, and cysts are benign (noncancerous) growths within or along the vocal folds. Vocal nodules are sometimes called "singer's nodes" because they are a frequent problem among professional singers. They form in pairs on opposite sides of the vocal folds as the result of too much pressure or friction, such as the way a callus forms on the foot from a shoe that is too tight. A vocal polyp typically occurs only on one side of the vocal fold. A vocal cyst is a hard mass of tissue encased in a membrane sac inside the vocal fold. The most common treatments for nodules, polyps, and cysts are voice rest, voice therapy, and surgery to remove the tissue.

- **Vocal fold hemorrhage.** Vocal fold hemorrhage occurs when a blood vessel on the surface of the vocal fold ruptures and the tissues fill with blood. If you lose your voice suddenly during strenuous vocal use (such as yelling), you may have a vocal fold hemorrhage. Sometimes, a vocal fold hemorrhage will cause hoarseness to develop quickly over a short amount of time and only affect your singing but not your speaking voice. Vocal fold hemorrhage must be treated immediately with total voice rest and a trip to the doctor.

- **Vocal fold paralysis.** Vocal fold paralysis is a voice disorder that occurs when one or both of the vocal folds do not open or close properly. It can be caused by injury to the head, neck, or chest; lung or thyroid cancer; tumors of the skull base, neck, or chest; or infection (for example, Lyme disease). People with certain neurological conditions, such as multiple sclerosis or Parkinson disease or who have sustained a stroke, may experience vocal fold paralysis. In many cases, however, the cause is unknown. Vocal fold paralysis is treated with voice therapy and, in some cases, surgery.

- **Neurological diseases and disorders.** Neurological conditions that affect areas of the brain that control muscles in the throat or larynx can also cause hoarseness. Hoarseness is sometimes a symptom of Parkinson disease or a stroke. Spasmodic dysphonia is a rare neurological disease that causes hoarseness and can also affect breathing. Treatment in these cases will depend upon the type of disease or disorder.

- **Other causes.** Thyroid problems and injury to the larynx can cause hoarseness. Hoarseness may sometimes be a symptom of laryngeal cancer, which is why it is so important to see your doctor if you are hoarse for more than three weeks. Hoarseness is also the most common symptom of a disease called "recurrent respiratory papillomatosis" (RRP), or "laryngeal papillomatosis," which causes noncancerous tumors to grow in the larynx and other air passages leading from the nose and mouth into the lungs.

Section 39.2

Spasmodic Dysphonia

This section includes text excerpted from "Spasmodic Dysphonia," National Institute on Deafness and Other Communication Disorders (NIDCD), March 6, 2017.

What Is Spasmodic Dysphonia?

Spasmodic dysphonia is a neurological disorder affecting the voice muscles in the larynx, or voice box. When we speak, air from the lungs is pushed between two elastic structures—called "vocal folds" or "vocal cords"—with sufficient pressure to cause them to vibrate, producing voice (see figure 39.1). In spasmodic dysphonia, the muscles inside the vocal folds experience sudden involuntary movements—called "spasms"—which interfere with the ability of the folds to vibrate and produce voice.

Spasmodic dysphonia causes voice breaks and can give the voice a tight, strained quality. People with spasmodic dysphonia may have occasional breaks in their voice that occur once every few sentences. Usually, however, the disorder is more severe and spasms may occur on every other word, making a person's speech very difficult for others to understand. At first, symptoms may be mild and occur only occasionally, but they may worsen and become more frequent over time. Spasmodic dysphonia is a chronic condition that continues throughout a person's life.

Spasmodic dysphonia can affect anyone. It is a rare disorder, occurring in roughly 1 to 4 people per 100,000 people. The first signs of spasmodic dysphonia are found most often in people between 30 and 50 years of age. It affects women more than men.

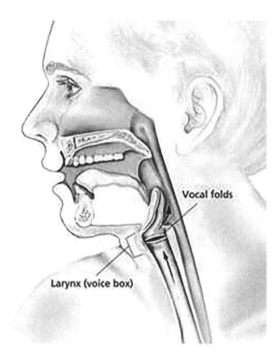

Figure 39.1. Parts of the Throat Involved in Spasmodic Dysphonia

What Are the Types of Spasmodic Dysphonia?

- Adductor spasmodic dysphonia is the most common form of spasmodic dysphonia. It is characterized by spasms that cause the vocal folds to slam together and stiffen. These spasms make it difficult for the vocal folds to vibrate and produce sounds. Words are often cut off or are difficult to start because of muscle spasms. Therefore, speech may be choppy. The voice of someone with adductor spasmodic dysphonia is commonly described as strained or strangled and full of effort. The spasms are usually absent—and the voice sounds normal—while laughing, crying, or shouting. Stress often makes the muscle spasms more severe.

- Abductor spasmodic dysphonia is characterized by spasms that cause the vocal folds to open. The vocal folds cannot vibrate when they are open too far. The open position also allows air to escape from the lungs during speech. As a result, the voice often sounds weak and breathy. As with adductor spasmodic dysphonia, the spasms are often absent during activities such as laughing, crying, or shouting.

- Mixed spasmodic dysphonia, a combination of the above two types, is very rare. Because both the muscles that open and the muscles that close the vocal folds are not working properly, it has features of both adductor and abductor spasmodic dysphonia.

What Causes Spasmodic Dysphonia

The cause of spasmodic dysphonia is unknown. Because the voice can sound normal or near normal at times, spasmodic dysphonia was once thought to be psychogenic, or originating in a person's mind, rather than from a physical cause. In rare cases, psychogenic forms of spasmodic dysphonia do exist; however, in most instances, the muscle spasms are caused by abnormalities in the central nervous system (CNS) (the brain).

A disorder that involves involuntary muscle contractions is also called a "dystonia"; therefore, another name for spasmodic dysphonia is laryngeal dystonia. Spasmodic dysphonia is considered a form of focal dystonia, a neurological disorder that affects muscle tone in one part of the body. Writer's cramp is another type of focal dystonia. Other dystonias can affect multiple regions of the body or the entire body.

Spasmodic dysphonia may co-occur with other dystonias that cause involuntary and repetitious movement of muscles, such as the eyes; face, body, arms, and legs; jaws, lips, and tongue; or neck.

Spasmodic dysphonia is thought to be caused by abnormal functioning in an area of the brain called the "basal ganglia." The basal ganglia consist of several clusters of nerve cells deep inside the brain. They help coordinate movements of the muscles throughout the body. Some research has found abnormalities in other regions of the brain, including the brainstem, the stalk-like part of the brain that connects to the spinal cord.

Symptoms of spasmodic dysphonia generally develop gradually and with no obvious explanation. Some people with spasmodic dysphonia also have vocal tremor, a shaking of the larynx and vocal folds that causes the voice to shake. Although the risk factors for spasmodic dysphonia have not been identified, the voice symptoms can begin following an upper respiratory infection, injury to the larynx, voice overuse, or stress.

In some cases, spasmodic dysphonia may run in families. Although 14 genes have been recently associated with various dystonias, only mutations in one gene, named *"THAP1,"* have been associated with forms of whole body dystonia that begin in childhood and appear with spasmodic dysphonia. This genetic defect does not seem to be associated with the more usual form of focal spasmodic dysphonia that begins in adults, however.

How Is Spasmodic Dysphonia Diagnosed?

Diagnosis of spasmodic dysphonia is sometimes difficult because individuals with spasmodic dysphonia often have symptoms similar to other voice disorders. The diagnosis of spasmodic dysphonia usually is made following careful examination by a team that includes an otolaryngologist, a doctor who specializes in diseases of the ear, nose, throat, head, and neck; a speech-language pathologist, a health professional trained to evaluate and treat speech, language, and voice disorders; and a neurologist, a doctor who specializes in nervous system disorders.

The otolaryngologist examines the vocal folds for other possible causes of the voice disorder. A small lighted tube is passed through the nose and into the back of the throat—a procedure called "fiberoptic nasolaryngoscopy"—allowing the otolaryngologist to evaluate vocal fold structure and movement during speech and other activities. The speech-language pathologist evaluates the types of voice symptoms to see if they are characteristic of spasmodic dysphonia or other voice disorders and voice quality. The neurologist evaluates the patient for signs of other muscle movement disorders.

What Treatment Is Available for Spasmodic Dysphonia?

There is currently no cure for spasmodic dysphonia; therefore, treatment can only help reduce its symptoms. The most common treatment for spasmodic dysphonia is the injection of very small amounts of botulinum toxin directly into the affected muscles of the larynx. Botulinum toxin is produced by Clostridium botulinum, the same bacterium that occurs in improperly canned foods and honey. The toxin weakens muscles by blocking the nerve impulse to the muscle. Botulinum toxin injections generally improve the voice for a period of three to four months, after which the voice symptoms gradually return. Reinjections are necessary to maintain a good speaking voice. Initial side effects, including a temporary weak, breathy voice and occasional swallowing difficulties, usually subside after a few days to a few weeks. Botulinum toxin will relieve symptoms of most cases of adductor spasmodic dysphonia and is helpful in many cases of abductor spasmodic dysphonia.

Behavioral therapy (voice therapy) is another form of treatment that may work to reduce symptoms in mild cases. Other people may benefit from psychological counseling to help them accept and live with their voice problem.

In some cases, augmentative and alternative devices can help people with spasmodic dysphonia to communicate more easily. For example, some devices can help amplify a person's voice in person or over the phone. Special software can be added to a computer or handheld device, such as a personal digital assistant (PDA) or cell phone, to translate text into synthetic speech.

When more conventional measures have failed, surgery on the larynx may be performed. Long-term benefits and effects of this procedure are unknown.

Section 39.3

Vocal Cord Paralysis

This section includes text excerpted from "Vocal Fold Paralysis,"
National Institute on Deafness and Other Communication Disorders
(NIDCD), March 6, 2017.

What Is Vocal Fold Paralysis?

Vocal fold paralysis (also known as "vocal cord paralysis") is a voice
disorder that occurs when one or both of the vocal folds do not open
or close properly. Single vocal fold paralysis is a common disorder.
Paralysis of both vocal folds is rare and can be life threatening.

The vocal folds are two elastic bands of muscle tissue located in
the larynx (voice box) directly above the trachea (windpipe) (see figure
39.2). When you breathe, your vocal folds remain apart and when you
swallow, they are tightly closed. When you use your voice, however,
air from the lungs causes your vocal folds to vibrate between open and
closed positions.

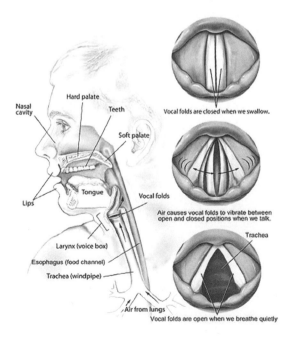

Figure 39.2. *Structures Involved in Speech and Voice Production*

If you have vocal fold paralysis, the paralyzed fold or folds may remain open, leaving the air passages and lungs unprotected. You could have difficulty swallowing, or food or liquids could accidentally enter the trachea and lungs, causing serious health problems.

What Causes Vocal Fold Paralysis

Vocal fold paralysis may be caused by injury to the head, neck, or chest; lung or thyroid cancer; tumors of the skull base, neck, or chest; or infection (for example, Lyme disease). People with certain neurological conditions, such as multiple sclerosis or Parkinson disease or who have sustained a stroke, may experience vocal fold paralysis. In many cases, however, the cause is unknown.

What Are the Symptoms?

Symptoms of vocal fold paralysis include changes in the voice, such as hoarseness or a breathy voice; difficulties with breathing, such as shortness of breath or noisy breathing; and swallowing problems, such as choking or coughing when you eat because food is accidentally entering the windpipe instead of the esophagus (the muscular tube that connects the throat to the stomach). Changes in voice quality, such as loss of volume or pitch, also may occur. Damage to both vocal folds, although rare, usually causes serious problems with breathing.

How Is Vocal Fold Paralysis Diagnosed?

Vocal fold paralysis is usually diagnosed by an otolaryngologist—a doctor who specializes in ear, nose, and throat disorders. He or she will ask you about your symptoms and when the problems began in order to help determine their cause. The otolaryngologist will also listen to your voice to identify breathiness or hoarseness. Using an endoscope—a tube with a light at the end—your doctor will look directly into the throat at the vocal folds. Some doctors also use a procedure called "laryngeal electromyography," which measures the electrical impulses of the nerves in the larynx, to better understand the areas of paralysis.

How Is Vocal Fold Paralysis Treated?

The most common treatments for vocal fold paralysis are voice therapy and surgery. Some people's voices will naturally recover sometime during the first year after diagnosis, which is why doctors often delay surgery for at least a year. During this time, your doctor will likely refer you to a speech-language pathologist for voice therapy, which may involve exercises to strengthen the vocal folds or improve breath control while speaking. You might also learn how to use your voice differently, for example, by speaking more slowly or opening your mouth wider when you speak. Several surgical procedures are available, depending on whether one or both of your vocal folds are paralyzed.

The most common procedures change the position of the vocal fold. These may involve inserting a structural implant or stitches to reposition the laryngeal cartilage and bring the vocal folds closer together. These procedures usually result in a stronger voice. Surgery is followed by additional voice therapy to help fine-tune the voice.

When both vocal folds are paralyzed, a tracheotomy may be required to help breathing. In a tracheotomy, an incision is made in the front of the neck and a breathing tube is inserted through an opening, called a "stoma," into the trachea. Rather than occurring through the nose and mouth, breathing now happens through the tube. Following surgery, therapy with a speech-language pathologist helps you learn how to use the voice and how to properly care for the breathing tube.

Section 39.4

Taking Care of Your Voice

This section includes text excerpted from "Taking Care of Your Voice," National Institute on Deafness and Other Communication Disorders (NIDCD), March 6, 2017.

What Is Voice?

The sound of your voice is produced by vibration of the vocal folds, which are two bands of smooth muscle tissue that are positioned opposite each other in the larynx. The larynx is located between the base of the tongue and the top of the trachea, which is the passageway to the lungs.

When you are not speaking, the vocal folds are open so that you can breathe. When it is time to speak, however, the brain orchestrates a series of events. The vocal folds snap together while air from the lungs blows past, making them vibrate. The vibrations produce sound waves that travel through the throat, nose, and mouth, which act as resonating cavities to modulate the sound. The quality of your voice—its pitch, volume, and tone—is determined by the size and shape of the vocal folds and the resonating cavities. This is why people's voices sound so different.

Many people use their voices for their work. Singers, teachers, doctors, lawyers, nurses, sales people, and public speakers are among those who make great demands on their voices. This puts them at risk for developing voice problems. An estimated 17.9 million adults in the U.S. report problems with their voice. Some of these disorders can be avoided by taking care of your voice.

How Do You Know When Your Voice Is Not Healthy?

If you answer "yes" to any of the following questions, you may have a voice problem:

- Has your voice become hoarse or raspy?

- Have you lost your ability to hit some high notes when singing?

- Does your voice suddenly sound deeper?

- Does your throat often feel raw, achy, or strained?

- Has it become an effort to talk?

- Do you find yourself repeatedly clearing your throat?

If you think you have a voice problem, consult a doctor to determine the underlying cause. A doctor who specializes in diseases or disorders of the ears, nose, and throat, and who can best diagnose a voice disorder, is an otolaryngologist, sometimes called an "ENT doctor." Your otolaryngologist may refer you to a speech-language pathologist. A speech-language pathologist can help you improve the way you use your voice.

What Causes Voice Problems

Causes of voice problems include:

- Upper respiratory infections

- Inflammation caused by gastroesophageal reflux (sometimes called "acid reflux," "heartburn," or "gastroesophageal reflux disease" (GERD))

- Vocal misuse and overuse

- Growths on the vocal folds, such as vocal nodules or laryngeal papillomatosis

- Cancer of the larynx

- Neurological diseases (such as spasmodic dysphonia or vocal fold paralysis)

- Psychological trauma

Most voice problems can be reversed by treating the underlying cause or through a range of behavioral and surgical treatments.

Tips to Prevent Voice Problems

Stay hydrated:

- Drink plenty of water. Six to eight glasses a day is recommended.

- Limit your intake of drinks that contain alcohol or caffeine, which can cause the body to lose water and make the vocal folds and larynx dry. Alcohol also irritates the mucous membranes that line the throat.

- Use a humidifier in your home. This is especially important in winter or in dry climates. 30 percent humidity is recommended.

- Avoid or limit use of medications that dry out the vocal folds, including some common cold and allergy medications. If you have voice problems, ask your doctor which medications would be safest for you to use.

Maintain a healthy lifestyle and diet:

- Do not smoke, and avoid secondhand smoke. Smoke irritates the vocal folds. Also, cancer of the vocal folds is seen most often in individuals who smoke.

- Avoid eating spicy foods. Spicy foods can cause stomach acid to move into the throat or esophagus, causing heartburn or GERD.

- Include plenty of whole grains, fruits, and vegetables in your diet. These foods contain vitamins A, E, and C. They also help keep the mucus membranes that line the throat healthy.

- Wash your hands often to prevent getting a cold or the flu.

- Get enough rest. Physical fatigue has a negative effect on voice.

- Exercise regularly. Exercise increases stamina and muscle tone. This helps provide good posture and breathing, which are necessary for proper speaking.

- If you have persistent heartburn or GERD, talk to your doctor about diet changes or medications that can help reduce flare-ups.

- Avoid mouthwash or gargles that contain alcohol or irritating chemicals. If you still wish to use a mouthwash that contains alcohol, limit your use to oral rinsing. If gargling is necessary, use a salt water solution.

- Avoid using mouthwash to treat persistent bad breath. Halitosis (bad breath) may be the result of a problem that mouthwash cannot cure, such as low grade infections in the nose, sinuses, tonsils, gums, or lungs, as well as from gastric acid reflux from the stomach.

Use your voice wisely:

- Try not to overuse your voice. Avoid speaking or singing when your voice is hoarse or tired.

- Rest your voice when you are sick. Illness puts extra stress on your voice.

- Avoid using the extremes of your vocal range, such as screaming or whispering. Talking too loudly and too softly can stress your voice.

- Practice good breathing techniques when singing or talking. Support your voice with deep breaths from the chest, and do not rely on your throat alone. Singers and speakers are often taught exercises that improve this kind of breath control. Talking from the throat, without supporting breath, puts a great strain on the voice.

- Avoid cradling the phone when talking. Cradling the phone between the head and shoulder for extended periods of time can cause muscle tension in the neck.

- Consider using a microphone when appropriate. In relatively static environments, such as exhibit areas, classrooms, or exercise rooms, a lightweight microphone and an amplifier-speaker system can be of great help.

- Avoid talking in noisy places. Trying to talk above noise causes strain on the voice.

- Consider voice therapy. A speech-language pathologist who is experienced in treating voice problems can teach you how to use your voice in a healthy way.

What Research on Voice Is the National Institute on Deafness and Other Communication Disorders Supporting?

The National Institute on Deafness and Other Communication Disorders (NIDCD) supports research that includes laboratory studies to understand diseases and stresses that can harm the voice, and clinical research to test new ways to diagnose, treat, or cure voice disorders.

Researchers are exploring how the brain controls the muscles and nerves of the larynx and tongue, and how these structures move to produce speech. This information may help other scientists design better treatments for conditions such as vocal fold paralysis and spasmodic dysphonia, which can damage the voice. It may also help researchers design new rehabilitation strategies to improve the quality of life for people challenged by severe voice disorders.

Another area of interest to researchers is developing replacement tissues to repair damaged vocal folds. NIDCD-funded scientists are testing human-made and biological materials and stem cell technologies that may eventually be used to engineer new vocal fold tissues, as well as methods to encourage nerve regrowth to treat laryngeal paralysis.

Researchers are also looking at new ways to assess vocal disorders and testing new methods of voice therapy for people with growths on the vocal folds. Research continues to explore ways to prevent scarring of the vocal fold after injury and to treat vocal scarring when it occurs. Additional ongoing research studies aim to understand the mechanisms of laryngeal papillomatosis caused by human papillomavirus (HPV) and to develop new drug treatments for the disorder.

New techniques to combat age-related weakness in the laryngeal muscles have the potential to prevent voice disorders in the aging population. Some results from NIDCD-funded researchers showed that, in an animal model of the aging voice, vocal training exercises helped the muscles of the larynx stay strong.

Because teachers have a high incidence of vocal disorders, the NIDCD is supporting the development of an educational website for teachers to support healthy behaviors and protection of their voices. The NIDCD is also supporting research into the effectiveness of voice hygiene education and voice production training for teachers.

Section 39.5

Statistics on Voice, Speech, and Language Disorders

This section contains text excerpted from the following sources: Text in this section begins with excerpts from "Statistics on Voice, Speech, and Language," National Institute on Deafness and Other Communication Disorders (NIDCD), July 11, 2016; Text under the heading "About 1 in 12 Children Has a Disorder Related to Voice, Speech, Language, or Swallowing" is excerpted from "About 1 in 12 Children Has a Disorder Related to Voice, Speech, Language, or Swallowing," National Institute on Deafness and Other Communication Disorders (NIDCD), July 11, 2015. Reviewed April 2019.

The functions, skills, and abilities of voice, speech, and language are related. Some dictionaries and textbooks use the terms almost interchangeably. But, for scientists and medical professionals, it is important to distinguish among them.

Head trauma can have an adverse effect on all 3. Males who are between 15 and 24 years of age tend to be more vulnerable because of their high-risk lifestyles. Young children and individuals over 75 years of age are also more susceptible to head injury. Falls around the home are the leading cause of injury for infants, toddlers, and elderly people. Violent shaking of an infant or toddler is another significant cause. The leading causes for adolescents and adults are automobile and motorcycle accidents, but injuries that occur during violent crimes are also a major source. Approximately 200,000 Americans die each year from their injuries. An additional half million or more are hospitalized. About 10 percent of the surviving individuals have mild to moderate problems that threaten their ability to live independently. Another 200,000 have serious problems that may require institutionalization or some other form of close supervision.

Voice
Statistics

- Approximately 7.5 million people in the United States have trouble using their voices.

- Spasmodic dysphonia (a voice disorder caused by involuntary movements of one or more muscles of the larynx or voice box) can affect anyone. The first signs of this disorder are found most often in individuals between 30 and 50 years of age. More women appear to be affected by spasmodic dysphonia than men.

- Laryngeal papillomatosis is a rare disease consisting of tumors that grow inside the larynx (voice box), vocal cords, or the air passages leading from the nose into the lungs. It is caused by the human papillomavirus (HPV). Although scientists are uncertain about how people are infected with HPV, they have identified more than 60 types of HPVs. Between 60 and 80 percent of laryngeal papillomatosis cases occur in children, usually before the age of 3.

- A cleft palate is the fourth most common birth defect, affecting approximately 1 of every 700 live births. Velocardiofacial syndrome (which can include a cleft palate, as well as heart defects, a characteristic facial appearance, minor learning problems, and speech and feeding problems) occurs in approximately 5 to 8 percent of children born with a cleft palate. It is estimated that over 130,000 individuals in the United States have this syndrome.

Voice Summary Report

Voice (or vocalization) is the sound produced by humans and other vertebrates using the lungs and the vocal folds in the larynx, or voice box. Voice is not always produced as speech, however. Infants babble and coo; animals bark, moo, whinny, growl, and meow; and adult humans laugh, sing, and cry. Voice is generated by airflow from the lungs as the vocal folds are brought close together. When air is pushed past the vocal folds with sufficient pressure, the vocal folds vibrate. If the vocal folds in the larynx did not vibrate normally, speech could only be produced as a whisper. Your voice is as unique as your fingerprint. It helps define your personality, mood, and health.

Approximately 7.5 million people in the United States have trouble using their voices. Disorders of the voice involve problems with pitch, loudness, and quality. Pitch is the highness or lowness of a sound based on the frequency of the sound waves. Loudness is the perceived volume (or amplitude) of the sound, while quality refers to the character or distinctive attributes of a sound. Many people who have normal speaking skills have great difficulty communicating when their vocal apparatus fails. This can occur if the nerves controlling the larynx are impaired because of an accident, a surgical procedure, a viral infection, or cancer.

Speech
Statistics

- The prevalence of speech sound disorder in young children is eight to nine percent. By the first grade, roughly five percent of children have noticeable speech disorders; the majority of these speech disorders have no known cause.

- Usually by 6 months of age an infant babbles or produces repetitive syllables, such as "ba, ba, ba" or "da, da, da." Babbling soon turns into a type of nonsense speech called "jargon" that often has the tone and cadence of human speech but does not contain real words. By the end of their first year, most children have mastered the ability to say a few simple words. By 18 months of age, most children can say 8 to 10 words and by age 2, are putting words together in crude sentences such as "more milk." At ages 3, 4, and 5, a child's vocabulary rapidly increases, and he or she begins to master the rules of language.

- It is estimated that more than three million Americans stutter. Stuttering affects individuals of all ages but occurs most frequently in young children between the ages of two and six who are developing language. Boys are three times more likely to stutter than girls. Most children, however, outgrow their stuttering, and it is estimated that fewer than one percent of adults stutter.

- Autism is one of the most common developmental disabilities, affecting individuals of all races and ethnic and socioeconomic backgrounds. Current estimates suggest that approximately 400,000 individuals in the United States have autism. Autism is 3 to 4 times more likely to affect boys than girls and occurs in individuals of all levels of intelligence. Approximately 75 percent are of low intelligence, while 10 percent may demonstrate high intelligence in specific areas, such as math.

Speech Summary Report

Humans express thoughts, feelings, and ideas orally to one another through a series of complex movements that alter and mold the basic tone created by voice into specific, decodable sounds. Speech is produced by precisely coordinated muscle actions in the head, neck, chest, and abdomen. Speech development is a gradual process that requires years of practice. During this process, a child learns how to regulate these muscles to produce understandable speech.

However, by the first grade, roughly 5 percent of children have noticeable speech disorders; the majority of these speech disorders have no known cause. One category of speech disorder is fluency disorder, or stuttering, which is characterized by a disruption in the flow of speech. It includes repetitions of speech sounds, hesitations before and during speaking, and the prolonged emphasis of speech sounds. More than 15 million individuals in the world stutter, most of whom began stuttering at a very early age. The majority of speech sound disorders in the preschool years occur in children who are developing normally in all other areas. Speech disorders also may occur in children who have developmental disabilities.

Children with specific speech sound disorders, which has also been termed "articulation disorder" or "phonological disorder," have clinically significant difficulties producing the speech sounds of their language expected for their age. The extent of these patterns of errors will affect the intelligibility of their speech to some degree and, in some cases, rendering the speech unintelligible to those unfamiliar with the child. Few publications provide summaries of prevalence estimates of this condition (Law et al. 2000; Shriberg, Tomblin, and McSweeny 1999). All these estimates have focused on children in the early school years and the prevalence estimates range from 2 percent among the oldest children who were 8 years of age, to 24.6 percent among the youngest who were 5 years of age. Much of this variability can be attributed to different diagnostic standards. The median prevalence estimate across these studies falls in the range of 8 to 9 percent. These studies all showed a greater rate of impairment in boys than girls with male to female ratios ranging from 1.5 to 2.4. Speech sound disorders have been shown to occur with a specific language impairment (SLI), particularly among children referred for clinical services. Risk factors for speech sound disorders consist of family histories of speech sound disorder (Lewis, Ekelman, and Aram 1989) and chronic otitis media (Shriberg LD et al. 2000).

Language
Statistics

* Between 6 and 8 million people in the United States have some form of language impairment.

* Research suggests that the first six months are the most crucial to a child's development of language skills. For a person to become fully competent in any language, exposure must begin as early as possible, preferably before school age.

* Anyone can acquire aphasia (a loss of the ability to use or understand language), but most people who have aphasia are in their middle to late years. Men and women are equally affected. It is estimated that approximately 80,000 individuals acquire aphasia each year. About 1 million persons in the United States currently have aphasia.

* More than 160 cases of Landau-Kleffner syndrome (LKS)—a childhood disorder involving loss of the ability to understand and use spoken language—have been reported from 1957 through 1990. Approximately 80 percent of children with LKS have 1 or more epileptic seizures that usually occur at night. Most children outgrow the seizures, and electrical brain activity on the electroencephalogram (EEG) usually returns to normal by the age of 15.

About 1 in 12 Children Has a Disorder Related to Voice, Speech, Language, or Swallowing

Nearly 1 in 12 children between the ages of 3 and 17 has had a disorder related to voice, speech, language, or swallowing in the past 12 months, according to results of the first nationally representative survey of these disorders among children in the United States. Data from a supplement to the 2012 National Health Interview Survey

451

(NHIS) also reveal that more than half of children with a communication or swallowing disorder receive intervention services.

The findings are published in a data brief released June 9, 2015, by the Center for Disease Control and Prevention's (CDC) National Center for Health Statistics (NCHS).

The analysis was done by researchers from NCHS and from the National Institute on Deafness and Other Communication Disorders (NIDCD), part of the National Institutes of Health (NIH), which collaborated on the development of the supplemental questions regarding children's communications disorders and co-funded the study.

Among the 7.7 percent of children with a communication or swallowing disorder, speech problems are most prevalent (5.0 percent), followed by language problems (3.3 percent), voice problems (1.4 percent), and swallowing problems (0.9 percent). More than one-third (34 percent) of children between the ages of 3 and 10 have multiple voice, speech, language or swallowing disorders, while about one quarter (25.4 percent) of children between the ages of 11 and 17 have more than 1 of these disorders.

To determine the prevalence of communication disorders among children, researchers analyzed information about a child randomly selected from each family participating in the NHIS; the data were collected from a parent or other adult living in the household. The NHIS is a nationally representative survey conducted annually and using personal household interviews to gather information about a range of health topics. Questions were asked about the child's experience in the past year. Based on the analysis, researchers found that young children between the ages of three and six, boys, and non-Hispanic Black children are more likely than other children to have one of these communication or swallowing disorders.

Early diagnosis and intervention services have shown to be effective in treating communication and swallowing disorders, leading to better quality of life and, in some cases, better academic success. Of the children who were reported to have had a communication or swallowing disorder, more than half (55.2 percent) had received treatment in the past year. Treatments include, for example, speech-language therapy or other intervention services. According to the data brief, children who have speech problems or language problems are more likely to receive intervention services, 67.6 percent and 66.8 percent, respectively, compared to those who have voice disorder (22.8 percent) or swallowing problems (12.7 percent).

The data brief also highlights demographic differences among children with communication and swallowing disorders.

- Boys are more likely than girls to have a communication disorder, 9.6 percent compared to 5.7 percent.

- The prevalence of communication disorders is highest among children between the ages of 3 and 6 (11.0 percent), compared to 9.3 percent of children between the ages of 7 and 10, and 4.9 percent of children between the ages of 11 and 17.

- Nearly 1 in 10 (9.6 percent) Black children has a communication disorder, compared to 7.8 percent of White children, and 6.9 percent of Hispanic children.

The researchers also reported demographic differences among children who had received services to improve their communication or swallowing disorders.

- White children with communication or swallowing disorders are more likely to receive intervention services, compared to Hispanic and Black children, at 60.1 percent, 47.3 percent and 45.8 percent, respectively.

- Boys are more likely than girls to receive intervention services, at 59.4 percent and 47.8 percent, respectively.

"While it is encouraging that more than half of children with communication and swallowing disorders have received some form of intervention services, increasing the number of children, particularly Black and Hispanic children, who receive intervention services is critical to helping children reach their full potential," said Howard J. Hoffman, M.A., co-author of the data brief and NIDCD director of epidemiology and statistics.

Part Seven

Cancers of the Ears, Nose, and Throat

Chapter 40

Head and Neck Cancers: Questions and Answers

What Are the Cancers of the Head and Neck?

Cancers that are known collectively as "head and neck cancers" usually begin in the squamous cells that line the moist, mucosal surfaces inside the head and neck (for example, inside the mouth, the nose, and the throat). These squamous cell cancers are often referred to as "squamous cell carcinomas" of the head and neck. Head and neck cancers can also begin in the salivary glands, but salivary gland cancers are relatively uncommon. Salivary glands contain many different types of cells that can become cancerous, so there are many different types of salivary gland cancer.

Cancers of the head and neck are further categorized by the area of the head or neck in which they begin.

- **Oral cavity:** Includes the lips, the front two-thirds of the tongue, the gums, the lining inside the cheeks and lips, the floor (bottom) of the mouth under the tongue, the hard palate (bony top of the mouth), and the small area of the gum behind the wisdom teeth.

- **Pharynx:** The pharynx (throat) is a hollow tube about five inches long that starts behind the nose and leads to the

---

This chapter includes text excerpted from "Head and Neck Cancers," National Cancer Institute (NCI), May 29, 2017.

esophagus. It has three parts: the nasopharynx (the upper part of the pharynx, behind the nose); the oropharynx (the middle part of the pharynx, including the soft palate [the back of the mouth], the base of the tongue, and the tonsils); the hypopharynx (the lower part of the pharynx).

- **Larynx:** The larynx, also called the "voicebox," is a short passageway formed by cartilage, just below the pharynx in the neck. The larynx contains the vocal cords. It also has a small piece of tissue, called the "epiglottis," which moves to cover the larynx to prevent food from entering the air passages.

- **Paranasal sinuses and nasal cavity:** The paranasal sinuses are small hollow spaces in the bones of the head surrounding the nose. The nasal cavity is the hollow space inside the nose.

- **Salivary glands:** The major salivary glands are on the floor of the mouth and near the jawbone. The salivary glands produce saliva.

What Causes Cancers of the Head and Neck

Alcohol and tobacco use (including smokeless tobacco, sometimes called "chewing tobacco" or "snuff") are the two most important risk factors for head and neck cancers, especially cancers of the oral cavity, oropharynx, hypopharynx, and larynx. At least 75 percent of head and neck cancers are caused by tobacco and alcohol use. People who use both tobacco and alcohol are at greater risk of developing these cancers than people who use either tobacco or alcohol alone. Tobacco and alcohol use are not risk factors for salivary gland cancers.

Infection with cancer-causing types of human papillomavirus (HPV), especially HPV type 16, is a risk factor for some types of head and neck cancers, particularly oropharyngeal cancers that involve the tonsils or the base of the tongue. In the United States, the incidence of oropharyngeal cancers caused by HPV infection is increasing, while the incidence of oropharyngeal cancers related to other causes is falling. Other risk factors for cancers of the head and neck include the following:

- **Paan (betel quid).** Immigrants from Southeast Asia who use paan (betel quid) in the mouth should be aware that this habit has been strongly associated with an increased risk of oral cancer.

- **Preserved or salted foods.** Consumption of certain preserved or salted foods during childhood is a risk factor for nasopharyngeal cancer.

- **Oral health.** Poor oral hygiene and missing teeth may be weak risk factors for cancers of the oral cavity. Use of mouthwash that has a high alcohol content is a possible, but not proven, risk factor for cancers of the oral cavity.

- **Occupational exposure.** Occupational exposure to wood dust is a risk factor for nasopharyngeal cancer. Certain industrial exposures, including exposures to asbestos and synthetic fibers, have been associated with cancer of the larynx, but the increase in risk remains controversial. People working in certain jobs in the construction, metal, textile, ceramic, logging, and food industries may have an increased risk of cancer of the larynx. Industrial exposure to wood or nickel dust or formaldehyde is a risk factor for cancers of the paranasal sinuses and nasal cavity.

- **Radiation exposure.** Radiation to the head and neck, for noncancerous conditions or cancer, is a risk factor for cancer of the salivary glands.

- **Epstein-Barr virus infection (EBV).** Infection with the Epstein-Barr virus is a risk factor for nasopharyngeal cancer and cancer of the salivary glands.

- **Ancestry.** Asian ancestry, particularly Chinese ancestry, is a risk factor for nasopharyngeal cancer.

What Are the Symptoms of Head and Neck Cancers?

The symptoms of head and neck cancers may include a lump or a sore that does not heal, a sore throat that does not go away, difficulty in swallowing, and a change or hoarseness in the voice. These symptoms may also be caused by other, less serious conditions. It is important to check with a doctor or dentist about any of these symptoms. Symptoms that may affect specific areas of the head and neck include the following:

- **Oral cavity.** A white or red patch on the gums, the tongue, or the lining of the mouth; a swelling of the jaw that causes dentures to fit poorly or become uncomfortable; and unusual bleeding or pain in the mouth

- **Pharynx.** Trouble breathing or speaking; pain when swallowing; pain in the neck or the throat that does not go away; frequent headaches, pain, or ringing in the ears; or trouble hearing

- **Larynx.** Pain when swallowing, or ear pain

- **Paranasal sinuses and nasal cavity.** Sinuses that are blocked and do not clear; chronic sinus infections that do not respond to treatment with antibiotics; bleeding through the nose; frequent headaches, swelling or other trouble with the eyes; pain in the upper teeth; or problems with dentures

- **Salivary glands.** Swelling under the chin or around the jawbone; numbness or paralysis of the muscles in the face; or pain in the face, the chin, or the neck that does not go away.

How Common Are Head and Neck Cancers?

Head and neck cancers account for approximately 4 percent of all cancers in the United States. These cancers are more than twice as common among men as they are among women. Head and neck cancers are also diagnosed more often among people over the age of 50 than they are among younger people.

Researchers estimated that more than 65,000 men and women in this country would be diagnosed with head and neck cancers in 2017.

How Can I Reduce My Risk of Developing Head and Neck Cancers?

People who are at risk of head and neck cancers—particularly those who use tobacco—should talk with their doctor about ways that they may be able to reduce their risk. They should also discuss with their doctor how often to have checkups. In addition, ongoing clinical trials are testing the effectiveness of various medications in preventing head and neck cancers in people who have a high risk of developing these diseases.

Avoiding oral HPV infection may reduce the risk of HPV-associated head and neck cancers. However, it is not yet known whether the U.S. Food and Drug Administration (FDA)-approved HPV vaccines Gardasil, Gardasil 9, and Cervarix prevent HPV infection of the oral cavity, and none of these vaccines have yet been approved for the prevention of oropharyngeal cancer.

How Are Head and Neck Cancers Diagnosed?

To find the cause of the signs or symptoms of a problem in the head and neck area, a doctor evaluates a person's medical history, performs a physical examination, and orders diagnostic tests. The exams and tests may vary depending on the symptoms. Examination of a sample of tissue under a microscope is always necessary to confirm a diagnosis of cancer.

If the diagnosis is cancer, the doctor will want to learn the stage (or extent) of disease. Staging is a careful attempt to find out whether cancer has spread and if so, to which parts of the body. Staging may involve an examination under anesthesia (in an operating room), X-rays and other imaging procedures, and laboratory tests. Knowing the stage of the disease helps the doctor plan treatment.

How Are Head and Neck Cancers Treated?

The treatment plan for an individual patient depends on a number of factors, including the exact location of the tumor, the stage of cancer, and the person's age and general health. Treatment for head and neck cancer can include surgery, radiation therapy, chemotherapy, targeted therapy, or a combination of treatment.

People who are diagnosed with HPV-positive oropharyngeal cancer may be treated differently than people with oropharyngeal cancers that are HPV-negative. A search has shown that patients with HPV-positive oropharyngeal tumors have a better prognosis and may do just as well on less intense treatment.

The patient and the doctor should consider treatment options carefully. They should discuss each type of treatment and how it might change the way the patient looks, talks, eats, or breathes.

What Are the Side Effects of Treatment?

Surgery for head and neck cancers often changes the patient's ability to chew, swallow, or talk. The patient may look different after surgery, and the face and neck may be swollen. The swelling usually goes away within a few weeks. However, if lymph nodes are removed, the flow of lymph in the area where they were removed may be slower and lymph could collect in the tissues, causing additional swelling; this swelling may last for a long time.

After a laryngectomy (surgery to remove the larynx) or other surgery in the neck, parts of the neck and throat may feel numb because nerves have been cut. If lymph nodes in the neck were removed, the shoulder and neck may become weak and stiff.

Patients who receive radiation to the head and neck may experience redness, irritation, and sores in the mouth; a dry mouth or thickened saliva; difficulty in swallowing; changes in taste; or nausea. Other problems that may occur during treatment are a loss of taste, which may decrease appetite and affect nutrition, and earaches (caused by the hardening of ear wax). Patients may also notice some swelling or drooping of the skin under the chin and changes in the texture of the skin. The jaw may feel stiff, and patients may not be able to open their mouth as wide as before treatment.

Patients should report any side effects to their doctor or nurse and discuss how to deal with them.

What Rehabilitation or Support Options Are Available for Patients with Head and Neck Cancers?

The goal of treatment for head and neck cancers is to control the disease, but doctors are also concerned about preserving the function of the affected areas as much as they can and helping the patient return to normal activities as soon as possible after treatment. Rehabilitation is a very important part of this process. The goals of rehabilitation depend on the extent of the disease and the treatment that a patient has received.

Depending on the location of cancer and the type of treatment, rehabilitation may include physical therapy, dietary counseling, speech therapy, and/or learning how to care for a stoma. A stoma is an opening into the windpipe through which a patient breathes after a laryngectomy, which is surgery to remove the larynx. The U.S. National Library of Medicine (NLM) has more information about laryngectomy in MedlinePlus.

Sometimes, especially with cancer of the oral cavity, a patient may need reconstructive and plastic surgery to rebuild bones or tissues. However, reconstructive surgery may not always be possible because of damage to the remaining tissue from the original surgery or from radiation therapy. If reconstructive surgery is not possible, a prosthodontist may be able to make a prosthesis (an artificial dental and/or facial part) to restore satisfactory swallowing, speech, and appearance. Patients will receive special training on how to use the device.

Patients who have trouble speaking after treatment may need speech therapy. Often, a speech-language pathologist will visit the patient in the hospital to plan therapy and teach speech exercises or alternative methods of speaking. Speech therapy usually continues after the patient returns home.

Eating may be difficult after treatment for head and neck cancer. Some patients receive nutrients directly into a vein after surgery or need a feeding tube until they can eat on their own. A feeding tube is a flexible plastic tube that is passed into the stomach through the nose or an incision in the abdomen. A nurse or speech-language pathologist can help patients learn how to swallow again after surgery.

Is Follow-Up Care Necessary? What Does It Involve?

Regular follow-up care is very important after treatment for head and neck cancer to make sure that cancer has not returned, or that a second primary (new) cancer has not developed. Depending on the type of cancer, medical checkups could include exams of the stoma, if one has been created, and of the mouth, neck, and throat. Regular dental exams may also be necessary.

From time to time, the doctor may perform a complete physical exam, blood tests, X-rays, and computed tomography (CT), positron emission tomography (PET), or magnetic resonance imaging (MRI) scans. The doctor may monitor thyroid and pituitary gland functions, especially if the head or neck was treated with radiation. Also, the doctor is likely to counsel patients to stop smoking. Research has shown that continued smoking by a patient with head and neck cancer may reduce the effectiveness of treatment and increase the chance of a second primary cancer.

How Can People Who Have Had Head and Neck Cancers Reduce Their Risk of Developing a Second Primary (New) Cancer?

People who have been treated for head and neck cancers have an increased chance of developing new cancer, usually in the head, neck, esophagus, or lungs. The chance of a second primary cancer varies depending on the site of original cancer, but it is higher for people who use tobacco and drink alcohol.

Especially because patients who smoke have a higher risk of a second primary cancer, doctors encourage patients who use tobacco to quit. Information about tobacco cessation is available from National Cancer Institute's (NCI) Cancer Information Service (CIS) at 800-4-CANCER (800-422-6237) and in the NCI fact sheet "Where To Get Help When You Decide To Quit Smoking." The federal government's main resource to help people quit using tobacco is BeTobaccoFree.gov. The government also sponsors Smokefree Women, a website to help women quit using tobacco, and Smokefree Teen, which is designed to help teens understand the decisions they make and how those decisions fit into their lives. The toll-free number 800-QUIT-NOW (800-784-8669) also serves as a single point of access to state-based telephone quitlines.

Chapter 41

Oropharyngeal Cancer

Oropharyngeal cancer is a disease in which malignant (cancer) cells form in the tissues of the oropharynx. The oropharynx is the middle part of the pharynx (throat), behind the mouth. The pharynx is a hollow tube about five inches long that starts behind the nose and ends where the trachea (windpipe) and esophagus (the tube from the throat to the stomach) begin. Air and food pass through the pharynx on the way to the trachea or the esophagus.

The oropharynx includes the following:

- Soft palate

- Side and back walls of the throat

- Tonsils

- Back one-third of the tongue

Oropharyngeal cancer is a type of head and neck cancer. Sometimes, more than one cancer can occur in the oropharynx and in other parts of the oral cavity, nose, pharynx, larynx (voice box), trachea, or esophagus at the same time. Most oropharyngeal cancers are squamous cell carcinomas (SCC). Squamous cells are the thin, flat cells that line the inside of the oropharynx.

This chapter includes text excerpted from "Oropharyngeal Cancer Treatment (Adult) (PDQ®)—Patient Version," National Cancer Institute (NCI), March 28, 2019.

Risks of Oropharyngeal Cancer

Smoking or being infected with human papillomavirus can increase the risk of oropharyngeal cancer. Anything that increases your risk of getting a disease is called a "risk factor." Having a risk factor does not mean that you will get cancer; not having risk factors does not mean that you will not get cancer. Talk with your doctor if you think you may be at risk.

The most common risk factors for oropharyngeal cancer include the following:

- A history of smoking cigarettes for more than 10 years and other tobacco use

- Personal history of head and neck cancer

- Heavy alcohol use

- Being infected with human papillomavirus (HPV), especially HPV type 16. The number of cases of oropharyngeal cancers linked to HPV infection is increasing.

- Chewing betel quid, a stimulant commonly used in parts of Asia

Signs and Symptoms of Oropharyngeal Cancer

These and other signs and symptoms may be caused by oropharyngeal cancer or by other conditions. Check with your doctor if you have any of the following:

- A sore throat that does not go away

- Trouble swallowing

- Trouble opening the mouth fully

- Trouble moving the tongue

- Weight loss for no known reason

- Ear pain

- A lump in the back of the mouth, throat, or neck

- A white patch on the tongue or lining of the mouth that does not go away

- Coughing up blood

Sometimes, oropharyngeal cancer does not cause early signs or symptoms.

Diagnosing Oropharyngeal Cancer

The following tests and procedures may be used:

- **Physical exam and history:** An exam of the body to check general signs of health, including checking for signs of disease, such as swollen lymph nodes in the neck or anything else that seems unusual. The medical doctor or dentist does a complete exam of the mouth and neck and looks under the tongue and down the throat with a small, long-handled mirror to check for abnormal areas. An exam of the eyes may be done to check for vision problems that are caused by nerves in the head and neck. A history of the patient's health habits and past illnesses and treatments will also be taken.

- **Positron emission tomography-computed technology scan (PET-CT):** A procedure that combines the pictures from a positron emission tomography (PET) scan and a computed tomography (CT) scan. The PET and CT scans are done at the same time with the same machine. The combined scans give more detailed pictures of areas inside the body than either scan gives by itself. A PET-CT scan may be used to help diagnose disease, such as cancer, plan treatment, or find out how well treatment is working.

  - **Computed technology (CT) scan (computed axial tomography (CAT) scan):** A procedure that makes a series of detailed pictures of areas inside the body, such as the head and neck, taken from different angles. The pictures are made by a computer linked to an X-ray machine. A dye is injected into a vein or swallowed to help the organs or tissues show up more clearly. This procedure is also called "computed tomography," "computerized tomography," or "computerized axial tomography."

  - **Positron emission tomography (PET) scan:** A procedure to find malignant tumor cells in the body. A small amount of radioactive glucose (sugar) is injected into a vein. The PET scanner rotates around the body and makes a picture of where glucose is being used in the body. Malignant tumor cells show up brighter in the picture because they are more active and take up more glucose than normal cells do.

- **Magnetic resonance imaging (MRI):** A procedure that uses a magnet, radio waves, and a computer to make a series of

467

detailed pictures of areas inside the body. This procedure is also called "nuclear magnetic resonance imaging" (NMRI).

- **Biopsy:** The removal of cells or tissues so they can be viewed under a microscope by a pathologist to check for signs of cancer. A fine-needle biopsy is usually done to remove a sample of tissue using a thin needle.

The following procedures may be used to remove samples of cells or tissue:

- **Endoscopy:** A procedure to look at organs and tissues inside the body to check for abnormal areas. An endoscope is inserted through an incision (cut) in the skin or opening in the body, such as the mouth or nose. An endoscope is a thin, tube-like instrument with a light and a lens for viewing. It may also have a tool to remove abnormal tissue or lymph node samples, which are checked under a microscope for signs of disease. The nose, throat, back of the tongue, esophagus, stomach, larynx, windpipe, and large airways will be checked. The type of endoscopy is named for the part of the body that is being examined. For example, pharyngoscopy is an exam to check the pharynx.

- **Laryngoscopy:** A procedure in which the doctor checks the larynx with a mirror or with a laryngoscope. A laryngoscope is a thin, tube-like instrument with a light and a lens for viewing. It may also have a tool to remove abnormal tissue or lymph node samples, which are checked under a microscope for signs of disease.

If cancer is found, the following test may be done to study the cancer cells:

- **Human papillomavirus (HPV) test:** A laboratory test used to check the sample of tissue for certain types of HPV infection. This test is done because oropharyngeal cancer can be caused by HPV.

Stages of Oropharyngeal Cancer

After oropharyngeal cancer has been diagnosed, tests are done to find out if cancer cells have spread within the oropharynx or to other parts of the body. The process used to find out if cancer has spread within the oropharynx or to other parts of the body is called "staging."

The information gathered from the staging process determines the stage of the disease. It is important to know the stage in order to plan treatment. The results of some of the tests used to diagnose oropharyngeal cancer are often used to stage the disease.

Stage 0 (Carcinoma in Situ)

In stage 0, abnormal cells are found in the lining of the oropharynx. These abnormal cells may become cancer and spread into nearby normal tissue. Stage 0 is also called "carcinoma in situ."

Stage I

In stage I, cancer has formed and is two centimeters or smaller and is found in the oropharynx only.

Stage II

In stage II, the cancer is larger than two centimeters but not larger than four centimeters and is found in the oropharynx only.

Stage III

In stage III, the cancer is either:

- Four centimeters or smaller; cancer has spread to one lymph node on the same side of the neck as the tumor, and the lymph node is three centimeters or smaller.
- Larger than four centimeters or has spread to the epiglottis (the flap that covers the trachea during swallowing). Cancer may have spread to one lymph node on the same side of the neck as the tumor, and the lymph node is three centimeters or smaller.

Stage IV

Stage IV is divided into stage IVA, IVB, and IVC.

- In stage IVA, cancer:
  - Has spread to the larynx, front part of the roof of the mouth, lower jaw, or muscles that move the tongue or are used for chewing. Cancer may have spread to one lymph node on the same side of the neck as the tumor, and the lymph node is three centimeters or smaller.

469

- Has spread to one lymph node on the same side of the neck as the tumor (the lymph node is larger than three centimeters but not larger than six centimeters) or to more than one lymph node anywhere in the neck (the lymph nodes are six centimeters or smaller), and one of the following is true:

  - Tumor in the oropharynx is any size and may have spread to the epiglottis (the flap that covers the trachea during swallowing).

  - Tumor has spread to the larynx, front part of the roof of the mouth, lower jaw, or muscles that move the tongue or are used for chewing.

- In stage IVB, the tumor:

  - Surrounds the carotid artery or has spread to the muscle that opens the jaw, the bone attached to the muscles that move the jaw, nasopharynx, or base of the skull. Cancer may have spread to one or more lymph nodes, which can be any size.

  - May be any size and has spread to one or more lymph nodes that are larger than six centimeters.

- In stage IVC, the tumor may be any size and has spread beyond the oropharynx to other parts of the body, such as the lung, bone, or liver.

Treatment Options Overview

Different types of treatment are available for patients with oropharyngeal cancer. Some treatments are standard (the currently used treatment), and some are being tested in clinical trials. A treatment clinical trial is a research study meant to help improve current treatments or obtain information on new treatments for patients with cancer. When clinical trials show that a new treatment is better than the standard treatment, the new treatment may become the standard treatment. Patients may want to think about taking part in a clinical trial. Some clinical trials are open only to patients who have not started treatment.

Patients with oropharyngeal cancer should have their treatment planned by a team of doctors with expertise in treating head and neck cancer.

The patient's treatment will be overseen by a medical oncologist, a doctor who specializes in treating people with cancer. Because the oropharynx helps in breathing, eating, and talking, patients may need special help adjusting to the side effects of cancer and its treatment. The medical oncologist may refer the patient to other health professionals with special training in the treatment of patients with head and neck cancer. These may include the following specialists:

- Head and neck surgeon
- Radiation oncologist
- Plastic surgeon
- Dentist
- Dietitian
- Psychologist
- Rehabilitation specialist
- Speech therapist

Surgery

Surgery (removing the cancer in an operation) is a common treatment of all stages of oropharyngeal cancer. A surgeon may remove the cancer and some of the healthy tissue around the cancer. After the surgeon removes all the cancer that can be seen at the time of the surgery, some patients may be given chemotherapy or radiation therapy after surgery to kill any cancer cells that are left. Treatment given after the surgery, to lower the risk that the cancer will come back, is called "adjuvant therapy."

New types of surgery, including transoral robotic surgery, are being studied for the treatment of oropharyngeal cancer. Transoral robotic surgery may be used to remove cancer from hard-to-reach areas of the mouth and throat. Cameras attached to a robot give a 3-dimensional (3D) image that a surgeon can see. Using a computer, the surgeon guides very small tools at the ends of the robot arms to remove the cancer. This procedure may also be done using an endoscope.

Radiation Therapy

Radiation therapy is a cancer treatment that uses high-energy X-rays or other types of radiation to kill cancer cells or keep them from growing. There are two types of radiation therapy:

- **External radiation therapy** uses a machine outside the body to send radiation toward the cancer. Certain ways of giving radiation therapy can help keep radiation from damaging nearby healthy tissue. These types of radiation therapy include the following.

- Intensity-modulated radiation therapy (IMRT): IMRT is a type of 3-dimensional (3-D) radiation therapy that uses a computer to make pictures of the size and shape of the tumor. Thin beams of radiation of different intensities (strengths) are aimed at the tumor from many angles.

- Stereotactic body radiation therapy (SBRT): Stereotactic body radiation therapy is a type of external radiation therapy. Special equipment is used to place the patient in the same position for each radiation treatment. Once a day for several days, a radiation machine aims a larger than usual dose of radiation directly at the tumor. By having the patient in the same position for each treatment, there is less damage to nearby healthy tissue. This procedure is also called "stereotactic external-beam radiation therapy" and "stereotaxic radiation therapy."

- **Internal radiation therapy** uses a radioactive substance sealed in needles, seeds, wires, or catheters that are placed directly into or near the cancer.

In advanced oropharyngeal cancer, dividing the daily dose of radiation into smaller-dose treatments improves the way the tumor responds to treatment. This is called "hyperfractionated radiation therapy."

The way the radiation therapy is given depends on the type and stage of the cancer being treated. External radiation therapy is used to treat oropharyngeal cancer. Radiation therapy may work better in patients who have stopped smoking before beginning treatment. If the thyroid or pituitary gland are part of the radiation treatment area, the patient has an increased risk of hypothyroidism (too little thyroid hormone). A blood test to check the thyroid hormone level in the body should be done before and after treatment.

Chemotherapy

Chemotherapy is a cancer treatment that uses drugs to stop the growth of cancer cells, either by killing the cells or by stopping them from dividing. When chemotherapy is taken by mouth or injected into a vein or muscle, the drugs enter the bloodstream and can reach cancer cells throughout the body (systemic chemotherapy). When chemotherapy is placed directly into the cerebrospinal fluid; an organ; or a body cavity, such as the abdomen, the drugs mainly affect cancer cells in those areas (regional chemotherapy). The way the chemotherapy is given depends on the type and stage of the cancer being treated. Systemic chemotherapy is used to treat oropharyngeal cancer.

Targeted Therapy

Targeted therapy is a type of treatment that uses drugs or other substances to attack specific cancer cells. Targeted therapies usually cause less harm to normal cells than chemotherapy or radiation therapy do. Monoclonal antibodies are a type of targeted therapy being used in the treatment of oropharyngeal cancer.

Monoclonal antibody therapy is a cancer treatment that uses antibodies made in the laboratory from a single type of immune system cell. These antibodies can identify substances on cancer cells or normal substances in the blood or tissues that may help cancer cells grow. The antibodies attach to the substances and kill the cancer cells, block their growth, or keep them from spreading. Monoclonal antibodies are given by infusion. They may be used alone or to carry drugs, toxins, or radioactive material directly to cancer cells.

Cetuximab is a type of monoclonal antibody that works by binding to a protein on the surface of the cancer cells and stops the cells from growing and dividing. It is used in the treatment of recurrent oropharyngeal cancer. Other types of monoclonal antibody therapy are being studied in the treatment of oropharyngeal cancer. Nivolumab is being studied in the treatment of stage III and IV oropharyngeal cancer.

Follow-Up Tests May Be Needed

Some of the tests that were done to diagnose the cancer or to find out the stage of the cancer may be repeated. Some tests will be repeated in order to see how well the treatment is working. Decisions about whether to continue, change, or stop treatment may be based on the results of these tests.

Some of the tests will continue to be done from time to time after treatment has ended. The results of these tests can show if your condition has changed or if the cancer has recurred. These tests are sometimes called "follow-up tests" or "check-ups." Following treatment, it is important to have careful head and neck exams to look for signs that the cancer has come back. Check-ups will be done every 6 to 12 weeks in the first year, every 3 months in the second year, every 3 to 4 months in the third year, and every 6 months thereafter.

Chapter 42

Nasopharyngeal Cancer

Nasopharyngeal cancer is a disease in which malignant (cancer) cells form in the tissues of the nasopharynx:

The nasopharynx is the upper part of the pharynx (throat) behind the nose. The pharynx is a hollow tube, about five inches long, that starts behind the nose and ends at the top of the trachea (windpipe) and esophagus (the tube that goes from the throat to the stomach). Air and food pass through the pharynx on the way to the trachea or the esophagus. The nostrils lead into the nasopharynx. An opening on each side of the nasopharynx leads into an ear. Nasopharyngeal cancer most commonly starts in the squamous cells that line the nasopharynx.

Risk of Nasopharyngeal Cancer

Ethnic background and being exposed to the Epstein-Barr virus can affect the risk of nasopharyngeal cancer:

Anything that increases your risk of getting a disease is called a "risk factor." Having a risk factor does not mean that you will get cancer; not having risk factors does not mean that you will not get cancer. Talk with your doctor if you think you may be at risk. Risk factors for nasopharyngeal cancer include the following:

- Having Chinese or Asian ancestry

This chapter includes text excerpted from "Nasopharyngeal Cancer Treatment (Adult) (PDQ®)–Patient Version," National Cancer Institute (NCI), July 6, 2018.

- Being exposed to the Epstein-Barr virus (EBV). The Epstein-Barr virus has been associated with certain cancers, including nasopharyngeal cancer and some lymphomas.

- Drinking large amounts of alcohol

Signs of Nasopharyngeal Cancer

These and other signs and symptoms may be caused by nasopharyngeal cancer or by other conditions. Check with your doctor if you have any of the following:

- A lump in the nose or neck

- A sore throat

- Trouble breathing or speaking

- Nosebleeds

- Trouble hearing

- Pain or ringing in the ear

- Headaches

Diagnosing Nasopharyngeal Cancer

Tests that examine the nose and throat are used to detect (find) and diagnose nasopharyngeal cancer.

The following tests and procedures may be used:

- **Physical exam and history:** An exam of the body to check general signs of health, including checking for signs of disease, such as swollen lymph nodes in the neck or anything else that seems unusual. A history of the patient's health habits and past illnesses and treatments will also be taken.

- **Neurological exam:** A series of questions and tests to check the brain, spinal cord, and nerve function. The exam checks a person mental status, coordination, and ability to walk normally, and how well the muscles, senses, and reflexes work. This may also be called a "neuro exam" or a "neurologic exam."

- **Biopsy:** The removal of cells or tissues so they can be viewed under a microscope by a pathologist to check for signs of cancer. The tissue sample is removed during one of the following procedures.

- **Nasoscopy:** A procedure to look inside the nose for abnormal areas. A nasoscope is inserted through the nose. A nasoscope is a thin, tube-like instrument with a light and a lens for viewing. It may also have a tool to remove tissue samples, which are checked under a microscope for signs of cancer.

- **Upper endoscopy:** A procedure to look at the inside of the nose, throat, esophagus, stomach, and duodenum (first part of the small intestine, near the stomach). An endoscope is inserted through the mouth and into the esophagus, stomach, and duodenum. An endoscope is a thin, tube-like instrument with a light and a lens for viewing. It may also have a tool to remove tissue samples. The tissue samples are checked under a microscope for signs of cancer.

- **Magnetic resonance imaging (MRI):** A procedure that uses a magnet, radio waves, and a computer to make a series of detailed pictures of areas inside the body. This procedure is also called "nuclear magnetic resonance imaging" (NMRI).

- **Computed tomography scan (CT):** A procedure that makes a series of detailed pictures of areas inside the body, taken from different angles. The pictures are made by a computer linked to an X-ray machine. A dye may be injected into a vein or swallowed to help the organs or tissues show up more clearly. This procedure is also called "CT," "computerized tomography," or "computerized axial tomography."

- **Positron emission tomography scan (PET):** A procedure to find malignant tumor cells in the body. A small amount of radioactive glucose (sugar) is injected into a vein. The PET scanner rotates around the body and makes a picture of where glucose is being used in the body. Malignant tumor cells show up brighter in the picture because they are more active and take up more glucose than normal cells do. PET scans may be used to find nasopharyngeal cancers that have spread to the bone. Sometimes, a PET scan and a CT scan are done at the same time. If there is any cancer, this increases the chance that it will be found.

- **Blood chemistry studies:** A procedure in which a blood sample is checked to measure the amounts of certain substances released into the blood by organs and tissues in the body. An unusual (higher or lower than normal) amount of a substance can be a sign of disease.

- **Complete blood count (CBC):** A procedure in which a sample of blood is drawn and checked for the following:

  - The number of red blood cells, white blood cells, and platelets

  - The amount of hemoglobin (the protein that carries oxygen) in the red blood cells

  - The portion of the blood sample made up of red blood cells

- **Epstein-Barr virus (EBV) test:** A blood test to check for antibodies to the Epstein-Barr virus and deoxyribonucleic acid (DNA) markers of the Epstein-Barr virus. These are found in the blood of patients who have been infected with EBV.

- **Hearing test:** A procedure to check whether soft and loud sounds and low- and high-pitched sounds can be heard. Each ear is checked separately.

Stages of Nasopharyngeal Cancer
Stage 0 (Carcinoma in Situ)

In stage 0, abnormal cells are found in the lining of the nasopharynx. These abnormal cells may become cancer and spread into nearby normal tissue. Stage 0 is also called "carcinoma in situ."

Stage I

In stage I, cancer has formed and the cancer:

- Is found in the nasopharynx only

- Has spread from the nasopharynx to the oropharynx and/or to the nasal cavity

The oropharynx is the middle part of the throat and includes the soft palate, the base of the tongue, and the tonsils.

Stage II

In stage II nasopharyngeal cancer, the cancer:

- Is found in the nasopharynx only or has spread from the nasopharynx to the oropharynx and/or to the nasal cavity.

Cancer has spread to one or more lymph nodes on one side of the neck and/or to lymph nodes behind the pharynx. The affected lymph nodes are six centimeters or smaller.

- Is found in the parapharyngeal space. Cancer may have spread to one or more lymph nodes on one side of the neck and/or to lymph nodes behind the pharynx. The affected lymph nodes are six centimeters or smaller.

The parapharyngeal space is a fat-filled, triangular area near the pharynx, between the base of the skull and the lower jaw.

Stage III

In stage III nasopharyngeal the cancer:

- Is found in the nasopharynx only or has spread from the nasopharynx to the oropharynx and/or to the nasal cavity. Cancer has spread to one or more lymph nodes on both sides of the neck. The affected lymph nodes are six centimeters or smaller.
- Is found in the parapharyngeal space. Cancer has spread to one or more lymph nodes on both sides of the neck. The affected lymph nodes are six centimeters or smaller.
- Has spread to nearby bones or sinuses. Cancer may have spread to one or more lymph nodes on one or both sides of the neck and/ or to lymph nodes behind the pharynx. The affected lymph nodes are six centimeters or smaller.

Stage IV

Stage IV nasopharyngeal cancer is divided into stages IVA, IVB, and IVC.

- **Stage IVA:** Cancer has spread beyond the nasopharynx and may have spread to the cranial nerves, the hypopharynx (bottom part of the throat), areas in and around the side of the skull or jawbone, and/or the bone around the eye. Cancer may also have spread to one or more lymph nodes on one or both sides of the neck and/or to lymph nodes behind the pharynx. The affected lymph nodes are six centimeters or smaller.
- **Stage IVB:** Cancer has spread to lymph nodes between the collarbone and the top of the shoulder and/or the affected lymph nodes are larger than six centimeters.

- **Stage IVC:** Cancer has spread beyond nearby lymph nodes to other parts of the body.

Treatment Options Overview

There are different types of treatment for patients with nasopharyngeal cancer.

Different types of treatment are available for patients with nasopharyngeal cancer. Some treatments are standard (the currently used treatment), and some are being tested in clinical trials. A treatment clinical trial is a research study meant to help improve current treatments or obtain information on new treatments for patients with cancer. When clinical trials show that a new treatment is better than the standard treatment, the new treatment may become the standard treatment. Patients may want to think about taking part in a clinical trial. Some clinical trials are open only to patients who have not started treatment.

Radiation Therapy

Radiation therapy is a cancer treatment that uses high-energy X-rays or other types of radiation to kill cancer cells or keep them from growing. There are two types of radiation therapy.

- **External radiation therapy** uses a machine outside the body to send radiation toward the cancer. Certain ways of giving radiation therapy can help keep radiation from damaging nearby healthy tissue. These types of radiation therapy include the following:

  - Intensity-modulated radiation therapy (IMRT): IMRT is a type of 3-dimensional (3-D) radiation therapy that uses a computer to make pictures of the size and shape of the tumor. Thin beams of radiation of different intensities (strengths) are aimed at the tumor from many angles. Compared to standard radiation therapy, intensity-modulated radiation therapy may be less likely to cause dry mouth.

  - Stereotactic radiation therapy: A rigid head frame is attached to the skull to keep the head still during the radiation treatment. A machine aims radiation directly at the tumor. The total dose of radiation is divided into several smaller doses given over several days. This procedure is also called "stereotactic external-beam radiation therapy" and "stereotaxic radiation therapy."

- **Internal radiation therapy** uses a radioactive substance sealed in needles, seeds, wires, or catheters that are placed directly into or near the cancer.

The way the radiation therapy is given depends on the type and stage of the cancer being treated. External and internal radiation therapy are used to treat nasopharyngeal cancer. External radiation therapy to the thyroid or the pituitary gland may change the way the thyroid gland works. A blood test to check the thyroid hormone level in the blood is done before and after therapy to make sure the thyroid gland is working properly. It is also important that a dentist checks the patients teeth, gums, and mouth and fixes any existing problems before radiation therapy begins.

Chemotherapy

Chemotherapy is a cancer treatment that uses drugs to stop the growth of cancer cells, either by killing the cells or by stopping them from dividing. When chemotherapy is taken by mouth or injected into a vein or muscle, the drugs enter the bloodstream and can reach cancer cells throughout the body (systemic chemotherapy). When chemotherapy is placed directly into the cerebrospinal fluid; an organ; or a body cavity, such as the abdomen, the drugs mainly affect cancer cells in those areas (regional chemotherapy). The way the chemotherapy is given depends on the type and stage of the cancer being treated.

Chemotherapy may be given after radiation therapy to kill any cancer cells that are left. Treatment given after radiation therapy, to lower the risk that the cancer will come back, is called "adjuvant therapy."

Surgery

Surgery is a procedure to find out whether cancer is present, to remove cancer from the body, or to repair a body part. Surgery is also called an "operation." Surgery is sometimes used for nasopharyngeal cancer that does not respond to radiation therapy. If cancer has spread to the lymph nodes, the doctor may remove lymph nodes and other tissues in the neck.

Side Effects of the Treatment

Patients may want to think about taking part in a clinical trial.

Some clinical trials only include patients who have not yet received treatment. Other trials test treatments for patients whose cancer has not gotten better. There are also clinical trials that test new ways to stop cancer from recurring or reduce the side effects of cancer treatment.

Patients can enter clinical trials before, during, or after starting their cancer treatment. Some clinical trials only include patients who have not yet received treatment. Other trials test treatments for patients whose cancer has not gotten better. There are also clinical trials that test new ways to stop cancer from recurring or reduce the side effects of cancer treatment.

Follow-Up Tests May Be Needed

Some of the tests that were done to diagnose cancer or to find out the stage of cancer may be repeated. Some tests will be repeated in order to see how well the treatment is working. Decisions about whether to continue, change, or stop treatment may be based on the results of these tests.

Some of the tests will continue to be done from time to time after treatment has ended. The results of these tests can show if your condition has changed or if cancer has recurred. These tests are sometimes called "follow-up tests" or "check-ups."

Treatment Options for Recurrent Nasopharyngeal Cancer

Treatment of recurrent nasopharyngeal cancer may include the following:

- Intensity-modulated radiation therapy, stereotactic radiation therapy, or internal radiation therapy
- Surgery
- Chemotherapy
- A clinical trial of chemotherapy
- A clinical trial of stereotactic radiation therapy

Chapter 43

Paranasal Sinus and Nasal Cavity Cancer

Paranasal sinus and nasal cavity cancer is a disease in which malignant (cancer) cells form in the tissues of the paranasal sinuses and nasal cavity.

Paranasal Sinuses

"Paranasal" means near the nose. The paranasal sinuses are hollow, air-filled spaces in the bones around the nose. The sinuses are lined with cells that make mucus, which keeps the inside of the nose from drying out during breathing.

There are several paranasal sinuses named after the bones that surround them:

- The frontal sinuses are in the lower forehead, above the nose

- The maxillary sinuses are in the cheekbones on either side of the nose

- The ethmoid sinuses are beside the upper nose, between the eyes

- The sphenoid sinuses are behind the nose, in the center of the skull

This chapter includes text excerpted from "Paranasal Sinus and Nasal Cavity Cancer Treatment (Adult) (PDQ®)—Patient Version," National Cancer Institute (NCI), March 28, 2019.

Nasal Cavity

The nose opens into the nasal cavity, which is divided into two nasal passages. Air moves through these passages during breathing. The nasal cavity lies above the bone that forms the roof of the mouth and curves down at the back to join the throat. The area just inside the nostrils is called the "nasal vestibule." A small area of special cells in the roof of each nasal passage sends signals to the brain to give the sense of smell.

Together, the paranasal sinuses and the nasal cavity filter and warm the air, and make it moist before it goes into the lungs. The movement of air through the sinuses and other parts of the respiratory system help make sounds for talking. Paranasal sinus and nasal cavity cancer is a type of head and neck cancer.

Different types of cells in the paranasal sinus and nasal cavity may become malignant.

The most common type of paranasal sinus and nasal cavity cancer is squamous cell carcinoma. This type of cancer forms in the thin, flat cells lining the inside of the paranasal sinuses and the nasal cavity.

Other types of paranasal sinus and nasal cavity cancer include the following:

- **Melanoma:** Cancer that starts in cells called "melanocytes," the cells that give skin its natural color

- **Sarcoma:** Cancer that starts in muscle or connective tissue

- **Inverting papilloma:** Benign tumors that form inside the nose. A small number of these change into cancer.

- **Midline granulomas:** Cancer of tissues in the middle part of the face

Being exposed to certain chemicals or dust in the workplace can increase the risk of paranasal sinus and nasal cavity cancer.

Anything that increases your chance of getting a disease is called a "risk factor." Having a risk factor does not mean that you will get cancer; not having risk factors does not mean that you will not get cancer. Talk with your doctor if you think you may be at risk. Risk factors for paranasal sinus and nasal cavity cancer include the following:

- Being exposed to certain workplace chemicals or dust, such as those found in the following jobs:

  - Furniture-making

  - Sawmill work

- Woodworking (carpentry)
- Shoemaking
- Metal-plating
- Flour mill or bakery work
- Being infected with human papillomavirus (HPV)
- Being male and older than 40 years of age
- Smoking

Signs of Paranasal Sinus and Nasal Cavity Cancer

Signs of paranasal sinus and nasal cavity cancer include sinus problems and nosebleeds.

These and other signs and symptoms may be caused by paranasal sinus and nasal cavity cancer or by other conditions. There may be no signs or symptoms in the early stages. Signs and symptoms may appear as the tumor grows. Check with your doctor if you have any of the following:

- Blocked sinuses that do not clear, or sinus pressure
- Headaches or pain in the sinus areas
- A runny nose
- Nosebleeds
- A lump or sore inside the nose that does not heal
- A lump on the face or roof of the mouth
- Numbness or tingling in the face
- Swelling or other trouble with the eyes, such as double vision or the eyes pointing in different directions
- Pain in the upper teeth, loose teeth, or dentures that no longer fit well
- Pain or pressure in the ear

Diagnosing Paranasal Sinus and Nasal Cavity Cancer

The following tests and procedures may be used:

- **Physical exam and history:** An exam of the body to check general signs of health, including checking for signs of disease, such as lumps or anything else that seems unusual. A history of the patient's health habits and past illnesses and treatments will also be taken.

- **Physical exam of the nose, face, and neck:** An exam in which the doctor looks into the nose with a small, long-handled mirror to check for abnormal areas and checks the face and neck for lumps or swollen lymph nodes.

- **X-rays of the head and neck:** An X-ray is a type of energy beam that can go through the body and onto film, making a picture of areas inside the body.

- **Magnetic resonance imaging (MRI):** A procedure that uses a magnet, radio waves, and a computer to make a series of detailed pictures of areas inside the body. This procedure is also called "nuclear magnetic resonance imaging" (NMRI).

- **Biopsy:** The removal of cells or tissues so they can be viewed under a microscope by a pathologist to check for signs of cancer. There are three types of biopsy:

  - **Fine-needle aspiration (FNA) biopsy:** The removal of tissue or fluid using a thin needle.

  - **Incisional biopsy:** The removal of part of an area of tissue that does not look normal.

  - **Excisional biopsy:** The removal of an entire area of tissue that does not look normal.

- **Nasoscopy:** A procedure to look inside the nose for abnormal areas. A nasoscope is inserted into the nose. A nasoscope is a thin, tube-like instrument with a light and a lens for viewing. A special tool on the nasoscope may be used to remove samples of tissue. The tissues samples are viewed under a microscope by a pathologist to check for signs of cancer.

- **Laryngoscopy:** A procedure in which the doctor checks the larynx (voice box) with a mirror or a laryngoscope to check for abnormal areas. A laryngoscope is a thin, tube-like instrument with a light and a lens for viewing the inside of the throat and voice box. It may also have a tool to remove tissue samples, which are checked under a microscope for signs of cancer.

Stages of Paranasal Sinus and Nasal Cavity Cancer

After paranasal sinus and nasal cavity cancer has been diagnosed, tests are done to find out if cancer cells have spread within the paranasal sinuses and nasal cavity or to other parts of the body.

The process used to find out if cancer has spread within the paranasal sinuses and nasal cavity or to other parts of the body is called "staging." The information gathered from the staging process determines the stage of the disease. It is important to know the stage in order to plan treatment. The following tests and procedures may be used in the staging process:

- **Endoscopy:** A procedure to look at organs and tissues inside the body to check for abnormal areas. An endoscope is inserted through an opening in the body, such as the nose or mouth. An endoscope is a thin, tube-like instrument with a light and a lens for viewing. It may also have a tool to remove tissue or lymph node samples, which are checked under a microscope for signs of disease.

- **Computed tomography (CT) scan (computerized axial tomography (CAT) scan):** A procedure that makes a series of detailed pictures of areas inside the body, taken from different angles. The pictures are made by a computer linked to an X-ray machine. A dye may be injected into a vein or swallowed to help the organs or tissues show up more clearly. This procedure is also called "computed tomography," "computerized tomography," or "computerized axial tomography."

- **Chest X-ray:** An X-ray of the organs and bones inside the chest. An X-ray is a type of energy beam that can go through the body and onto film, making a picture of areas inside the body.

- **Magnetic resonance imaging (MRI) with gadolinium:** A procedure that uses a magnet, radio waves, and a computer to make a series of detailed pictures of areas inside the body. Sometimes a substance called "gadolinium" is injected into a vein. The gadolinium collects around the cancer cells, so they show up brighter in the picture. This procedure is also called "nuclear magnetic resonance imaging" (NMRI).

- **Positron emission tomography scan (PET):** A procedure to find malignant tumor cells in the body. A small amount of radioactive glucose (sugar) is injected into a vein. The PET scanner rotates around the body and makes a picture of where glucose is being used in the body. Malignant tumor cells show up brighter in the picture because they are more active and take up more glucose than normal cells do.

- **Bone scan:** A procedure to check if there are rapidly dividing cells, such as cancer cells, in the bone. A very small amount of radioactive material is injected into a vein and travels through the bloodstream. The radioactive material collects in the bones with cancer and is detected by a scanner.

Stages of Maxillary Sinus Cancer
Stage 0 (Carcinoma in Situ)

In stage 0, abnormal cells are found in the innermost lining of the maxillary sinus. These abnormal cells may become cancer and spread into nearby normal tissue. Stage 0 is also called "carcinoma in situ."

Stage I

In stage I, cancer has formed in the mucous membranes of the maxillary sinus.

Stage II

In stage II, cancer has spread to bone around the maxillary sinus, including the roof of the mouth and nose, but not to the bone at the back of the maxillary sinus or the base of the skull.

Stage III

In stage III, cancer has spread to any of the following:

- The bone at the back of the maxillary sinus
- Tissues under the skin
- The eye socket
- The base of the skull
- The ethmoid sinuses

Or:

Cancer has spread to one lymph node on the same side of the neck as the cancer and the lymph node is three centimeters or smaller. Cancer has also spread to any of the following:

- The lining of the maxillary sinus
- Bones around the maxillary sinus, including the roof of the mouth and the nose
- Tissues under the skin
- The eye socket
- The base of the skull
- The ethmoid sinuses

Stage IV

Stage IV is divided into stage IVA, IVB, and IVC.

Stage IVA

In stage IVA, cancer has spread:

- To one lymph node on the same side of the neck as the cancer, and the lymph node is larger than three centimeters but not larger than six centimeters.
- To more than one lymph node on the same side of the neck as the original tumor, and the lymph nodes are not larger than six centimeters.
- To lymph nodes on the opposite side of the neck as the original tumor or on both sides of the neck, and the lymph nodes are not larger than six centimeters.

Stage IVB

In stage IVB, cancer has spread to any of the following:

- The back of the eye
- The brain
- The middle parts of the skull
- The nerves in the head that go to the brain
- The upper part of the throat behind the nose
- The base of the skull

And cancer may be found in one or more lymph nodes of any size, anywhere in the neck or cancer is found in a lymph node larger than six centimeters. Cancer may also be found anywhere in or near the maxillary sinus.

Stage IVC

In stage IVC, cancer may be anywhere in or near the maxillary sinus, may have spread to lymph nodes, and has spread to organs far away from the maxillary sinus, such as the lungs.

Stages of Nasal Cavity and Ethmoid Sinus Cancer
Stage 0 (Carcinoma in Situ)

In stage 0, abnormal cells are found in the innermost lining of the nasal cavity or ethmoid sinus. These abnormal cells may become cancer and spread into nearby normal tissue. Stage 0 is also called "carcinoma in situ."

Stage I

In stage I, cancer has formed and is found in only one area (of either the nasal cavity or the ethmoid sinus) and may have spread into bone.

Stage II

In stage II, cancer is found in two areas (of either the nasal cavity or the ethmoid sinus) that are near each other or has spread to an area next to the sinuses. Cancer may also have spread into bone.

Stage III

In stage III, cancer has spread to any of the following:

- The eye socket
- The maxillary sinus
- The roof of the mouth
- The bone between the eyes

Or:

Cancer has spread to one lymph node on the same side of the neck as the cancer, and the lymph node is three centimeters or smaller. Cancer has also spread to any of the following:

- The nasal cavity

- The ethmoid sinus
- The eye socket
- The maxillary sinus
- The roof of the mouth
- The bone between the eyes

Stage IV

Stage IV is divided into stage IVA, IVB, and IVC.

Stage IVA

In stage IVA, cancer has spread:

- To one lymph node on the same side of the neck as the cancer, and the lymph node is larger than three centimeters but not larger than six centimeters.
- To more than one lymph node on the same side of the neck as the original tumor, and the lymph nodes are not larger than six centimeters.
- To lymph nodes on the opposite side of the neck as the original tumor or on both sides of the neck, and the lymph nodes are not larger than six centimeters.

And cancer has spread to any of the following:

- The nasal cavity
- The ethmoid sinus
- The eye socket
- The maxillary sinus
- The roof of the mouth
- The bone between the eyes

Or:
Cancer has spread to any of the following:

- The front of the eye
- The skin of the nose or cheek
- Front parts of the skull

- The base of the skull
- The sphenoid or frontal sinuses

And cancer may have spread to one or more lymph nodes six centimeters or smaller, anywhere in the neck.

Stage IVB

In stage IVB, cancer has spread to any of the following:

- The back of the eye
- The brain
- The middle parts of the skull
- The nerves in the head that go to the brain
- The upper part of the throat behind the nose
- The base of the skull

And cancer may be found in one or more lymph nodes of any size, anywhere in the neck, or cancer is found in a lymph node larger than six centimeters. Cancer may also be found anywhere in or near the nasal cavity and ethmoid sinus.

Stage IVC

In stage IVC, cancer may be anywhere in or near the nasal cavity and ethmoid sinus, may have spread to lymph nodes, and has spread to organs far away from the nasal cavity and ethmoid sinus, such as the lungs.

Treatment Options Overview

Different types of treatment are available for patients with paranasal sinus and nasal cavity cancer. Some treatments are standard (the currently used treatment), and some are being tested in clinical trials. A treatment clinical trial is a research study meant to help improve current treatments or obtain information on new treatments for patients with cancer. When clinical trials show that a new treatment is better than the standard treatment, the new treatment may become the standard treatment. Patients may want to think about taking part in a clinical trial. Some clinical trials are open only to patients who have not started treatment.

Patients with paranasal sinus and nasal cavity cancer should have their treatment planned by a team of doctors with expertise in treating head and neck cancer.

Treatment will be overseen by a medical oncologist, a doctor who specializes in treating people with cancer. The medical oncologist works with other doctors who are experts in treating patients with head and neck cancer and who specialize in certain areas of medicine and rehabilitation. Patients who have paranasal sinus and nasal cavity cancer may need special help adjusting to breathing problems or other side effects of the cancer and its treatment. If a large amount of tissue or bone around the paranasal sinuses or nasal cavity is taken out, plastic surgery may be done to repair or rebuild the area. The treatment team may include the following specialists:

- Radiation oncologist
- Neurologist
- Oral surgeon or head and neck surgeon
- Plastic surgeon
- Dentist
- Nutritionist
- Speech and language pathologist
- Rehabilitation specialist

Surgery

Surgery (removing the cancer in an operation) is a common treatment for all stages of paranasal sinus and nasal cavity cancer. A doctor may remove the cancer and some of the healthy tissue and bone around the cancer. If the cancer has spread, the doctor may remove lymph nodes and other tissues in the neck.

After the doctor removes all the cancer that can be seen at the time of the surgery, some patients may be given chemotherapy or radiation therapy after surgery to kill any cancer cells that are left. Treatment given after the surgery, to lower the risk that the cancer will come back, is called "adjuvant therapy."

Radiation Therapy

Radiation therapy is a cancer treatment that uses high-energy X-rays or other types of radiation to kill cancer cells or keep them from growing. There are two types of radiation therapy:

- External radiation therapy uses a machine outside the body to send radiation toward the cancer. The total dose of radiation therapy is sometimes divided into several smaller, equal doses delivered over a period of several days. This is called "fractionation."

• Internal radiation therapy uses a radioactive substance sealed in needles, seeds, wires, or catheters that are placed directly into or near the cancer.

The way the radiation therapy is given depends on the type and stage of the cancer being treated. External and internal radiation therapy are used to treat paranasal sinus and nasal cavity cancer. External radiation therapy to the thyroid or the pituitary gland may change the way the thyroid gland works. The thyroid hormone levels in the blood may be tested before and after treatment.

Chemotherapy

Chemotherapy is a cancer treatment that uses drugs to stop the growth of cancer cells, either by killing the cells or by stopping them from dividing. When chemotherapy is taken by mouth or injected into a vein or muscle, the drugs enter the bloodstream and can reach cancer cells throughout the body (systemic chemotherapy). When chemotherapy is placed directly into the cerebrospinal fluid; an organ; or a body cavity, such as the abdomen, the drugs mainly affect cancer cells in those areas (regional chemotherapy). Combination chemotherapy is treatment using more than one anticancer drug. The way the chemotherapy is given depends on the type and stage of the cancer being treated.

Patients may want to think about taking part in a clinical trial. For some patients, taking part in a clinical trial may be the best treatment choice. Clinical trials are part of the cancer research process. Clinical trials are done to find out if new cancer treatments are safe and effective or better than the standard treatment.

Many of today's standard treatments for cancer are based on earlier clinical trials. Patients who take part in a clinical trial may receive the standard treatment or be among the first to receive a new treatment. Patients who take part in clinical trials also help improve the way cancer will be treated in the future. Even when clinical trials do not lead to effective new treatments, they often answer important questions and help move research forward. Patients can enter clinical trials before, during, or after starting their cancer treatment. Some clinical trials only include patients who have not yet received treatment. Other trials test treatments for patients whose cancer has not gotten better.

There are also clinical trials that test new ways to stop cancer from recurring or reduce the side effects of cancer treatment.

Follow-up tests may be needed. Some of the tests that were done to diagnose the cancer or to find out the stage of the cancer may be repeated. Some tests will be repeated in order to see how well the treatment is working. Decisions about whether to continue, change, or stop treatment may be based on the results of these tests. Some of the tests will continue to be done from time to time after treatment has ended. The results of these tests can show if your condition has changed or if the cancer has recurred (come back). These tests are sometimes called "follow-up tests" or "check-ups."

Treatment Options for Recurrent Paranasal Sinus and Nasal Cavity Cancer

Recurrent paranasal sinus and nasal cavity cancer is cancer that has recurred after it has been treated. The cancer may come back in the paranasal sinuses and nasal cavity or in other parts of the body.

Treatment of recurrent paranasal sinus and nasal cavity cancer depends on where cancer is found in the paranasal sinuses and nasal cavity.

If cancer is in the maxillary sinus, treatment may include the following:

- Surgery followed by radiation therapy

- Radiation therapy followed by surgery

- Chemotherapy as palliative therapy to relieve symptoms and improve the quality of life (QOL)

- A clinical trial of chemotherapy

If cancer is in the ethmoid sinus, treatment may include the following:

- Surgery and/or radiation therapy

- Chemotherapy as palliative therapy to relieve symptoms and improve the quality of life

- A clinical trial of chemotherapy

- If cancer is in the sphenoid sinus, treatment is the same as for nasopharyngeal cancer and may include radiation therapy with or without chemotherapy.

If cancer is in the sphenoid sinus, treatment is the same as for nasopharyngeal cancer and may include radiation therapy with or without chemotherapy.

If cancer is in the nasal cavity, treatment may include the following:

- Surgery and/or radiation therapy

- Chemotherapy as palliative therapy to relieve symptoms and improve the quality of life

- A clinical trial of chemotherapy

- For inverting papilloma, treatment is usually surgery with or without radiation therapy.

For melanoma and sarcoma, treatment may include the following:

- Surgery

- Chemotherapy as palliative therapy to relieve symptoms and improve the quality of life

For midline granuloma, treatment is usually radiation therapy.

If cancer is in the nasal vestibule, treatment may include the following:

- Surgery and/or radiation therapy

- Chemotherapy as palliative therapy to relieve symptoms and improve the quality of life

- A clinical trial of chemotherapy

Chapter 44

What You Need to Know about Esophageal Cancer

Esophageal cancer is a disease in which malignant (cancer) cells form in the tissues of the esophagus. The esophagus is the hollow, muscular tube that moves food and liquid from the throat to the stomach. The wall of the esophagus is made up of several layers of tissue, including mucous membrane, muscle, and connective tissue. Esophageal cancer starts on the inside lining of the esophagus and spreads outward through the other layers as it grows.

The two most common forms of esophageal cancer are named for the type of cells that become malignant (cancerous):

- **Squamous cell carcinoma:** Cancer that forms in the thin, flat cells lining the inside of the esophagus. This cancer is most often found in the upper and middle part of the esophagus but can occur anywhere along the esophagus. This is also called "epidermoid carcinoma."

- **Adenocarcinoma:** Cancer that begins in glandular cells. Glandular cells in the lining of the esophagus produce and release fluids, such as mucus. Adenocarcinomas usually form in the lower part of the esophagus, near the stomach.

This chapter includes text excerpted from "Esophageal Cancer Treatment (PDQ®)—Patient Version," National Cancer Institute (NCI), March 7, 2019.

Risk of Esophageal Cancer

Anything that increases your risk of getting a disease is called a "risk factor." Having a risk factor does not mean that you will get cancer; not having risk factors does not mean that you will not get cancer. Talk with your doctor if you think you may be at risk. Risk factors include the following:

- Tobacco use

- Heavy alcohol use

- Barrett esophagus: A condition in which the cells lining the lower part of the esophagus have changed or been replaced with abnormal cells that could lead to cancer of the esophagus. Gastric reflux (heartburn) is the most common cause of Barrett esophagus.

- Older age

Signs and Symptoms of Esophageal Cancer

These and other signs and symptoms may be caused by esophageal cancer or by other conditions. Check with your doctor if you have any of the following:

- Painful or difficult swallowing

- Weight loss

- Pain behind the breastbone

- Hoarseness and cough

- Indigestion and heartburn

- A lump under the skin

Diagnosing Esophageal Cancer

Tests that examine the esophagus are used to detect (find) and diagnose esophageal cancer.

The following tests and procedures may be used:

- **Physical exam and history:** An exam of the body to check general signs of health, including checking for signs of disease, such as lumps or anything else that seems unusual. A history of the patient's health habits and past illnesses and treatments will also be taken.

- **Chest X-ray:** An X-ray of the organs and bones inside the chest. An X-ray is a type of energy beam that can go through the body and onto film, making a picture of areas inside the body.

- **Esophagoscopy:** A procedure to look inside the esophagus to check for abnormal areas. An esophagoscope is inserted through the mouth or nose and down the throat into the esophagus. An esophagoscope is a thin, tube-like instrument with a light and a lens for viewing. It may also have a tool to remove tissue samples, which are checked under a microscope for signs of cancer. When the esophagus and stomach are looked at, it is called an "upper endoscopy."

- **Biopsy:** The removal of cells or tissues so they can be viewed under a microscope by a pathologist to check for signs of cancer. The biopsy is usually done during an esophagoscopy. Sometimes, a biopsy shows changes in the esophagus that are not cancer but may lead to cancer.

Stages of Esophageal Cancer

After esophageal cancer has been diagnosed, tests are done to find out if cancer cells have spread within the esophagus or to other parts of the body.

The process used to find out if cancer cells have spread within the esophagus or to other parts of the body is called "staging." The information gathered from the staging process determines the stage of the disease. It is important to know the stage in order to plan treatment. The following tests and procedures may be used in the staging process.

- **Endoscopic ultrasound (EUS):** A procedure in which an endoscope is inserted into the body, usually through the mouth or rectum. For esophageal cancer, the endoscope is inserted through the mouth. An endoscope is a thin, tube-like instrument with a light and a lens for viewing. A probe at the end of the endoscope is used to bounce high-energy sound waves (ultrasound) off internal tissues or organs and make echoes. The echoes form a picture of body tissues called a "sonogram." A biopsy may also be done. This procedure is also called "endosonography."

- **Computed tomography (CT scan):** A procedure that makes a series of detailed pictures of areas inside the body, such as the chest, abdomen, and pelvis, taken from different angles.

The pictures are made by a computer linked to an X-ray machine. A dye may be injected into a vein or swallowed to help the organs or tissues show up more clearly. This procedure is also called "computed tomography," "computerized tomography," or "computerized axial tomography."

- **Positron emission tomography (PET) scan:** A procedure to find malignant tumor cells in the body. A small amount of radioactive glucose (sugar) is injected into a vein. The PET scanner rotates around the body and makes a picture of where glucose is being used in the body. Malignant tumor cells show up brighter in the picture because they are more active and take up more glucose than normal cells do. A PET scan and CT scan may be done at the same time. This is called a "PET-CT."

- **Magnetic resonance imaging (MRI):** A procedure that uses a magnet, radio waves, and a computer to make a series of detailed pictures of areas inside the body. This procedure is also called "nuclear magnetic resonance imaging" (NMRI).

- **Thoracoscopy:** A surgical procedure to look at the organs inside the chest to check for abnormal areas. An incision (cut) is made between two ribs and a thoracoscope is inserted into the chest. A thoracoscope is a thin, tube-like instrument with a light and a lens for viewing. It may also have a tool to remove tissue or lymph node samples, which are checked under a microscope for signs of cancer. In some cases, this procedure may be used to remove part of the esophagus or lung.

- **Laparoscopy:** A surgical procedure to look at the organs inside the abdomen to check for signs of disease. Small incisions (cuts) are made in the wall of the abdomen and a laparoscope (a thin, lighted tube) is inserted into one of the incisions. Other instruments may be inserted through the same or other incisions to perform procedures, such as removing organs or taking tissue samples to be checked under a microscope for signs of disease.

- **Ultrasound exam:** A procedure in which high-energy sound waves (ultrasound) are bounced off internal tissues or organs, such as those in the neck, and make echoes. The echoes form a sonogram. The picture can be printed to be looked at later.

Stages of Squamous Cell Carcinoma of the Esophagus

The following stages are used for squamous cell carcinoma of the esophagus.

Stage 0 (High-Grade Dysplasia)

In stage 0, cancer has formed in the inner lining of the esophagus wall. Stage 0 is also called "high-grade dysplasia."

Stage I Squamous Cell Carcinoma of the Esophagus

Stage I is divided into stages IA and IB, depending on where the cancer has spread.

- **Stage IA:** Cancer has spread into the mucosa layer or thin muscle layer of the esophagus wall. The cancer cells are grade 1, or the grade is not known.

- **Stage IB:** Cancer has spread into the mucosa layer, thin muscle layer, or submucosa layer of the esophagus wall. The cancer cells are any grade, or the grade is not known.

Stage II Squamous Cell Carcinoma of the Esophagus

Stage II is divided into stages IIA and IIB, depending on where the cancer has spread.

- **Stage IIA:** Cancer has spread:
  - Into the thick muscle layer of the esophagus wall. The cancer cells are grade 2 or 3, or the grade is not known.
  - Into the connective tissue layer of the esophagus wall. The tumor is in the lower esophagus.
  - Into the connective tissue layer of the esophagus wall. The tumor is in either the upper or middle esophagus.

- **Stage IIB:** Cancer has spread:
  - Into the connective tissue layer of the esophagus wall. The cancer cells are grade 2 or 3. The tumor is in either the upper or middle esophagus.
  - Into the connective tissue layer of the esophagus wall. The grade of the cancer cells is not known, or it is not known where the tumor has formed in the esophagus.

- Into the mucosa layer, thin muscle layer, or submucosa layer of the esophagus wall. Cancer is found in one or two lymph nodes near the tumor.

Stage III Squamous Cell Carcinoma of the Esophagus

Stage III is divided into stages IIIA and IIIB, depending on where the cancer has spread.

- **Stage IIIA:** Cancer has spread:

  - Into the mucosa layer, thin muscle layer, or submucosa layer of the esophagus wall. Cancer is found in three to six lymph nodes near the tumor.

  - Into the thick muscle layer of the esophagus wall. Cancer is found in one or two lymph nodes near the tumor.

- **Stage IIIB:** Cancer has spread:

  - Into the thick muscle layer or the connective tissue layer of the esophagus wall. Cancer is found in one to six lymph nodes near the tumor.

  - Into the diaphragm, pleura, sac around the heart, azygos vein, or peritoneum. Cancer may be found in one or two lymph nodes near the tumor.

Stage IV Squamous Cell Carcinoma of the Esophagus

Stage IV is divided into stages IVA and IVB, depending on where the cancer has spread.

- **Stage IVA:** Cancer has spread:

  - Into the diaphragm, pleura, sac around the heart, azygos vein, or peritoneum. Cancer is found in three to six lymph nodes near the tumor.

  - Into nearby structures, such as the aorta, airway, or spine. Cancer may be found in one to six lymph nodes near the tumor.

  - To seven or more lymph nodes near the tumor

- **Stage IVB:** Cancer has spread to other parts of the body, such as the liver.

Stages of Adenocarcinoma of the Esophagus

The following stages are used for adenocarcinoma of the esophagus:

Stage 0 (High-Grade Dysplasia)

In stage 0, cancer has formed in the inner lining of the esophagus wall. Stage 0 is also called "high-grade dysplasia."

Stage I Adenocarcinoma of the Esophagus

Stage I is divided into stages IA, IB, and IC, depending on where the cancer has spread.

- **Stage IA:** Cancer has spread into the mucosa layer or thin muscle layer of the esophagus wall. The cancer cells are grade 1, or the grade is not known.
- **Stage IB:** Cancer has spread:
  - Into the mucosa layer or thin muscle layer of the esophagus wall. The cancer cells are grade 2.
  - Into the submucosa layer of the esophagus wall. The cancer cells are grade 1 or 2, or the grade is not known.
- **Stage IC:** Cancer has spread:
  - Into the mucosa layer, thin muscle layer, or submucosa layer of the esophagus wall. The cancer cells are grade 3.
  - Into the thick muscle layer of the esophagus wall. The cancer cells are grade 1 or 2.

Stage II Adenocarcinoma of the Esophagus

Stage II is divided into stages IIA and IIB, depending on where the cancer has spread.

- **Stage IIA:** Cancer has spread into the thick muscle layer of the esophagus wall. The cancer cells are grade 3, or the grade is not known.
- **Stage IIB:** Cancer has spread:
  - Into the connective tissue layer of the esophagus wall
  - Into the mucosa layer, thin muscle layer, or submucosa layer of the esophagus wall. Cancer is found in one or two lymph nodes near the tumor.

Stage III Adenocarcinoma of the Esophagus

Stage III is divided into stages IIIA and IIIB, depending on where the cancer has spread.

- **Stage IIIA:** Cancer has spread:
  - Into the mucosa layer, thin muscle layer, or submucosa layer of the esophagus wall. Cancer is found in three to six lymph nodes near the tumor.
  - Into the thick muscle layer of the esophagus wall. Cancer is found in one or two lymph nodes near the tumor.
- **Stage IIIB:** Cancer has spread:
  - Into the thick muscle layer of the esophagus wall. Cancer is found in three to six lymph nodes near the tumor.
  - Into the connective tissue layer of the esophagus wall. Cancer is found in one to six lymph nodes near the tumor.
  - Into the diaphragm, pleura, sac around the heart, azygos vein, or peritoneum. Cancer may be found in one or two lymph nodes near the tumor.

Stage IV Adenocarcinoma of the Esophagus

Stage IV is divided into stages IVA and IVB, depending on where the cancer has spread.

- **Stage IVA:** Cancer has spread:
  - Into the diaphragm, pleura, sac around the heart, azygos vein, or peritoneum. Cancer is found in three to six lymph nodes near the tumor.
  - Into nearby structures, such as the aorta, airway, or spine. Cancer may be found in one to six lymph nodes near the tumor.
  - To seven or more lymph nodes near the tumor
- **Stage IVB:** Cancer has spread to other parts of the body, such as the liver.

Treatment Options Overview

Different types of treatment are available for patients with esophageal cancer. Some treatments are standard (the currently used treatment), and some are being tested in clinical trials. A treatment clinical trial is a research study meant to help improve current treatments or obtain information on new treatments for patients with cancer. When clinical trials show that a new treatment is better than the standard treatment, the new treatment may become the standard treatment. Patients may want to think about taking part in a clinical trial. Some clinical trials are open only to patients who have not started treatment.

Patients have special nutritional needs during treatment for esophageal cancer.

Many people with esophageal cancer find it hard to eat because they have trouble swallowing. The esophagus may be narrowed by the tumor or as a side effect of treatment. Some patients may receive nutrients directly into a vein. Others may need a feeding tube (a flexible plastic tube that is passed through the nose or mouth into the stomach) until they are able to eat on their own.

Surgery

Surgery is the most common treatment for cancer of the esophagus. Part of the esophagus may be removed in an operation called an "esophagectomy."

The doctor will connect the remaining healthy part of the esophagus to the stomach so the patient can still swallow. A plastic tube or part of the intestine may be used to make the connection. Lymph nodes near the esophagus may also be removed and viewed under a microscope to see if they contain cancer. If the esophagus is partly blocked by the tumor, an expandable metal stent (tube) may be placed inside the esophagus to help keep it open.

Small, early-stage cancer and high-grade dysplasia of the esophagus may be removed by endoscopic resection. An endoscope is inserted through a small incision in the skin or through an opening in the body, such as the mouth. A tool attached to the endoscope is used to remove tissue.

Radiation Therapy

Radiation therapy is a cancer treatment that uses high-energy X-rays or other types of radiation to kill cancer cells or keep them from growing. There are two types of radiation therapy:

1. External radiation therapy uses a machine outside the body to send radiation toward the cancer.

2. Internal radiation therapy uses a radioactive substance sealed in needles, seeds, wires, or catheters that are placed directly into or near the cancer.

The way the radiation therapy is given depends on the type and stage of the cancer being treated. External and internal radiation therapy are used to treat esophageal cancer.

A plastic tube may be inserted into the esophagus to keep it open during radiation therapy. This is called "intraluminal intubation and dilation."

Chemotherapy

Chemotherapy is a cancer treatment that uses drugs to stop the growth of cancer cells, either by killing the cells or by stopping them from dividing. When chemotherapy is taken by mouth or injected into a vein or muscle, the drugs enter the bloodstream and can reach cancer cells throughout the body (systemic chemotherapy). When chemotherapy is placed directly into the cerebrospinal fluid; an organ; or a body cavity, such as the abdomen, the drugs mainly affect cancer cells in those areas (regional chemotherapy). The way the chemotherapy is given depends on the type and stage of the cancer being treated.

Chemoradiation Therapy

Chemoradiation therapy combines chemotherapy and radiation therapy to increase the effects of both.

Laser Therapy

Laser therapy is a cancer treatment that uses a laser beam (a narrow beam of intense light) to kill cancer cells.

Electrocoagulation

Electrocoagulation is the use of an electric current to kill cancer cells.

Treatment for Esophageal Cancer May Cause Side Effects

For some patients, taking part in a clinical trial may be the best treatment choice. Clinical trials are part of the cancer research process.

Clinical trials are done to find out if new cancer treatments are safe and effective or better than the standard treatment.

Many of standard treatments for cancer are based on earlier clinical trials. Patients who take part in a clinical trial may receive the standard treatment or be among the first to receive a new treatment. Patients who take part in clinical trials also help improve the way cancer will be treated in the future. Even when clinical trials do not lead to effective new treatments, they often answer important questions and help move research forward.

Patients can enter clinical trials before, during, or after starting their cancer treatment. Some clinical trials only include patients who have not yet received treatment. Other trials test treatments for patients whose cancer has not gotten better. There are also clinical trials that test new ways to stop cancer from recurring or reduce the side effects of cancer treatment. Clinical trials are taking place in many parts of the country. Information about clinical trials supported by the National Cancer Institute (NCI) can be found on the NCI's clinical trials search webpage.

Follow-Up Tests May Be Needed

Some of the tests that were done to diagnose cancer or to find out the stage of the cancer may be repeated. Some tests will be repeated in order to see how well the treatment is working. Decisions about whether to continue, change, or stop treatment may be based on the results of these tests.

Some of the tests will continue to be done from time to time after treatment has ended. The results of these tests can show if your condition has changed or if cancer has recurred. These tests are sometimes called "follow-up tests" or "check-ups."

Chapter 45

Hypopharyngeal Cancer

Hypopharyngeal cancer is a disease in which malignant (cancer) cells form in the tissues of the hypopharynx.

The hypopharynx is the bottom part of the pharynx (throat). The pharynx is a hollow tube, about five inches long, that starts behind the nose, goes down the neck, and ends at the top of the trachea (windpipe) and esophagus (the tube that goes from the throat to the stomach). Air and food pass through the pharynx on the way to the trachea or the esophagus.

Most hypopharyngeal cancers form in squamous cells—the thin, flat cells lining the inside of the hypopharynx. The hypopharynx has three different areas. Cancer may be found in one or more of these areas.

Hypopharyngeal cancer is a type of head and neck cancer.

Risk of Hypopharyngeal Cancer

Use of tobacco products and heavy drinking can affect the risk of developing hypopharyngeal cancer.

Anything that increases your risk of getting a disease is called a "risk factor." Having a risk factor does not mean that you will get cancer; not having risk factors does not mean that you will not get

This chapter includes text excerpted from "Hypopharyngeal Cancer Treatment (Adult) (PDQ®)–Patient Version," National Cancer Institute (NCI), May 1, 2018.

cancer. Talk with your doctor if you think you may be at risk. Risk factors include the following:

- Smoking tobacco

- Chewing tobacco

- Heavy alcohol use

- Eating a diet without enough nutrients

- Having Plummer-Vinson syndrome

Signs and Symptoms of Hypopharyngeal Cancer

These and other signs and symptoms may be caused by hypopharyngeal cancer or by other conditions. Check with your doctor if you have any of the following:

- A sore throat that does not go away

- Ear pain

- A lump in the neck

- Painful or difficult swallowing

- A change in voice

Diagnosing Hypopharyngeal Cancer

Tests that examine the throat and neck are used to help detect (find) and diagnose hypopharyngeal cancer.

The following tests and procedures may be used.

- **Physical exam of the throat**: An exam in which the doctor feels for swollen lymph nodes in the neck and looks down the throat with a small, long-handled mirror to check for abnormal areas.

- **Computed tomography (CT scan)**: A procedure that makes a series of detailed pictures of areas inside the body, taken from different angles. The pictures are made by a computer linked to an X-ray machine. A dye may be injected into a vein or swallowed to help the organs or tissues show up more clearly. This procedure is also called "computed tomography," "computerized tomography," or "computerized axial tomography."

- **Positron emission tomography scan (PET scan)**: A procedure to find malignant tumor cells in the body. A small amount of radioactive glucose (sugar) is injected into a vein. The PET scanner rotates around the body and makes a picture of where glucose is being used in the body. Malignant tumor cells show up brighter in the picture because they are more active and take up more glucose than normal cells do. A PET scan and CT scan may be done at the same time. This is called a "PET-CT."

- **Magnetic resonance imaging (MRI scan)**: A procedure that uses a magnet, radio waves, and a computer to make a series of detailed pictures of areas inside the body. This procedure is also called "nuclear magnetic resonance imaging" (NMRI).

- **Bone scan**: A procedure to check if there are rapidly dividing cells, such as cancer cells, in the bone. A very small amount of radioactive material is injected into a vein and travels through the bloodstream. The radioactive material collects in the bones with cancer and is detected by a scanner.

- **Barium esophagogram**: An X-ray of the esophagus. The patient drinks a liquid that contains barium (a silver-white metallic compound). The liquid coats the esophagus and X-rays are taken.

- **Endoscopy**: A procedure used to look at areas in the throat that cannot be seen with a mirror during the physical exam of the throat. An endoscope (a thin, lighted tube) is inserted through the nose or mouth to check the throat for anything that seems unusual. Tissue samples may be taken for biopsy.

- **Esophagoscopy**: A procedure to look inside the esophagus to check for abnormal areas. An esophagoscope (a thin, lighted tube) is inserted through the mouth or nose and down the throat into the esophagus. Tissue samples may be taken for biopsy.

- **Bronchoscopy**: A procedure to look inside the trachea and large airways in the lung for abnormal areas. A bronchoscope (a thin, lighted tube) is inserted through the nose or mouth into the trachea and lungs. Tissue samples may be taken for biopsy.

- **Biopsy**: The removal of cells or tissues so they can be viewed under a microscope to check for signs of cancer.

Stages of Hypopharyngeal Cancer

After hypopharyngeal cancer has been diagnosed, tests are done to find out if cancer cells have spread within the hypopharynx or to other parts of the body.

The process used to find out if cancer has spread within the hypopharynx or to other parts of the body is called "staging." The information gathered from the staging process determines the stage of the disease. It is important to know the stage of the disease in order to plan treatment. The results of some of the tests used to diagnose hypopharyngeal cancer are often also used to stage the disease.

The following stages are used for hypopharyngeal cancer.

Stage 0 (Carcinoma in Situ)

In stage 0, abnormal cells are found in the lining of the hypopharynx. These abnormal cells may become cancer and spread into nearby normal tissue. Stage 0 is also called "carcinoma in situ."

Stage I

In stage I, cancer has formed in one area of the hypopharynx only, and/or the tumor is two centimeters or smaller.

Stage II

In stage II, the tumor is either:

- Larger than two centimeters but not larger than four centimeters and has not spread to the Larynx (voice box)

- Found in more than one area of the hypopharynx or in nearby tissues

Stage III

In stage III, the tumor:

- It is larger than four centimeters or has spread to the larynx (voice box) or esophagus. Cancer may have spread to one lymph node on the same side of the neck as the tumor, and the lymph node is three centimeters or smaller.

- Has spread to one lymph node on the same side of the neck as the tumor, and the lymph node is three centimeters or smaller. The cancer is found:

  - In one area of the hypopharynx and/or is two centimeters or smaller

    - In more than one area of the hypopharynx or in nearby tissues, or is larger than two centimeters but not larger than four centimeters and has not spread to the larynx

Stage IV

Stage IV is divided into stage IVA, IVB, and IVC as follows:

- In stage IVA, cancer:
- Has spread to cartilage around the thyroid or trachea, the bone under the tongue, the thyroid, or nearby soft tissue. Cancer may have spread to one lymph node on the same side of the neck as the tumor, and the lymph node is three centimeters or smaller.
- Has spread to one lymph node on the same side of the neck as the tumor (the lymph node is larger than three centimeters but not larger than six centimeters) or to lymph nodes anywhere in the neck (affected lymph nodes are six centimeters or smaller), and one of the following is true:
  - Cancer is found in one area of the hypopharynx and/or is two centimeters or smaller.
  - Cancer is found in more than one area of the hypopharynx or in nearby tissues, or is larger than two centimeters but not larger than four centimeters and has not spread to the larynx (voice box).
  - Cancer has spread to the larynx or esophagus and is larger than four centimeters.
  - Cancer has spread to cartilage around the thyroid or trachea, the bone under the tongue, the thyroid, or nearby soft tissue.
- In stage IVB, the tumor:
  - Has spread to muscles around the upper part of the spinal column, the carotid artery, or the lining of the chest cavity and may have spread to lymph nodes which can be any size
  - May be any size and has spread to one or more lymph nodes that are larger than six centimeters.
- In stage IVC, the tumor may be any size and has spread beyond the hypopharynx to other parts of the body.

Treatment Options Overview

There are different types of treatment for patients with hypopharyngeal cancer:

Different types of treatment are available for patients with hypopharyngeal cancer. Some treatments are standard (the currently used treatment), and some are being tested in clinical trials. A treatment clinical trial is a research study meant to help improve current treatments or obtain information on new treatments for patients with cancer. When clinical trials show that a new treatment is better than the standard treatment, the new treatment may become the standard treatment. Patients may want to think about taking part in a clinical trial. Some clinical trials are open only to patients who have not started treatment.

Surgery

Surgery (removing the cancer in an operation) is a common treatment for all stages of hypopharyngeal cancer. The following surgical procedures may be used:

- **Laryngopharyngectomy**: Surgery to remove the larynx (voice box) and part of the pharynx (throat).

- **Partial laryngopharyngectomy**: Surgery to remove part of the larynx and part of the pharynx. A partial laryngopharyngectomy prevents loss of the voice.

- **Neck dissection**: Surgery to remove lymph nodes and other tissues in the neck.

After the doctor removes all the cancer that can be seen at the time of the surgery, some patients may be given chemotherapy or radiation therapy after surgery to kill any cancer cells that are left. Treatment given after the surgery, to lower the risk that the cancer will come back, is called "adjuvant therapy."

Radiation Therapy

Radiation therapy is a cancer treatment that uses high-energy X-rays or other types of radiation to kill cancer cells or keep them from growing. There are two types of radiation therapy:

- External radiation therapy uses a machine outside the body to send radiation toward the cancer.

- Internal radiation therapy uses a radioactive substance sealed in needles, seeds, wires, or catheters that are placed directly into or near the cancer.

The way the radiation therapy is given depends on the type and stage of the cancer being treated. External radiation therapy is used to treat hypopharyngeal cancer.

Radiation therapy may work better in patients who have stopped smoking before beginning treatment. External radiation therapy to the thyroid or the pituitary gland may change the way the thyroid gland works. A blood test to check the thyroid hormone level in the body may be done before and after therapy to make sure the thyroid gland is working properly.

Chemotherapy

Chemotherapy is a cancer treatment that uses drugs to stop the growth of cancer cells, either by killing the cells or by stopping the cells from dividing. When chemotherapy is taken by mouth or injected into a vein or muscle, the drugs enter the bloodstream and can reach cancer cells throughout the body (systemic chemotherapy). When chemotherapy is placed directly into the cerebrospinal fluid, an organ, or a body cavity such as the abdomen, the drugs mainly affect cancer cells in those areas (regional chemotherapy). The way the chemotherapy is given depends on the type and stage of the cancer being treated.

Chemotherapy may be used to shrink the tumor before surgery or radiation therapy. This is called "neoadjuvant chemotherapy."

Treatment for Hypopharyngeal Cancer May Cause Side Effects

Patients may want to think about taking part in a clinical trial.

For some patients, taking part in a clinical trial may be the best treatment choice. Clinical trials are part of the cancer research process. Clinical trials are done to find out if new cancer treatments are safe and effective or better than the standard treatment.

Many of standard treatments for cancer are based on earlier clinical trials. Patients who take part in a clinical trial may receive the standard treatment or be among the first to receive a new treatment. Patients who take part in clinical trials also help improve the way cancer will be treated in the future. Even when clinical trials do not lead to effective new treatments, they often answer important questions and help move research forward.

Patients can enter clinical trials before, during, or after starting their cancer treatment. Some clinical trials only include patients who have not yet received treatment. Other trials test treatments for patients whose cancer has not gotten better. There are also clinical trials that test new ways to stop cancer from recurring (coming back) or reduce the side effects of cancer treatment.

Follow-Up Tests May Be Needed

Some of the tests that were done to diagnose the cancer or to find out the stage of the cancer may be repeated. Some tests will be repeated in order to see how well the treatment is working. Decisions about whether to continue, change, or stop treatment may be based on the results of these tests.

Some of the tests will continue to be done from time to time after treatment has ended. The results of these tests can show if your condition has changed or if the cancer has recurred (come back). These tests are sometimes called "follow-up tests" or "check-ups."

For hypopharyngeal cancer, follow-ups to check for recurrence should include careful head and neck exams once a month in the first year after treatment ends, every two months in the second year, every three months in the third year, and every six months thereafter.

Chapter 46

Laryngeal Cancer

Laryngeal cancer is a disease in which malignant (cancer) cells form in the tissues of the larynx.

The larynx is a part of the throat, between the base of the tongue and the trachea. The larynx contains the vocal cords, which vibrate and make sound when the air is directed against them. The sound echoes through the pharynx, mouth, and nose to make a person's voice. There are three main parts of the larynx:

- **Supraglottis:** The upper part of the larynx above the vocal cords, including the epiglottis.

- **Glottis:** The middle part of the larynx where the vocal cords are located.

- **Subglottis:** The lower part of the larynx between the vocal cords and the trachea (windpipe).

Most laryngeal cancers form in squamous cells—the thin, flat cells lining the inside of the larynx.

Laryngeal cancer is a type of head and neck cancer. Use of tobacco products and drinking too much alcohol can affect the risk of laryngeal cancer. Anything that increases your risk of getting a disease is called a "risk factor." Having a risk factor does not mean that you will get

This chapter includes text excerpted from "Laryngeal Cancer Treatment (Adult) (PDQ®)—Patient Version," National Cancer Institute (NCI), April 5, 2019.

cancer; not having risk factors does not mean that you will not get cancer. Talk with your doctor if you think you may be at risk.

Signs and Symptoms of Laryngeal Cancer

Signs and symptoms of laryngeal cancer include a sore throat and ear pain.

These and other signs and symptoms may be caused by laryngeal cancer or by other conditions. Check with your doctor if you have any of the following:

- A sore throat or cough that does not go away

- Trouble or pain when swallowing

- Ear pain

- A lump in the neck or throat

- A change or hoarseness in the voice

Diagnosing Laryngeal Cancer

The following tests and procedures may be used:

- **Physical exam of the throat and neck:** An exam to check the throat and neck for abnormal areas. The doctor will feel the inside of the mouth with a gloved finger and examine the mouth and throat with a small long-handled mirror and light. This will include checking the insides of the cheeks and lips; the gums; the back, roof, and floor of the mouth; the top, bottom, and sides of the tongue; and the throat. The neck will be felt for swollen lymph nodes. A history of the patient's health habits and past illnesses and medical treatments will also be taken.

- **Biopsy:**The removal of cells or tissues so they can be viewed under a microscope by a pathologist to check for signs of cancer. The sample of tissue may be removed during one of the following procedures:

  - **Laryngoscopy:** A procedure in which the doctor checks the larynx (voice box) with a mirror or a laryngoscope to check for abnormal areas. A laryngoscope is a thin, tube-like instrument with a light and a lens for viewing the inside of the throat and voice box. It may also have a tool to remove tissue samples, which are checked under a microscope for signs of cancer.

- **Endoscopy:** A procedure to look at organs and tissues inside the body, such as the throat, esophagus, and trachea, to check for abnormal areas. An endoscope (a thin, lighted tube with a light and a lens for viewing) is inserted through an opening in the body, such as the mouth. A special tool on the endoscope may be used to remove samples of tissue.

- **Computed tomography (CT) scan:** A procedure that makes a series of detailed pictures of areas inside the body, taken from different angles. The pictures are made by a computer linked to an X-ray machine. A dye may be injected into a vein or swallowed to help the organs or tissues show up more clearly. This procedure is also called "computed tomography," "computerized tomography," or "computerized axial tomography."

- **Magnetic resonance imaging (MRI):** A procedure that uses a magnet, radio waves, and a computer to make a series of detailed pictures of areas inside the body. This procedure is also called "nuclear magnetic resonance imaging" (NMRI).

- **Positron emission tomography scan (PET):** A procedure to find malignant tumor cells in the body. A small amount of radioactive glucose (sugar) is injected into a vein. The PET scanner rotates around the body and makes a picture of where glucose is being used in the body. Malignant tumor cells show up brighter in the picture because they are more active and take up more glucose than normal cells do.

- **Positron emission tomography-computed tomography scan (PET-CT):** A procedure that combines the pictures from a positron emission tomography (PET) scan and a computed tomography (CT) scan. The PET and CT scans are done at the same time with the same machine. The combined scans give more detailed pictures of areas inside the body than either scan gives by itself. A PET-CT scan may be used to help diagnose disease, such as cancer; plan treatment; or find out how well treatment is working.

- **Bone scan:** A procedure to check if there are rapidly dividing cells, such as cancer cells, in the bone. A very small amount of radioactive material is injected into a vein and travels through the bloodstream. The radioactive material collects in the bones with cancer and is detected by a scanner.

- **Barium swallow:** A series of X-rays of the esophagus and stomach. The patient drinks a liquid that contains barium (a silver-white metallic compound). The liquid coats the esophagus and stomach, and X-rays are taken. This procedure is also called an "upper GI series."

Stages of Laryngeal Cancer

After laryngeal cancer has been diagnosed, tests are done to find out if cancer cells have spread within the larynx or to other parts of the body.

The process used to find out if cancer has spread within the larynx or to other parts of the body is called "staging." The information gathered from the staging process determines the stage of the disease. It is important to know the stage of the disease in order to plan treatment. The results of some of the tests used to diagnose laryngeal cancer are often also used to stage the disease.

Stage 0 (Carcinoma in Situ)

In stage 0, abnormal cells are found in the lining of the larynx. These abnormal cells may become cancer and spread into nearby normal tissue. Stage 0 is also called "carcinoma in situ."

Stage I

In stage I, cancer has formed. Stage I laryngeal cancer depends on where cancer began in the larynx:

- **Supraglottis:** Cancer is in one area of the supraglottis only, and the vocal cords can move normally.

- **Glottis:** Cancer is in one or both vocal cords, and the vocal cords can move normally.

- **Subglottis:** Cancer is in the subglottis only.

Stage II

In stage II, cancer is in the larynx only. Stage II laryngeal cancer depends on where cancer began in the larynx:

- **Supraglottis:** Cancer is in more than one area of the supraglottis or surrounding tissues.

- **Glottis:** Cancer has spread to the supraglottis and/or the subglottis and/or the vocal cords cannot move normally.

- **Subglottis:** Cancer has spread to one or both vocal cords, which may not move normally.

Stage III

Stage III laryngeal cancer depends on whether cancer has spread from the supraglottis, glottis, or subglottis.

In stage III cancer of the supraglottis:

- Cancer is in the larynx only, and the vocal cords cannot move, and/or cancer is in tissues next to the larynx. Cancer may have spread to one lymph node on the same side of the neck as the original tumor, and the lymph node is three centimeters or smaller.

- Cancer is in one area of the supraglottis and in one lymph node on the same side of the neck as the original tumor; the lymph node is three centimeters or smaller, and the vocal cords can move normally.

- Cancer is in more than one area of the supraglottis or surrounding tissues and in one lymph node on the same side of the neck as the original tumor; the lymph node is three centimeters or smaller.

In stage III cancer of the glottis:

- Cancer is in the larynx only, and the vocal cords cannot move, and/or cancer is in tissues next to the larynx; cancer may have spread to one lymph node on the same side of the neck as the original tumor, and the lymph node is three centimeters or smaller.

- Cancer is in one or both vocal cords and in one lymph node on the same side of the neck as the original tumor; the lymph node is three centimeters or smaller, and the vocal cords can move normally.

- Cancer has spread to the supraglottis and/or the subglottis, and/ or the vocal cords cannot move normally. Cancer has also spread to one lymph node on the same side of the neck as the original tumor, and the lymph node is three centimeters or smaller.

In stage III cancer of the subglottis:

- Cancer is in the larynx, and the vocal cords cannot move; cancer may have spread to one lymph node on the same side of the neck as the original tumor, and the lymph node is three centimeters or smaller.

- Cancer is in the subglottis and in one lymph node on the same side of the neck as the original tumor; the lymph node is three centimeters or smaller.

- Cancer has spread to one or both vocal cords, which may not move normally. Cancer has also spread to one lymph node on the same side of the neck as the original tumor, and the lymph node is three centimeters or smaller.

Stage IV

Stage IV is divided into stage IVA, stage IVB, and stage IVC. Each substage is the same for cancer in the supraglottis, glottis, or subglottis.

- In stage IVA:

  - Cancer has spread through the thyroid cartilage and/or has spread to tissues beyond the larynx, such as the neck, trachea, thyroid, or esophagus. Cancer may have spread to one lymph node on the same side of the neck as the original tumor, and the lymph node is three centimeters or smaller.

  - Cancer has spread to one lymph node on the same side of the neck as the original tumor, and the lymph node is larger than three centimeters but not larger than six centimeters or has spread to more than one lymph node anywhere in the neck, with none larger than six centimeters. Cancer may have spread to tissues beyond the larynx, such as the neck, trachea, thyroid, or esophagus. The vocal cords may not move normally.

- In stage IVB:

  - Cancer has spread to the space in front of the spinal column, surrounds the carotid artery, or has spread to parts of the chest. Cancer may have spread to one or more lymph nodes anywhere in the neck, and the lymph nodes may be any size.

  - Cancer has spread to a lymph node that is larger than six centimeters and may have spread as far as the space in front of the spinal column, around the carotid artery, or to parts of the chest. The vocal cords may not move normally.

- In stage IVC, cancer has spread to other parts of the body, such as the lungs, liver, or bone.

Treatment Options Overview

Different types of treatment are available for patients with laryngeal cancer. Some treatments are standard (the currently used treatment), and some are being tested in clinical trials. A treatment clinical trial is a research study meant to help improve current treatments or obtain information on new treatments for patients with cancer. When clinical trials show that a new treatment is better than the standard treatment, the new treatment may become the standard treatment. Patients may want to think about taking part in a clinical trial. Some clinical trials are open only to patients who have not started treatment.

Radiation Therapy

Radiation therapy is a cancer treatment that uses high-energy X-rays or other types of radiation to kill cancer cells or keep them from growing. There are two types of radiation therapy:

- External radiation therapy uses a machine outside the body to send radiation toward the cancer.

- Internal radiation therapy uses a radioactive substance sealed in needles, seeds, wires, or catheters that are placed directly into or near the cancer.

The way the radiation therapy is given depends on the type and stage of the cancer being treated. External radiation therapy is used to treat laryngeal cancer.

Radiation therapy may work better in patients who have stopped smoking before beginning treatment. External radiation therapy to the thyroid or the pituitary gland may change the way the thyroid gland works. A blood test to check the thyroid hormone level in the body may be done before and after therapy to make sure the thyroid gland is working properly.

Hyperfractionated radiation therapy may be used to treat laryngeal cancer. Hyperfractionated radiation therapy is radiation treatment in which a smaller than usual total daily dose of radiation is divided into two doses, and the treatments are given twice a day. Hyperfractionated radiation therapy is given over the same period of time (days or weeks) as standard radiation therapy. New types of radiation therapy are being studied in the treatment of laryngeal cancer.

Surgery

Surgery (removing the cancer in an operation) is a common treatment for all stages of laryngeal cancer. The following surgical procedures may be used:

- **Cordectomy:** Surgery to remove the vocal cords only.

- **Supraglottic laryngectomy:** Surgery to remove the supraglottis only.

- **Hemilaryngectomy:** Surgery to remove half of the larynx (voice box). A hemilaryngectomy saves the voice.

- **Partial laryngectomy:** Surgery to remove part of the larynx (voice box). A partial laryngectomy helps keep the patient's ability to talk.

- **Total laryngectomy:** Surgery to remove the whole larynx. During this operation, a hole is made in the front of the neck to allow the patient to breathe. This is called a "tracheostomy."

- **Thyroidectomy:** The removal of all or part of the thyroid gland.

- **Laser surgery:** A surgical procedure that uses a laser beam (a narrow beam of intense light) as a knife to make bloodless cuts in tissue or to remove a surface lesion, such as a tumor in the larynx.

After the doctor removes all the cancer that can be seen at the time of the surgery, some patients may be given chemotherapy or radiation therapy after surgery to kill any cancer cells that are left. Treatment given after the surgery, to lower the risk that the cancer will come back, is called "adjuvant therapy."

Chemotherapy

Chemotherapy is a cancer treatment that uses drugs to stop the growth of cancer cells, either by killing the cells or by stopping the cells from dividing. When chemotherapy is taken by mouth or injected into a vein or muscle, the drugs enter the bloodstream and can reach cancer cells throughout the body (systemic chemotherapy). When chemotherapy is placed directly into the cerebrospinal fluid; an organ; or a body cavity, such as the abdomen, the drugs mainly affect cancer cells in those areas (regional chemotherapy). The way the chemotherapy is given depends on the type and stage of the cancer being treated.

Targeted Therapy

Targeted therapy is a type of treatment that uses drugs or other substances to attack specific cancer cells. Targeted therapies usually cause less harm to normal cells than chemotherapy or radiation therapy do.

Monoclonal antibodies are a type of targeted therapy being studied in the treatment of laryngeal cancer. Monoclonal antibody therapy is a cancer treatment that uses antibodies made in the laboratory from a single type of immune system cell. These antibodies can identify substances on cancer cells or normal substances in the blood or tissues that may help cancer cells grow. The antibodies attach to the substances and kill the cancer cells, block their growth, or keep them from spreading. Monoclonal antibodies are given by infusion. They may be used alone or to carry drugs, toxins, or radioactive material directly to cancer cells.

Cetuximab is a type of monoclonal antibody that is being studied in the treatment of laryngeal cancer. It works by binding to a protein on the surface of the cancer cells and stops the cells from growing and dividing.

Radiosensitizers

Radiosensitizers are drugs that make tumor cells more sensitive to radiation therapy. Combining radiation therapy with radiosensitizers may kill more tumor cells.

Patients may want to think about taking part in a clinical trial. For some patients, taking part in a clinical trial may be the best treatment choice. Clinical trials are part of the cancer research process. Clinical trials are done to find out if new cancer treatments are safe and effective or better than the standard treatment.

Many of today's standard treatments for cancer are based on earlier clinical trials. Patients who take part in a clinical trial may receive the standard treatment or be among the first to receive a new treatment. Patients who take part in clinical trials also help improve the way cancer will be treated in the future. Even when clinical trials do not lead to effective new treatments, they often answer important questions and help move research forward.

Patients can enter clinical trials before, during, or after starting their cancer treatment. Some clinical trials only include patients who have not yet received treatment. Other trials test treatments for patients whose cancer has not gotten better. There are also clinical trials that test new ways to stop cancer from recurring or reduce the side effects of cancer treatment.

Follow-up tests may be needed. Some of the tests that were done to diagnose the cancer or to find out the stage of the cancer may be repeated. Some tests will be repeated in order to see how well the treatment is working. Decisions about whether to continue, change, or stop treatment may be based on the results of these tests. Some of the tests will continue to be done from time to time after treatment has ended. The results of these tests can show if your condition has changed or if the cancer has recurred. These tests are sometimes called "follow-up tests" or "check-ups."

Treatment Options for Recurrent Laryngeal Cancer

Recurrent laryngeal cancer is cancer that has recurred after it has been treated. The cancer is most likely to come back in the first two to three years. It may come back in the larynx or in other parts of the body.

Treatment of recurrent laryngeal cancer may include the following:

- Surgery with or without radiation therapy

- Radiation therapy

- Chemotherapy

- A clinical trial of chemotherapy as palliative therapy to relieve symptoms caused by the cancer and improve quality of life

Chapter 47

Recent Research in Cancer of the Ear, Nose, and Throat

Chapter Contents

Section 47.1

Cetuximab with Radiation Found to Be Inferior to Standard Treatment in HPV-Positive Oropharyngeal Cancer

This section includes text excerpted from "Cetuximab with Radiation Found to Be Inferior to Standard Treatment in HPV-Positive Oropharyngeal Cancer," National Cancer Institute (NCI), August 14, 2018.

An interim analysis of data from a randomized clinical trial of patients with human papillomavirus (HPV)-positive oropharyngeal cancer found that treatment with radiation therapy and cetuximab is associated with worse overall and progression-free survival, compared to the current standard treatment with radiation and cisplatin. The trial was designed to see if cetuximab with radiation would be less toxic than cisplatin with radiation without compromising survival for patients with the disease.

The phase 3 trial, which closed enrollment in 2014, was funded by the National Cancer Institute's (NCI), part of the National Institutes of Health (NIH), and led by NRG Oncology, part of National Clinical Trials Network (NCTN). The data monitoring committee overseeing the trial recommended releasing the data after an interim data analysis showed that cetuximab with radiation was associated with inferior overall and progression-free survival, compared to cisplatin and radiation. The U.S. Food and Drug Administration (FDA) has previously approved cetuximab with radiation for patients with head and neck cancer, including oropharyngeal cancer. Cetuximab with radiation is an accepted standard of care, especially for patients who cannot tolerate cisplatin.

"The goal of this trial was to find an alternative to cisplatin that would be as effective at controlling the cancer, but with fewer side effects," said Andy Trotti, M.D., of the Moffitt Cancer Center in Tampa, Florida, a lead investigator of the trial. "We were surprised by the loss of tumor control with cetuximab."

There has been a lot of recent interest in the cancer clinical research community in evaluating the "de-escalation" of therapies for cancers that have a good prognosis, such as HPV-positive cancer of the oropharynx (the part of the throat at the back of the mouth, including the soft palate, the base of the tongue, and the tonsils). The goal is to improve patients' quality of life (QOL) and reduce long-term toxic effects without compromising treatment efficacy. HPV-positive oropharyngeal cancer is frequently diagnosed in individuals in their fifties and sixties and is associated with high survival rates, providing the incentive for this trial. Moreover, the incidence of this type of cancer has increased rapidly in recent years in the United States.

"Clinical trials designed to test less-toxic treatment strategies for patients without compromising clinical benefit are a very important area of interest for NCI and the cancer research community," said Shakun Malik, M.D., of NCI's Division of Cancer Treatment and Diagnosis (DCTD).

This trial's primary objective was to determine whether the substitution of cetuximab for cisplatin with radiation would result in comparable overall survival, while reducing toxic side effects with an improved long-term quality of life. The trial enrolled 849 patients with HPV-positive oropharyngeal cancer who were randomly assigned to receive either cetuximab or cisplatin with radiation. The study had 3 planned interim analyses.

The third and final interim analysis, done after a median follow-up of four and a half years, found that overall survival on the cetuximab arm was significantly inferior to the cisplatin arm. Overall rates of serious (grade 3–5) adverse events were similar for patients in both groups. However, as the researchers expected, toxic side effects were different, with adverse events of renal toxicity, hearing loss, and bone marrow suppression more common in patients in the cisplatin arm, while body rash was more common in the cetuximab arm. All patients in this trial had completed therapy at the time of this analysis.

"This trial is the first randomized clinical trial specifically designed for patients with HPV-positive oropharyngeal cancer, and it establishes cisplatin with radiation as the standard of care," said Maura Gillison, M.D, Ph.D., of the University of Texas MD Anderson Cancer Center in Houston, the other lead investigator of the trial.

About the National Cancer Institute (NCI): NCI leads the National Cancer Program and NIH's efforts to dramatically reduce the prevalence of cancer and improve the lives of cancer patients and their families, through research into prevention and cancer biology, the development of new interventions, and the training and mentoring of new researchers. For more information about cancer, please visit the NCI website at cancer.gov or call NCI's Contact Center (formerly known as the "Cancer Information Service") at 800-4-CANCER (800-422-6237).

About the National Institutes of Health (NIH): NIH, the nation's medical research agency, includes 27 institutes and centers and is a component of the U.S. Department of Health and Human Services (HHS). NIH is the primary federal agency conducting and supporting basic, clinical, and translational medical research and is investigating the causes, treatments, and cures for both common and rare diseases.

About NRG Oncology: NRG Oncology conducts practice-changing, multi-institutional clinical and translational research to improve the lives of patients with cancer. Founded in 2012, NRG Oncology is a Pennsylvania-based nonprofit corporation that integrates the research of the National Surgical Adjuvant Breast and Bowel Project (NSABP) Foundation, the Radiation Therapy Oncology Group (RTOG), and the Gynecologic Oncology Group (GOG). The research network seeks to carry out clinical trials with emphases on gender-specific malignancies, including gynecologic, breast, and prostate cancers, and on localized or locally advanced cancers of all types. NRG Oncology extensive research organization comprises multidisciplinary investigators, including medical oncologists, radiation oncologists, surgeons, physicists, pathologists, and statisticians, and encompasses more than 1,300 research sites located world-wide, with predominance in the United States and Canada. NRG Oncology is supported primarily through grants from the National Cancer Institute (NCI) and is one of five research groups in NCI's National Clinical Trials Network.

Section 47.2

Human Papillomavirus Vaccination Linked to Decreased Oral HPV Infections

This section includes text excerpted from "HPV Vaccination
Linked to Decreased Oral HPV Infections," National Cancer
Institute (NCI), June 5, 2017.

New study results suggest that vaccination against the human papillomavirus (HPV) may sharply reduce oral HPV infections that are a major risk factor for oropharyngeal cancer, a type of head and neck cancer.

The study of more than 2,600 young adults in the United States found that the prevalence of oral infection with 4 HPV types, including 2 high-risk or cancer-causing, types, was 88 percent lower in those who reported receiving at least 1 dose of an HPV vaccine than in those who said they were not vaccinated.

About 70 percent of oropharyngeal cancers are caused by high-risk HPV infection, and the incidence of HPV-positive oropharyngeal cancer has been increasing in the United States in recent decades. In the United States, more than half of oropharyngeal cancers are linked to a single high-risk HPV type, HPV 16, which is one of the types covered by U.S. Food and Drug Administration (FDA)-approved HPV vaccines.

"In an unvaccinated population, we would estimate that about a million young adults would have an oral HPV infection by one of these vaccine HPV types. If they had all been vaccinated, we could have prevented almost 900,000 of those infections," said senior study author Maura Gillison, M.D., Ph.D., of the University of Texas MD Anderson Cancer Center.

Dr. Gillison presented the new findings at a press briefing ahead of the 2017 annual American Society of Clinical Oncology (ASCO) meeting, held from June 2 to 6 in Chicago.

A Rapidly Rising Cancer

Oropharyngeal cancer "is the fastest-rising cancer among young white men in the United States," said Dr. Gillison, who was at Ohio State University (OSO) when she conducted the study.

"The HPV types that cause oropharyngeal cancers are primarily transmitted through sexual contact," explained lead study author Anil Chaturvedi, Ph.D., of NCI's Division of Cancer Epidemiology and Genetics (DCEG). The increased incidence of oropharyngeal cancers in white men has been linked to changes in sexual behaviors from the 1950s through the 1970s, he said. The exact reasons for the greater increase in oropharynx cancer incidence in men versus women are still unclear, Dr. Chaturvedi added.

Clinical trials have shown that FDA-approved HPV vaccines can prevent anogenital HPV infections and precancerous lesions that lead to HPV-associated cancers, including cervical and anal cancer. However, Dr. Gillison said, the potential impact of current HPV vaccines on oral HPV infections that lead to cancer has not yet been rigorously tested in clinical trials, and thus, the vaccines are not specifically approved for preventing cancers of the oropharynx.

From 2006 through 2014, most HPV-vaccinated individuals in the United States received Gardasil, an HPV vaccine that protects against infection from HPV types 6, 11, 16, and 18. In January 2015, the FDA approved an updated HPV vaccine, Gardasil 9, that protects against 5 additional HPV types.

Looking for a Link

To investigate the relationship between HPV vaccination and oral HPV infection, the researchers analyzed data for 2,627 young adults who participated in the National Health and Nutrition Examination Survey (NHANES), a national survey that assesses the health of a representative slice of the U.S. population.

Drs. Gillison, Chaturvedi, and their colleagues restricted their analysis to NHANES data from 2011 to 2014, focusing on men and women between 18 and 33 years of age "because they were the first group [in the United States] to receive the vaccine," Dr. Gillison said.

In the United States, routine vaccination against HPV, which causes nearly all cervical cancers, has been recommended since mid-2006 for 11- to 12-year-old girls and for females up to 26 years of age who have not previously been vaccinated. HPV vaccination has been recommended for males between 9 and 26 years of age since 2009.

The researchers analyzed mouth rinse samples (containing oral cells) from all study participants for the presence of 37 HPV types, including types 6, 11, 16, and 18, which are covered by Gardasil, Dr. Gillison said.

The prevalence of oral infections with these 4 HPV types was 1.61 percent in unvaccinated young adults versus 0.11 percent in vaccinated young adults—an 88 percent reduction in HPV prevalence with vaccination. Among men, the prevalence of oral infection with the 4 HPV types was 2.1 percent in unvaccinated individuals and 0.0 percent in vaccinated individuals.

By contrast, the prevalence of oral infection with 33 HPV types not covered by the vaccine was 4.0 percent in vaccinated groups and 4.7 percent in non-vaccinated groups, the researchers found, a difference that was not considered to be statistically meaningful.

Vaccination rates were low overall, with only 29.2 percent of women and 6.9 percent of men in the study population reporting having received at least 1 dose of an HPV vaccine before the age of 26.

Prevention Potential

Although the self-reported vaccination rates in this study were low, Dr. Gillison said, "there is considerable optimism because more data indicate that [roughly] 60 percent of girls and 50 percent of boys under age 18 have received more than 1 HPV vaccine dose."

"HPV vaccines are already strongly recommended for cancer prevention," Dr. Gillison continued. "Parents who choose to have their children vaccinated against HPV should realize that the vaccine may provide additional benefits, such as preventing oral HPV infections linked to oral cancers."

However, she and Dr. Chaturvedi noted, only a randomized clinical trial that follows people over time could definitively show a cause and effect relationship between HPV vaccination and a lasting reduction of high-risk oral HPV infections, which experts agree is a more meaningful indicator of vaccine effectiveness.

In July 2013, NCI researchers and their collaborators reported findings from the NCI-sponsored HPV Vaccine Trial in Costa Rica that suggested that HPV vaccination can reduce oral HPV infections in women.

"Our study builds on those results by showing a reduction in oral HPV prevalence in vaccinated men, the group that bears the greatest burden of HPV-associated oropharynx cancers," Dr. Chaturvedi said.

Section 47.3

Nivolumab Improves Survival for Patients with Recurrent Head and Neck Cancer

This section includes text excerpted from "Nivolumab Improves Survival for Patients with Recurrent Head and Neck Cancer," National Cancer Institute (NCI), January 4, 2017.

In patients with head and neck squamous cell carcinoma (HNSCC), the immune checkpoint inhibitor nivolumab (Opdivo) improved overall survival compared with standard chemotherapy, according to results from a large phase III trial.

The study, led by Robert L. Ferris, M.D., Ph.D., of the University of Pittsburgh Medical Center and Cancer Institute (UPMC), and Maura L. Gillison, M.D., Ph.D., of Ohio State University, was funded by Bristol-Myers Squibb, the manufacturer of nivolumab.

The findings were published October 10, 2016, in the *New England Journal of Medicine*. Based on results from the trial, the U.S. Food and Drug Administration (FDA) approved nivolumab for the treatment of HNSCC in November 2016.

HNSCC includes cancers that begin in the squamous cells that line the oral cavity, larynx, pharynx, salivary glands, and nose and nasal passages. Human papillomavirus (HPV) infection can increase the risk of many types of head and neck cancer, and in general, patients with HNSCC who are HPV-positive typically have better treatment outcomes than patients who are HPV-negative. Currently, there are no effective second-line therapy options for patients with HNSCC whose cancer has progressed or recurred despite treatment with platinum-based chemotherapy, and, typically, these patients have poor prognosis.

Earlier studies have shown that HNSCC tumor growth and metastasis depend on suppression of the immune system. Evidence suggests that immunotherapies may be able to overcome this negative interaction. In fact, earlier this year, the FDA granted accelerated approval for another immune checkpoint inhibitor, pembrolizumab (Keytruda), for the treatment of recurrent or metastatic HNSCC. Both nivolumab and pembrolizumab block the checkpoint molecule PD-1, allowing immune cells to attack cancer cells.

The new trial investigated whether, compared with standard chemotherapy, nivolumab could increase overall survival for patients with HNSCC whose cancer progressed within 6 months of treatment with platinum-based chemotherapy. Patients were randomly assigned to receive nivolumab (240 patients) or standard therapy with methotrexate, docetaxel, or cetuximab (121 patients). Patients were treated until their cancer progressed or if they experienced unacceptable side effects. The median length of treatment was 1.9 months in both groups.

After a median follow-up of 5.1 months, median overall survival was 7.5 months in the nivolumab group and 5.1 months in the standard therapy group. The estimated rate of overall survival at 1 year in the nivolumab group was more than twice that in the standard therapy group (36.0% versus 16.6%).

The effect of nivolumab on overall survival was independent of the percentage of tumor cells expressing PD-L1—a molecule sometimes used as a biomarker for tumor response to immunotherapy. Nivolumab increased overall survival for patients with both HPV-negative and HPV-positive tumors.

Although there was no difference in median progression-free survival between the groups, the estimated rate of progression-free survival at 6 months for the nivolumab group (19.7%) was greater than that in the standard therapy group (9.9%). The response rate for the nivolumab group was 13.3 percent, compared with 5.8 percent for the standard therapy group.

The rate of grade 3 or 4 treatment-related adverse events was less in the nivolumab group, with most common adverse events being fatigue, nausea, and rash. Patients who received nivolumab reported that their quality of life remained unchanged or improved slightly compared with what it was before treatment.

That "nivolumab has shown clinical benefit in these patients" is important, said Shakun Malik, M.D., of NCI's Cancer Therapy Evaluation Program, because although pembrolizumab was granted accelerated FDA approval for patients with HNSCC, "we do not know whether it improves survival." A randomized trial to investigate whether pembrolizumab improves survival is ongoing.

And the fact that "nivolumab has worked across the board in all patients, irrespective of PD-L1 expression" and HPV status, means that a broader group of patients with HNSCC may benefit, Dr. Malik said.

Part Eight

Additional Help and Information

Chapter 48

Glossary of Terms Related to the Ears, Nose, and Throat

adverse effect: An unexpected medical problem that happens during treatment with a drug or other therapy. Adverse effects may be mild, moderate, or severe, and may be caused by something other than the drug or therapy being given. Also called adverse event.

American Sign Language (ASL): Manual language with its own syntax and grammar, used primarily by people who are deaf.

anosmia: Absence of the sense of smell.

antibody: A protein made by plasma cells (a type of white blood cell (WBC)) in response to an antigen (a substance that causes the body to make a specific immune response). Each antibody can bind to only one specific antigen. The purpose of this binding is to help destroy the antigen. Some antibodies destroy antigens directly. Others make it easier for white blood cells to destroy the antigen. An antibody is a type of immunoglobulin.

aphasia: Total or partial loss of the ability to use or understand language; usually caused by stroke, brain disease, or injury.

assistive technology: Products, devices, or equipment that help maintain, increase, or improve the functional capabilities of people with disabilities.

This glossary contains terms excerpted from documents produced by several sources deemed reliable.

auditory nerve: Eighth cranial nerve that connects the inner ear to the brainstem and is responsible for hearing and balance.

auditory system: The outer, middle, and inner ear, along with the neurons and brain regions involved in hearing.

bacteria: A large group of single-cell microorganisms. Some cause infections and disease in animals and humans.

barotrauma: Injury to the middle ear caused by a reduction of air pressure.

benign paroxysmal positional vertigo (BPPV): Balance disorder that results in sudden onset of dizziness, spinning, or vertigo when moving the head.

biofilm: Communities of bacteria, such as the potentially antibiotic-resistant bacterial communities that are present in the middle ears of most children with chronic ear infections.

biomarker: A specific physical trait or a measurable biologically produced change in the body connected with a disease or health condition.

cetuximab: A drug used to treat certain types of head and neck cancer, and a certain type of colorectal cancer that has spread to other parts of the body. It is also being studied in the treatment of other types of cancer. Cetuximab binds to a protein called epidermal growth factor receptor (EGFR), which is on the surface of some types of cancer cells. This may stop cancer cells from growing. Cetuximab is a type of monoclonal antibody. Also called "Erbitux."

chemical senses: Taste and smell.

cholesteatoma: Accumulation of dead cells in the middle ear, caused by repeated middle ear infections.

cochlea: Snail-shaped structure in the inner ear that contains the organ of hearing.

cochlear implant: A medical device that bypasses damaged structures in the inner ear and directly stimulates the auditory nerve, allowing some people who are deaf or hard of hearing to learn to hear and interpret sounds and speech.

computed tomography (CT): A procedure for taking X-ray images from many different angles and then assembling them into a cross-section of the body. This technique is generally used to visualize bone.

cued speech: Method of communication that combines speech reading with a system of handshapes placed near the mouth to help deaf or hard-of-hearing individuals differentiate words that look similar on the lips (e.g., bunch versus punch) or are hidden (e.g., gag).

decibel: Unit that measures the intensity or loudness of sound.

deoxyribonucleic acid (DNA): The double-helix molecule that provides the basis of genetic heredity, about two nanometers in diameter but often several millimeters in length.

diabetes: A disease in which blood glucose (blood sugar) levels are above normal. There are two main types of diabetes. Type 1 diabetes is caused by a problem with the body's defense system, called the immune system.

ear wax: Yellow secretion from glands in the outer ear (cerumen) that keeps the skin of the ear dry and protected from infection.

electrocochleography: Technique that records electrical activity of the inner ear in response to sounds; used to help confirm the diagnosis of Ménière disease.

endocrinologist: A physician who specializes in diagnosing and treating disorders of the body's glands and hormones.

enlarged vestibular aqueducts (EVA): Vestibular aqueducts are narrow, bony canals that travel from the inner ear to inside the skull. A vestibular aqueduct is often considered enlarged if it is greater than 1.0 millimeter in size. Research suggests that most children with EVA will develop some degree of hearing loss.

epidemiology: The branch of medical science that investigates all the factors that determine the presence or absence of diseases and disorders in a population.

esophageal cancer: Cancer that forms in tissues lining the esophagus (the muscular tube through which food passes from the throat to the stomach). Two types of esophageal cancer are squamous cell carcinoma (cancer that begins in flat cells lining the esophagus) and adenocarcinoma (cancer that begins in cells that make and release mucus and other fluids).

esophageal stent: A tube placed in the esophagus to keep a blocked area open so the patient can swallow soft food and liquids. Esophageal stents are made of metal mesh, plastic, or silicone, and may be used in the treatment of esophageal cancer.

eustachian tube: A small passageway that connects the upper part of the throat to the middle ear; its job is to supply fresh air to the middle ear, drain fluid, and keep air pressure at a steady level between the nose and the ear.

gene expression: The process by which the information encoded in a gene is used to direct the assembly of a protein molecule; different subsets of genes are expressed in different cell types or under different conditions.

genetics: The study of particular genes, deoxyribonucleic acid (DNA), and heredity.

hair cells: Sensory cells of the inner ear, which are topped with hair-like structures (stereocilia) and which transform the mechanical energy of sound waves into nerve impulses.

hearing aid: An electronic device that brings amplified sound to the ear; it usually consists of a microphone, amplifier, and receiver.

hoarseness: Abnormally rough or harsh-sounding voice caused by vocal abuse and other disorders, such as gastroesophageal reflux, thyroid problems, or trauma to the larynx (voice box).

human immunodeficiency virus (HIV): HIV is the virus that infects and destroys the body's immune cells and causes a disease called AIDS, or acquired immunodeficiency syndrome.

hypertension: Also called high blood pressure, it is having blood pressure greater than 140 over 90 mmHg (millimeters of mercury). Long-term high blood pressure can damage blood vessels and organs, including the heart, kidneys, eyes, and brain.

hypopharyngeal cancer: Cancer that forms in tissues of the hypopharynx (the bottom part of the throat). The most common type is squamous cell carcinoma (cancer that begins in flat cells lining the hypopharynx).

immune system: A complex system of cellular and molecular components having the primary function of distinguishing self from not self and defense against foreign organisms or substances.

inner ear: Part of the ear that contains both the organ of hearing (the cochlea) and the organ of balance (the labyrinth).

labyrinth: Organ of balance located in the inner ear. The labyrinth consists of three semicircular canals and the vestibule.

labyrinthitis: Viral or bacterial infection or inflammation of the inner ear that can cause dizziness, loss of balance, and temporary hearing loss.

Landau-Kleffner syndrome: Childhood disorder of unknown origin which often extends into adulthood and can be identified by gradual or sudden loss of the ability to understand and use spoken language.

laryngeal cancer: Cancer that forms in tissues of the larynx (area of the throat that contains the vocal cords and is used for breathing, swallowing, and talking). Most laryngeal cancers are squamous cell carcinomas (cancer that begins in flat cells lining the larynx).

Laryngoscopy: Procedure used to see, directly or indirectly, the vocal folds (formerly known as vocal cords) and neighboring tissue in the larynx (voice box) or other parts of the throat.

larynx: The area of the throat containing the vocal cords and used for breathing, swallowing, and talking. Also called voice box.

magnetic resonance imaging (MRI): A noninvasive procedure that uses magnetic fields and radio waves to produce three-dimensional computerized images of areas inside the body.

Ménière disease: Inner ear disorder that can affect both hearing and balance. It can cause episodes of vertigo, hearing loss, tinnitus, and the sensation of fullness in the ear.

meningitis: Inflammation of the meninges, the membranes that envelop the brain and the spinal cord; may cause hearing loss or deafness.

middle ear: Part of the ear that includes the eardrum and three tiny bones of the middle ear, ending at the round window that leads to the inner ear.

middle-ear implant: Hearing aid consisting of an internal device that is surgically attached to one of the bones of the middle ear, thereby bypassing the ear canal and eardrum and strengthening the sound vibrations entering the inner ear. The implant is combined with an external audio processor unit that is worn behind the ear.

motion sickness: Dizziness, sweating, nausea, vomiting, and generalized discomfort experienced when an individual is in motion.

mutation: A change in a DNA sequence that can result from DNA copying mistakes made during cell division, exposure to ionizing radiation, exposure to chemical mutagens, or infection by viruses.

nasopharyngeal cancer: Cancer that forms in tissues of the nasopharynx (upper part of the throat behind the nose). Most nasopharyngeal cancers are squamous cell carcinomas (cancer that begins in flat cells lining the nasopharynx).

neurofibromatosis type 2 (NF2): Group of inherited disorders in which noncancerous tumors grow on several nerves that usually include the hearing nerve. The symptoms of NF2 include tumors on the hearing nerve which can affect hearing and balance. NF2 may occur in the teenage years with hearing loss. Also see acoustic neurinoma.

nivolumab: A drug used alone or with ipilimumab to treat a certain type of colorectal cancer that has mutations (changes) in genes involved in DNA repair. It is also used with ipilimumab in some patients to treat renal cell carcinoma (RCC) and melanoma. Nivolumab is also used alone in some patients to treat small cell lung cancer, nonsmall cell lung cancer, cancer of the head and neck, Hodgkin lymphoma, melanoma, RCC, urothelial carcinoma, and hepatocellular carcinoma.

noise-induced hearing loss: Hearing loss caused by exposure to harmful sounds, either very loud impulse sound(s) or repeated exposure to sounds over 90-decibel level over an extended period of time that damage the sensitive structures of the inner ear.

oropharyngeal cancer: Cancer that forms in tissues of the oropharynx (the part of the throat at the back of the mouth, including the soft palate, the base of the tongue, and the tonsils). Most oropharyngeal cancers are squamous cell carcinomas (cancer that begins in flat cells lining the oropharynx).

otitis externa: Inflammation of the outer part of the ear extending to the auditory canal.

otitis media: Inflammation of the middle ear caused by infection.

otitis media with effusion: Ear infection in which fluid remains trapped behind the eardrum inside the middle ear after the infection is over.

otoacoustic emissions: Low-intensity sounds produced by the inner ear that can be quickly measured with a sensitive microphone placed in the ear canal.

otolaryngologist: Physician/surgeon who specializes in diseases of the ears, nose, throat, and head and neck.

otosclerosis: Abnormal growth of bone of the inner ear. This bone prevents structures within the ear from working properly and causes hearing loss. For some people with otosclerosis, the hearing loss may become severe.

otoscope: A tool that doctors use to look into the ear; has a cylindrical handle and a top with a lighted conical viewer at one end that inserts into the ear and a magnifying lens at the other end that enlarges the viewing area.

ototoxic drugs: Drugs such as a special class of antibiotics, aminoglycoside antibiotics, that can damage the hearing and balance organs located in the inner ear for some individuals.

outer ear: External portion of the ear, consisting of the pinna, or auricle, and the ear canal.

papillomavirus: Group of viruses that can cause noncancerous wartlike tumors to grow on the surface of skin and internal organs, such as the respiratory tract; can be life-threatening.

paranasal sinus: One of many small hollow spaces in the bones around the nose. Paranasal sinuses are named after the bones that contain them: frontal (the lower forehead), maxillary (cheekbones), ethmoid (beside the upper nose), and sphenoid (behind the nose). The paranasal sinuses open into the nasal cavity (space inside the nose) and are lined with cells that make mucus to keep the nose from drying out during breathing.

paranasal sinus and nasal cavity cancer: Cancer that forms in tissues of the paranasal sinuses (small hollow spaces in the bones around the nose) or nasal cavity (the inside of the nose). The most common type of paranasal sinus and nasal cavity cancer is squamous cell carcinoma (cancer that begins in flat cells lining these tissues and cavities).

parosmia: Any disease or perversion of the sense of smell, especially the subjective perception of odors that do not exist.

pathogenesis: The development of a disease or condition, particularly the cellular and molecular origins and causes of disease development.

Pendred syndrome: Genetic disorder that causes early childhood hearing loss and sometimes progresses to total deafness; also often affects the thyroid gland and may affect balance.

perception (hearing): Process of knowing or being aware of information through the ear.

perilymph fistula: Leakage of inner ear fluid to the middle ear that occurs without apparent cause or that is associated with head trauma, physical exertion, or barotrauma.

phenotype: An individual's physical and behavioral characteristics.

phonology: Language-based sounds: in particular, phonemes, which are the units that make up words. `

presbycusis: Loss of hearing that gradually occurs because of changes in the inner ear in individuals as they grow older.

rhinitis: Inflammation of the mucous membranes of the nose, generally accompanied by discharge (runny nose) and usually caused by a virus infection (e.g., the common cold) or by an allergic reaction (e.g., hay fever).

sensorineural hearing loss: Hearing loss caused by damage to the sensory cells and/or nerve fibers of the inner ear.

sign language: Method of communication for people who are deaf or hard of hearing in which hand movements, gestures, and facial expressions convey grammatical structure and meaning.

sinusitis: Inflammation or infection of one of the air-filled nasal sinuses.

smell: To perceive odor or scent through stimuli affecting the olfactory nerves.

smell disorder: Inability to perceive odors. It may be temporary, caused by a head cold or swelling or blockage of the nasal passages. It can be permanent when any part of the olfactory region is damaged by factors such as brain injury, tumor, disease, or chronic rhinitis.

spasmodic dysphonia: Momentary disruption of voice caused by involuntary movements of one or more muscles of the larynx.

specific language impairment (SLI): Difficulty with language or the organized-symbol system used for communication in the absence of problems, such as mental retardation, hearing loss, or emotional disorders.

speech disorder: Any defect or abnormality that prevents an individual from communicating by means of spoken words. Speech disorders may develop from nerve injury to the brain, muscular paralysis, structural defects, hysteria, or mental retardation.

speech-language pathologist: Health professional trained to evaluate and treat people who have voice, speech, language, or swallowing disorders (including hearing impairment) that affect their ability to communicate.

speech processor: Part of a cochlear implant that converts speech sounds into electrical impulses to stimulate the auditory nerve, allowing an individual to understand sound and speech.

stapedectomy: Surgical procedure to improve hearing by removing a defective or damaged ear bone (the stapes) and replacing it with a tiny, piston-shaped artificial structure that permits sound waves to travel to the inner ear.

stereocilia: Tiny hair-like structures on the tops of sensory hair cells in the inner ear. A group of stereocilia on one hair cell is also called a hair cell bundle.

stroke: Also known as a cerebrovascular accident (CVA); caused by a lack of blood to the brain, resulting in the sudden loss of speech, language, or the ability to move a body part, and, if severe enough, death.

stuttering: A speech disorder in which sounds, syllables, or words are repeated or prolonged, disrupting the normal flow of speech.

sudden deafness: Loss of hearing that occurs quickly due to such causes as explosion, a viral infection, or the use of some drugs.

swallowing disorders: Any of a group of problems that interferes with the transfer of food from the mouth to the stomach.

tai chi: A form of traditional Chinese mind/body exercise and meditation that uses slow sets of body movements and controlled breathing. Tai chi is done to improve balance, flexibility, muscle strength, and overall health.

taste: Sensation produced by a stimulus applied to the gustatory nerve endings in the tongue. The four tastes are salt, sour, sweet, and bitter. Some scientists indicate the existence of a fifth taste, described as savory.

taste buds: Groups of cells located on the tongue that enable one to recognize different tastes.

taste disorder: Inability to perceive different flavors. Taste disorders may result from poor oral hygiene, gum disease, hepatitis, or medicines and chemotherapeutic drugs. Taste disorders may also be neurological.

tinnitus: Sensation of a ringing, roaring, or buzzing sound in the ears or head when no actual sound stimulus is present in the environment.

tongue: Large muscle on the floor of the mouth that manipulates food for chewing and swallowing. It is the main organ of taste, and assists in forming speech sounds.

tonotopic: The spatial arrangement of where sounds of different frequency are processed in the brain. For example, the auditory nerves that carry signals from adjacent portions of the cochlea project their information to adjacent portions of the auditory cortex.

tracheostomy: Surgical opening into the trachea (windpipe) to help someone breathe who has an obstruction or swelling in the larynx (voice box) or upper throat or who has had the larynx surgically removed.

tympanic membrane (eardrum): Thin, cone-shaped, and flexible structure that separates the external ear from the middle ear and transmits sound from outside the body to inside the ear.

tympanoplasty: Surgical repair of the eardrum (tympanic membrane) or bones of the middle ear.

Usher syndrome: Hereditary disease that affects hearing and vision and sometimes balance.

velocardiofacial syndrome: Inherited disorder characterized by cleft palate (opening in the roof of the mouth), heart defects, characteristic facial appearance, minor learning problems, and speech and feeding problems.

vertigo: Illusion of movement; a sensation as if the external world were revolving around an individual (objective vertigo) or as if the individual were revolving in space (subjective vertigo).

vestibular aqueducts: Narrow, bony, fluid-filled canals that extend from the membranous labyrinth into the inner ear and skull.

vestibular neuronitis: Irritation and swelling (inflammation) of the vestibular nerve that causes sudden dizziness; sometimes accompanied by nausea and vomiting, but not hearing loss.

vestibular system: System in the body that is responsible for maintaining balance, posture, and the body's orientation in space. This system also regulates locomotion and other movements and keeps objects in visual focus as the body moves.

vocal folds (vocal cords): Muscularized folds of mucous membrane that extend from the larynx (voice box) wall. The folds are enclosed in elastic vocal ligament and muscle that control the tension and rate of vibration of the folds as air passes through them.

vocal fold paralysis: Inability of one or both vocal folds (vocal cords) to move because of damage to the brain or nerves.

vocal nodule: Small, noncancerous growth on the vocal folds (formerly known as vocal cords); among the most common of voice disorders directly related to misusing or overusing the voice.

vocal tremor: Trembling or shaking of one or more of the muscles of the larynx, resulting in an unsteady-sounding voice.

voice: Sound produced by air passing out through the larynx and upper respiratory tract.

voice disorders: Group of problems involving abnormal pitch, loudness, or quality of the sound produced by the larynx (voice box).

Waardenburg syndrome: Hereditary disorder that is characterized by hearing impairment, a white shock of hair and/or distinctive blue color to one or both eyes, and wide-set inner corners of the eyes. Balance problems are also associated with some types of Waardenburg syndrome.

X-ray: A type of radiation used in the diagnosis and treatment of cancer and other diseases. In low doses, X-rays are used to diagnose diseases by making pictures of the inside of the body.

Chapter 49

Ear, Nose, and Throat Disorders: Resources for Information and Support

General Information

Agency for Healthcare Research and Quality (AHRQ)
Office of Communications and Knowledge Transfer (OCKT)
5600 Fishers Ln., Seventh Fl.
Phone: 301-427-1104
Website: www.ahrq.gov

American Academy of Otolaryngology-Head and Neck Surgery (AAO-HNS)
1650 Diagonal Rd.
Alexandria, VA 22314-2857
Phone: 703-836-4444
Website: www.entnet.org

American Head and Neck Society (AHNS)
11300 W. Olympic Blvd.
Ste. 600
Los Angeles, CA 90064
Phone: 310-437-0559
Fax: 310-437-0585
Website: www.ahns.info
E-mail: admin@ahns.info

Resources in this chapter were compiled from several sources deemed reliable; all contact information was verified and updated in April 2019.

Centers for Disease Control and Prevention (CDC)
1600 Clifton Rd.
Atlanta, GA 30329-4027
Toll-Free: 800-CDC-INFO
(800-232-4636)
Toll-Free TTY: 888-232-6348
Website: www.cdc.gov

Massachusetts Eye and Ear Infirmary (MEEI)
243 Charles St.
Boston, MA 02114
Phone: 617-523-7900
TDD: 617-523-5498
Website: www.meei.harvard.edu

National Cancer Institute (NCI)
9609 Medical Center Dr.
BG 9609, MSC 9760
Bethesda, MD 20892-9760
Toll-Free: 800-4-CANCER
(800-422-6237)
Phone: 301-435-3848
Website: www.cancer.gov
E-mail: cancergovstaff@mail.nih.gov

National Center on Deaf-Blindness (NCDB)
141 Middle Neck Rd.
Sands Point, NY 11050
Phone: 503-838-8754
Fax: 503-838-8150
Website: www.nationaldb.org
E-mail: info@nationaldb.org

National Heart, Lung, and Blood Institute (NHLBI)
Bldg. 31, 31 Center Dr.
Bethesda, MD 20892
Website: www.nhlbi.nih.gov
E-mail: nhlbiinfo@nhlbi.nih.gov

National Institute of Dental and Craniofacial Research (NIDCR)
Office of Communications and Health Education (OCHE)
Bldg. 31, Rm. 5B55
31 Center Dr. MSC 2190
Bethesda, MD 20892-2190
Phone: 301-496-4261
Fax: 301-496-9988
Website: www.nidr.nih.gov
E-mail: nidcrinfo@mail.nih.gov

National Institute of Diabetes, Digestive and Kidney Diseases (NIDDK)
Toll-Free: 800-860-8747
Toll-Free TTY: 866-569-1162
Website: www.niddk.nih.gov
E-mail: healthinfo@niddk.nih.gov

National Institute on Aging Information Center (NIA)
Bldg. 31, Rm. 5C27
31 Center Dr. MSC 2292
Bethesda, MD 20892
Toll-Free: 800-222-2225
Phone: 301-496-1752
Toll-Free TTY: 800-222-4225
Website: www.nia.nih.gov
E-mail: niaic@nia.nih.gov

National Organization for Rare Disorders (NORD)
55 Kenosia Ave.
Danbury, CT 06810
Toll-Free: 800-999-NORD
(800-999-6673)
Phone: 203-744-0100
Fax: 203-263-9938
Website: www.rarediseases.org

New York Eye and Ear Infirmary (NYEE)
310 E. 14th St.
New York, NY 10003
Phone: 212-979-4000
Website: www.nyee.edu

Acoustic Neuroma

Acoustic Neuroma Association (ANA)
600 Peachtree Pkwy
Ste. 108
Cumming, GA 30041
Phone: 770-205-8211
Fax: 770-205-0239
Website: www.anausa.org
E-mail: info@anausa.org

Hearing Loss

Alexander Graham Bell Association for the Deaf and Hard of Hearing (AG Bell)
3417 Volta Pl. N.W.
Washington, DC 20007
Phone: 202-337-5220
TTY: 202-337-5221
Fax: 202-337-8314
Website: www.agbell.org
E-mail: info@agbell.org

American Academy of Audiology (AAA)
11480 Commerce Park Dr.
Ste. 220
Reston, VA 20191
Toll-Free: 800-AAA-2336
(800-222-2336)
Phone: 703-790-8466
Fax: 703-790-8631
Website: www.audiology.org

American Association of the Deaf-Blind (AADB)
248 RAINBOW Dr. #14864
Livingston, TX 77399-2048
Website: www.aadb.org
E-mail: aadb-info@aadb.org

American Hearing Research Foundation (AHRF)
275 N. York St.
Ste. 201
Elmhurst, IL 60126
Phone: 630-617-5079
Website: www.american-hearing.org
E-mail: info@american-hearing.org

American Society for Deaf Children (ASDC)
P.O. Box 23
Woodbine, MD 21797
Toll-Free: 800-942-ASDC
(800-942-2732)
Website: www.deafchildren.org
E-mail: info@deafchildren.org

American Speech-Language-Hearing Association (ASHA)
2200 Research Blvd.
Rockville, MD 20850-3289
Toll-Free: 800-638-8255
Phone: 301-296-5700
TTY: 301-296-5650
Fax: 301-296-8580
Website: www.asha.org
E-mail: actioncenter@asha.org

Association of Late-Deafened Adults (ALDA)
8038 Macintosh Ln.
Ste. 2
Rockford, IL 61107-5336
Toll-Free: 866-402-ALDA
(866-402-2532)
Phone: 815-332-1515
Website: www.alda.org
E-mail: info@alda.org

Boys Town National Research Hospital (BTNRH)
555 N. 30th St.
Omaha, NE 68131
Phone: 531-355-6540
Websites: www.boystownhospital.org

Center for Hearing and Communication (CHC)
50 Bdwy. Sixth Fl.
Lower Manhattan (Financial District)
New York, NY 10004
Phone: 917-305-7700
TTY: 917-305-7999
Fax: 917-305-7888
Website: www.chchearing.org

Harvard Medical School Center for Hereditary Deafness (HMSCHD)
Website: www.hearing.harvard.edu
E-mail: hearing@hms.harvard.edu

HealthyHearing
P.O. Box 515381 #42919
Los Angeles, CA 90051-6681
Toll-Free: 800-567-1692
Website: www.healthyhearing.com

Hearing Industries Association (HIA)
777 Sixth St. N.W.
Office 09-114
Washington, DC 20001
Phone: 202-975-0905
Website: www.hearing.org

Hearing Loss Association of America (HLAA)
7910 Woodmont Ave.
Ste. 1200
Bethesda, MD 20814
Phone: 301-657-2248
Fax: 301-913-9413
Website: www.hearingloss.org

House Ear Institute (HEI)
201 S. Alvarado Ave.
Ste. 809, Los Angeles, CA 90057
Phone: 213-483-9930
Website: www.hei.org

John Tracy Center (JTC)
806 W. Adams Blvd.
Los Angeles, CA 90007
Phone: 213-748-5481
Fax: 213-749-1651
Website: www.jtc.org
E-mail: web@jtc.org

Laurent Clerc National Deaf Education Center
800 FL Ave. N.E.
Washington, DC 20002
Phone: 202-651-5855
Website: www3.gallaudet.edu
E-mail: clerc.center@gallaudet.edu

National Association of the Deaf (NAD)
8630 Fenton St.
Ste. 820
Silver Spring, MD 20910
Phone: 301-587-1788
TTY: 301-587-1789
Fax: 301-587-1791
Website: www.nad.org
E-mail: nad.info@nad.org

National Black Association for Speech-Language and Hearing (NBASLH)
191 Clarksville Rd.
Princeton Junction, NJ 08550
Phone: 609-799-4900
Website: www.nbaslh.org
E-mail: nbaslh@nbaslh.org

National Cued Speech Association (NCSA)
1300 Pennsylvania Ave. N.W.
Ste. 190-713
Washington, DC 20004
Toll-Free: 800-459-3529
Website: www.cuedspeech.org

National Family Association for Deaf-Blind (NFADB)
P.O. Box 1667
Sands Point, NY 11050
Toll-Free: 800-255-0411
Fax: 516-883-9060
Website: www.nfadb.org
E-mail: nfadbinfo@gmail.com

National Institute on Deafness and Other Communication Disorders (NIDCD) Clearinghouse
1 Communication Ave.
Bethesda, MD 20892-3456
Toll-Free: 800-241-1044
Toll-Free TTY: 800-241-1055
Fax: 301-770-8977
Website: www.nidcd.nih.gov
E-mail: nidcdinfo@nidcd.nih.gov

Raising Deaf Kids
Deafness and Family
Communication Center (DFCC)
3440 Market St.
Fourth Fl.
Philadelphia, PA 19104
Phone: 215-590-7440
TTY: 215-590-6817
Fax: 215-590-1335
Website: www.raisingdeafkids.org
E-mail: info@raisingdeafkids.org

The SEE Center (for the Advancement of Deaf Children)
10443 Los Alamitos Blvd.
Los Alamitos, CA 90720
Phone: 562-430-1467
Website: www.seecenter.org
E-mail: seecenter@seecenter.org

Starkey Hearing Foundation
6801 WA Ave. S.
Ste. 200
Minneapolis, MN 55439
Toll-Free: 866-354-3254
Fax: 952-828-6900
Website: www.
starkeyhearingfoundation.org
E-mail: info@starkeyfoundation.
org

Laryngeal Papillomatosis

International Recurrent Respiratory Papillomatosis (RRP) Information, Service, and Advocacy Center
International RRP ISA Center
P.O. Box 4330
Bellingham, WA 98227
Phone: 360-756-8185
Website: www.rrpwebsite.org
E-mail: webmaster@rrpwebsite.
org

Recurrent Respiratory Papillomatosis Foundation (RRPF)
Marlene and Bill Stern
P.O. Box 6643
Lawrenceville, NJ 08648
Phone: 609-530-1095
Toll-Free Fax: 866-498-7559
Website: www.rrpf.org

Nasal and Sinus Disorders

American Academy of Allergy, Asthma and Immunology (AAAAI)
555 E. Wells St.
Ste. 1100
Milwaukee, WI 53202-3823
Phone: 414-272-6071
Website: www.aaaai.org
E-mail: info@aaaai.org

American College of Allergy, Asthma and Immunology (ACAAI)
85 W. Algonquin Rd.
Ste. 550
Arlington Heights, IL 60005
Phone: 847-427-1200
Fax: 847-427-9656
Website: www.acaai.org
E-mail: mail@acaai.org

American Rhinologic Society (ARS)
P.O. Box 269
Oak Ridge, NJ 07438
Phone: 973-545-2735
Fax: 845-986-1527
Website: www.american-rhinologic.org
E-mail: membership@american-rhinologic.org

Joint Council of Allergy, Asthma, and Immunology
50 N. Brockway
Ste. 3-3
Palatine, IL 60067
Phone: 847-934-1918
Website: www.jcaai.org
E-mail: info@jcaai.org

Sleep Apnea

American Sleep Apnea Association (ASAA)
641 S St. N.W.
Third Fl.
Washington, DC 20001-5196
Toll-Free: 888-293-3650
Toll-Free Fax: 888-293-3650
Website: www.sleepapnea.org
E-mail: asaa@sleepapnea.org

National Center on Sleep Disorders Research (NCSDR)
National Heart, Lung, and Blood Institute (NHLBI)
6701 Rockledge Dr.
Ste. 7024
Bethesda, MD, 20892-7920
Phone: 301-435-0199
Fax: 301-480-3451
Website: www.nhlbi.nih.gov/health-pro/guidelines/current/obesity-guidelines/e_textbook/appndx/apndx7.htm

Smell and Taste Disorders

Monell Chemical Senses Center
3500 Market St.
Philadelphia, PA 19104-3308
Phone: 267-519-4700
Website: www.monell.org
E-mail: mcsc@monell.org

Rocky Mountain Taste and Smell Center (RMTSC)
University of Colorado Health Sciences Center (UCHSC)
4200 E. Ninth Ave.
Box B205
Denver, CO 80262
Phone: 303-315-6600
Fax: 303-315-8787

State University of New York (SUNY) Smell and Taste Disorders Clinic
750 E. Adams St.
Syracuse, NY 13210
Phone: 315-464-5588
Fax: 315-464-7712
Website: www.upstate.edu/ent/
smelltaste.shtml
E-mail: kurtzd@mail.upstate.
edu

University of Pennsylvania Smell and Taste Center
3400 Spruce St.
Ravdin Bldg. Fifth Fl.
Philadelphia, PA 19104
Phone: 215-662-6580
Fax: 215-349-5266
Website: www.med.upenn.edu/
stc

Spasmodic Dysphonia

National Spasmodic Dysphonia Association (NSDA)
300 Park Blvd.
Ste. 335
Itasca, IL 60143
Toll-Free: 800-795-NSDA
(800-795-6732)
Fax: 630-250-4505
Website: www.dysphonia.org
E-mail: nsda@dysphonia.org

Tinnitus

American Tinnitus Association (ATA) National Headquarters
P.O. Box 424049
Washington, DC 20042-4049
Toll-Free: 800-634-8978
Website: www.ata.org
E-mail: tinnitus@ata.org

Vestibular Disorders

Vestibular Disorders Association (VEDA)
5018 N.E. 15th Ave.
Portland, OR 97211
Toll-Free: 800-VESTIBU
(800-837-8428)
Fax: 503-229-8064
Website: www.vestibular.org
E-mail: info@vestibular.org

Vocal Disorders

American Academy of Otolaryngic Allergy (AAOA)
11130 Sunrise Valley Dr.
Ste. 100
Reston, VA 20191
Phone: 202-955-5010
Fax: 202-955-5016
Website: www.aaoallergy.org
E-mail: contact@aaoallergy.org

American Laryngological Association (ALA)
P.O. Box 941
Antioch, TN 37013-0941
Phone: 615-812-6170
Website: www.alahns.org

National Center for Voice and Speech (NCVS)
136 S. Main St.
Ste. 320
Salt Lake City, UT 84101-1623
Phone: 801-596-2012
Fax: 801-596-2013
Website: www.ncvs.org

Voice Foundation
219 N. Broad St. 10th Fl.
Philadelphia, PA 19107
Phone: 215-735-7999
Fax: 215-762-5572
Website: www.voicefoundation.org
E-mail: office@voicefoundation.org

Index

Index

575